The
Healthiest Diet in the World

A Cookbook and Mentor

The
Healthiest Diet in the World
A Cookbook and Mentor

Nikki and David Goldbeck

A DUTTON BOOK

A NOTE TO THE READER: The ideas, procedures, and suggestions contained in this book are not intended as a substitute for consulting with your physician. All matters regarding your health require medical supervision.

DUTTON
Published by the Penguin Group
Penguin Putnam Inc., 375 Hudson Street,
New York, New York 10014, U.S.A.
Penguin Books Ltd, 27 Wrights Lane,
London W8 5TZ, England
Penguin Books Australia Ltd, Ringwood,
Victoria, Australia
Penguin Books Canada Ltd, 10 Alcorn Avenue,
Toronto, Ontario, Canada M4V 3B2
Penguin Books (N.Z.) Ltd, 182–190 Wairau Road,
Auckland 10, New Zealand

Penguin Books Ltd, Registered Offices:
Harmondsworth, Middlesex, England

First published by Dutton, an imprint of Dutton NAL,
a member of Penguin Putnam Inc.

First Printing, September, 1998
10 9 8 7 6 5 4 3 2 1

 REGISTERED TRADEMARK—MARCA REGISTRADA

LIBRARY OF CONGRESS CATALOGING-IN-PUBLICATION DATA:
Goldbeck, Nikki.
    The healthiest diet in the world / Nikki and David Goldbeck.
        p.   cm.
    ISBN 0-525-94282-3
    1. Cookery (Natural foods)   2. Nutrition.   I. Goldbeck, David.
II. Title.
TX741.G65   1998
641.5'63—dc21   98-13025
                                                              CIP

Printed in the United States of America
Set in Sabon
Designed by Leonard Telesca

This book is printed on acid-free paper.

∞

Acknowledgments

We are grateful to the following people for sharing their research and helping us to evaluate data: Jed Fahey, faculty research associate at the Brassica Chemoprotection Laboratory at Johns Hopkins University; Mark Messina, researcher and author; Clare Hasler, director of the University of Illinois Functional Foods for Health Program; Patricia Murphy, Iowa State University; and Sidi Christen, postdoctoral researcher working with Bruce Ames at the University of California at Berkeley.

Our special thanks to Judy Fichetti, research librarian; Barry Samuels, for his knowledgeable advice and support; Elena Zang and Alan Hoffman, for providing the cover pottery; and for the assistance extended by ESHA Research, makers of The Food Processor® Nutritional Analysis Software Program.

Mark Larson, thank you for so willingly coming to our rescue and for the extraordinary cover you created. And finally, we couldn't have managed without our trusted friend and assistant, Cheryl Matthews.

Contents

Introduction ix

PART I Goldbecks' Golden Guidelines

PART II In Nikki's Kitchen: Healthiest Diet Recipes

Introduction

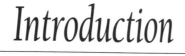

We have a rare opportunity in North America today to enjoy the healthiest diet in the world. We say this because no other people have ever had the resources available to them that we do right now. Our markets are filled with an abundance of wholesome foods, with more choices than any other continent. We have the capacity to keep foods safe from microbes and physical deterioration. The availability of organic food has grown from a fringe movement to a multibillion-dollar industry.*

Added to this is the significant progress that has been made during the last few decades regarding human nutrition. There is currently an unprecedented depth and breadth to our understanding of which foods nourish us best and how our bodies make use of them. What makes all of this so exciting is that we also have the creativity and skills to prepare these foods in many convenient, interesting, and satisfying ways.

The Marriage of Science and Art

The Healthiest Diet in the World was generated by our more than twenty-five years of work in the field of food and nutrition, which have taught us many things that we need to share on a broader scale than workshops or individual counseling allow. Our vision is to bring together the science and practice of nutrition with the art of cooking. We remain confident that the nourishment needed to keep us healthy can be provided by wholefoods—that is, foods that are as close to their natural state as possible.

To write this book, Nikki spent almost two years reading and analyzing pub-

---

*We recognize that problems do exist that keep this from being a "perfect diet," including the use of agricultural chemicals, growth hormones, food irradiation, and the like, which continue to pollute the food supply, water, and air. Moreover, lax industry practices and inadequate monitoring, particularly in a global food system, will cause occasional (perhaps inevitable) serious outbreaks of food poisoning.

lished research studies, transcripts, journals, and texts regarding various issues of human nutrition. We then designed a set of basic principles around what she found to be the most reliable, enduring, and reasonable scientific information that could be applied to the current food supply, contemporary life needs, and the historical human diet. These principles are organized into the eight Goldbecks' Golden Guidelines that form the first part of this book. Once the Guidelines were established, Nikki set about developing recipes, menus, tips, and techniques to bring these ideas to life (and to your lives). In Part II we take you "In Nikki's Kitchen" so that you can begin to experience this right away. An in-depth discussion of the research on which the Guidelines are based is contained in Part III: "Mentor."

A New Level of Cooking

The recipes provided in "In Nikki's Kitchen" represent a new level of cooking. In addition to relying on fresh wholefoods as we have always done, these recipes have several distinctive qualities:

• The recipes use very few concentrated fats. Instead, dishes have been designed to take advantage of the natural fat and moisture within foods, with attention to creating a healthier and more favorable balance of fats in the diet.

• The recipes focus on helping you achieve the high level of vegetable (and fruit) consumption that is recommended in the Guidelines.

• The recipes emphasize soy foods, legumes, yogurt and yogurt cheese, to entice you to eat more of these valuable foods.

• Moreover, the recipes and accompanying menus bring you the benefits of newly recognized elements within food such as phytochemicals, along with all the critical nutrients your body requires.

Of course, underlying all of this is our commitment to creating recipes that are easy to prepare and that we know you will enjoy.

Accentuating the Positive

Although you'll profit most by focusing on the recipes in "In Nikki's Kitchen," which support the Golden Guidelines, we don't take an all-or-nothing approach: You can improve the quality of *any* diet by integrating the material in this book as often as possible into whatever eating pattern you follow.

While the health effects of our Western diet are usually attributed to what it has too much of—fat, calories, salt, protein, sugar, refined carbohydrates—there is a tendency to overlook what it may be missing. Many people who come to Nikki for nutrition counseling are surprised by her lack of enthusiasm for low-fat or high-protein or low-carbohydrate regimes, or other similar trendy diets. She takes this approach because people who achieve the limited goals set by these programs usually only succeed in modifying a portion of their diets, such as their intake of fats or carbohydrates. For optimum health, they must also incorporate vegetables, beans, and other beneficial foods. We are being so bold as to call this book *The Healthiest Diet in the World* because it pays attention to the true variety and balance that a healthful diet demands.

When you read the Golden Guidelines, many of you may wonder, "Why no meat?" One reason is that the emphasis commonly given to meat tends to decrease consumption of other foods that are crucial to good health—most particularly, vegetables and legumes. As you will see, numerous other items also aren't included in this book. This doesn't mean they must be banned from your table. People who decide to eat foods that aren't promoted in the Guidelines—refined grains, processed sugars, additive-laden foods, meat, poultry, fish, milk, cheese, and larger amounts of concentrated fats and eggs than we counsel—don't need advice on how to cook more of them. What people do need to know more about are the areas of nutrition that we foster in our eight Golden Guidelines.

Getting Started

Goldbecks' Golden Guidelines are written for immediate access and action. We present each Guideline along with Basic Steps to start you on your way. As you come to The Next Step, a series of options appears to enable you to proceed as your interest or needs warrant. Those seeking more detail will find them in the chapters that parallel each Guideline, located in Part III.

When you delve into the chapters, along with the science you will discover a series of dialogue boxes where Nikki speaks to you in a more personal manner. Here she answers frequently asked questions and provides new insights into popular nutrition issues. This is why we have chosen to subtitle the book "A Cookbook and Mentor."

Practical Not Theoretical

Since the 1983 publication of our cookbook *American Wholefoods Cuisine*, Nikki has focused much of her attention on nutrition workshops and private counseling. She often works with those who are at risk or have already experienced a variety of conditions and illnesses, including heart disease, diabetes, cancer, eating disorders, and obesity. This has given her a rare perspective on the health-diet-cooking-lifestyle relationship. She has had the opportunity to come into contact with many people who are eager to embrace a healthy diet, and from them she has learned a great deal about what individuals are looking for and what common concerns and misconceptions they share.

Likewise, she has grown in her work as clients reveal the secrets of their successes, as well as the pitfalls, frustrations, and confusion they encounter along the way. Since, in addition to providing nourishment, food plays a strong cultural and social role in most people's lives, these experiences have helped Nikki develop food strategies that promote optimal health *and* fit comfortably into one's life.

Relax, Eat Happy

What is perhaps of greatest importance is that no diet can be considered successful if it creates anxiety. One particularly striking feature of the last quarter century has been the emergence of a genuine interest among people in improving health through nutrition. Unfortunately, a growing *hypersensitivity* to nutrition news has caused many of us to feel insecure and anxious about what we eat.

To achieve optimal nutrition people need to relax and fully enjoy what they eat. Because we are all individuals, and the circumstances and events of our lives differ, a healthful diet is most likely to be accomplished when there is a flexible course built on a sound foundation, rather than with a rigid formula, which is what most "diets" are. *The Healthiest Diet in the World* doesn't rely on a secret food or nutrient, or magical food combinations. Instead, we offer Guidelines, not rules, that leave room for variations in individual biochemical needs, food preferences, lifestyles, and cultural patterns. What we have discovered for ourselves and observed in others is that by paying attention to the areas covered in the eight Golden Guidelines, one can eat well and maintain good nutrition even in the context of a busy work schedule and an active family/social life.

Ultimately, what distinguishes our work is the synthesis of sound nutrition science, professional experience, and a historical viewpoint of the human food supply. In 1983, in *American Wholefoods Cuisine*, we described our convictions in the "Wholefoods Philosophy." Here is what we said then; it remains the foundation for our work today.

> *The human digestive system is essentially the same one our ancestors had 50,000 years ago. It is designed to digest and utilize the foods provided by our habitat. For the most part, these basic foodstuffs were discovered by our Stone Age ancestors in a hit-or-miss fashion. Those who ate best tended to live longest, and consequently their heirs and friends followed their example. The accepted diet became the one that maintained the species, and thus you might say it is a "Darwinian diet." Additionally, as certain foods became more constant in the diet, our bodies accommodated to these choices.*
>
> *Processed and fragmented foods, and those that add unnatural amounts of sugar, salt and fat, as well as modern food chemicals, are still very new to our system. We have seen many problems created by the fragmentation of wholefoods.*

The problem has always been to find the best mix of wholefoods in a modern context. That is the essence of this book.

Before we introduce the Golden Guidelines, we would like to offer a few encompassing principles:

1. Strive to consume as great a variety of unprocessed, intact foods as possible, giving preference to those grown without pesticides, herbicides, and other applied chemicals.

2. Don't become unduly influenced by every nutrition "breakthrough." If your diet is focused on a wide assortment of wholefoods, current research is likely to support what you're doing anyway, not undermine it.

3. Pay attention to total diet, not individual nutrients or foods. There is an interplay between food components that makes the sum of what we eat more relevant than any single item.

4. Set goals you can reach. The route to a sensible, health-enhancing diet needn't be severe or absolute. Choose where *you* want to go and how *you* want to get there.

5. Remember, *The Healthiest Diet in the World* will provide the greatest benefits if coupled with physical activity and a generous daily dose of fresh air and natural light.

We know that the Golden Guidelines and our new recipes will be your companions to achieving a nourishing diet and all that flows from it. But most of all, our wish is that this book will help you develop a new sense of joy and relaxation when it comes to mealtime.

—Nikki and David Goldbeck

PART I

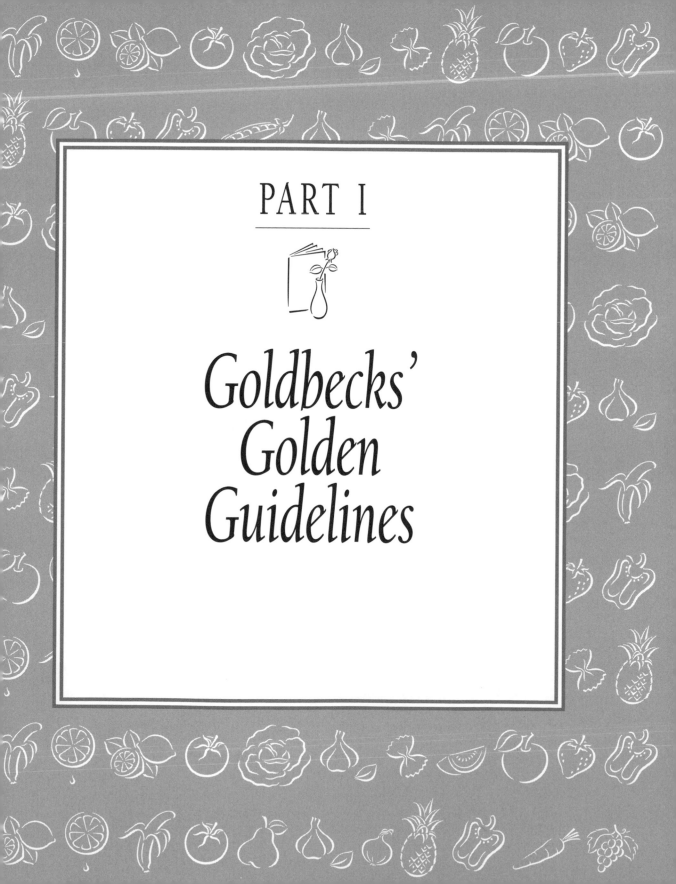

Goldbecks' Golden Guidelines

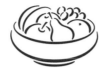

GOLDEN GUIDELINE #1:
CARBOHYDRATE COMPATIBILITY

Carbohydrates are intimately connected to the body's chemistry: They are not just the starches and sugars that we rely on for energy; they also influence how the body uses fats and proteins. In order to have a healthful diet, it's necessary to consume carbohydrates in a way that is compatible with your individual system and select carbohydrate-rich foods for their inherent health-protective nature. Carbohydrate compatibility will help with weight management, regulate blood sugar and insulin levels—which are implicated in such ailments as diabetes and heart disease—and reduce the risk of certain cancers.

There has probably never been a time in human history when dietary practices changed as radically as during the past 150 years. Widespread advocacy for reducing fat consumption has resulted in a greater proportion of calories coming from foods that are composed mainly of carbohydrates. In fact, this trend toward increased carbohydrate intake has become a central tenet of most government- and medically sanctioned dietary advice over the last decade. With the general shift toward carbohydrate-abundant diets, choosing carbohydrates properly is increasingly important for everyone because carbohydrates have such a broad reach. This is even more critical for the estimated 25 percent of the population who are carbohydrate sensitive. (After the Basic Steps below there is a self-check to help determine your carbohydrate compatibility.) If you fall into the carbohydrate-sensitive group, it means you should pay special attention to *which* carbohydrates you eat and *when* you eat them to obtain their benefits without ill effects.

None of this is meant to diminish the importance of carbohydrates. Foods that are abundant in carbohydrates have a profound influence on health. Carbohydrates are our most efficient source of energy. In addition, many carbohydrate-containing foods provide essential minerals, fibers, and other biologically active elements that foster well-being and offer protection against strokes, heart attacks, and certain cancers. (On the other hand, some carbohydrate-containing foods have little to offer beyond calories.)

Basic Steps

1. Determine your individual carbohydrate compatibility and then consume carbohydrates in accordance with your body's unique needs.

• Most people can tolerate at least 40 percent of calories from carbohydrates; those who handle carbohydrates well (based on the self-check that follows), should be able to go as high as 60 percent. To translate your calories from carbohydrate into grams of carbohydrate (which is how this nutrient is represented on food labels and in food reference tables), see Carbohydrate Intake as Percent of Calories, on page 270.

2. The best way to satisfy the need for carbohydrates is with legumes (beans), vegetables, whole grains, and fruit, *in this order.*

• Eat protein-rich foods such as soy products, legumes (which provide both protein and carbohydrates), and yogurt just before or along with your carbohydrates.

• If the Self-Check for Carbohydrate Compatibility leads you to believe that your ability to use carbohydrates is in any way impaired, give preference to foods with a low G-Force, which is a measure of how they influence blood sugar. In addition, couple foods with a high G-Force with other foods that reduce their impact. (To learn about G-Force and develop an understanding of how carbohydrates fit into your diet, see page 280.)

• Whether you're carbohydrate intolerant or not, try to keep intake of refined carbohydrates, such as white flour products, white rice, degermed cornmeal, and concentrated sweets to a minimum. The poorer your carbohydrate tolerance, the more important this advice is. (See Where Carbohydrates Come From, on page 266.)

3. Pay attention to the amount and type of fiber.

• Although there is disagreement as to how much fiber is optimal, here are the parameters:

One approach is the "age + 5" formula: Beginning at the age of two years, total daily fiber consumption should equal 5 grams added to age, until the age of twenty. By then 25 grams of daily fiber should continue for a lifetime.

Some health practitioners advise going beyond this and striving for 35 grams of fiber a day. Most controlled research studies designed to reduce cholesterol or study cancer-protective effects have used from 40 to 50 grams. There is no indication that these higher amounts are harmful, but some people suffer gastrointestinal reactions such as flatulence, cramping, bloating, loose stools, and diarrhea. A good approach is to increase fiber gradually, giving the body time to adapt. And don't forget: High-fiber diets must provide adequate fluids.

• Different types of fiber—water-soluble, water-insoluble, and resistant starch—elicit different outcomes. You can read about them in Friendly Fiber, on page 289.

4. Rather than eating two or three big meals, try several small meals interspersed with snacks over the course of the day.

• Despite the common three-meal-a-day pattern, in general most people fare better with several small meals interspersed with snacks. This plan is particularly helpful when you are carbohydrate intolerant. The preferred approach for everyone is to divide carbohydrate intake fairly evenly over the course of a day, and combine carbohydrates with protein-providing foods and the right fats (the subject of Golden Guideline #2). In this way, glucose is released gradually into the bloodstream, protecting against periods of excess or depletion. There is more tolerance for deviation from this pattern when eating carbohydrate foods with a low G-Force, such as legumes.

The Next Step

I. If the conditions described in the Self-Check for Carbohydrate Compatibility apply to you, monitor your carbohydrate intake more closely. The knowledge of how the body uses carbohydrates (discussed in Chapter 1, "Controversial Carbohydrates") will help you avoid problems by making compatible food choices.

★ SELF-CHECK FOR CARBOHYDRATE COMPATIBILITY ★

If you answer yes to any of the following, you need to monitor your carbohydrate intake more closely.

1. You are unable to maintain a healthy body weight or lose weight, if indicated, following a restricted-calorie program.
2. Your body carries a disproportionate amount of weight around the midsection.
3. Your blood tests indicate elevated triglycerides.
4. You have been diagnosed with hyperlipidemia—determined by elevated blood cholesterol, high low-density-lipoproteins (LDLs) and low high-density lipoproteins (HDLs)—that fails to respond to a restricted-fat diet.
5. You have elevated blood pressure that isn't responsive to weight loss and exercise.
6. You have been diagnosed with diabetes, hyperglycemia (elevated blood sugar levels), or hypoglycemia (frequent episodes of low blood sugar). A strong family history of these conditions should also be considered. (This means one or more parents or siblings, or several collateral relatives.)
7. You display other signs that you may be carbohydrate intolerant, including increased hunger following a high-carbohydrate meal; trouble controlling food intake triggered by carbohydrate-rich foods but improved by protein-rich foods; and overeating in response to alcohol.

II. If your body works in the highly efficient manner it's designed to, how it handles carbohydrates may be immaterial. In that case, you may only be interested in following the Basic Steps and enjoying the health-enhancing recipes found in "In Nikki's Kitchen."

GOLDEN GUIDELINE #2: THE RIGHT FAT VS. LOW-FAT

Just because a diet is low in fat doesn't make it sound. Fat is indispensable to a healthy diet; however, both the *amount* and *balance* are crucial. Wholefoods should be the primary source of the fat you eat to preserve the fat's integrity and avoid overconsumption.

Low-fat regimens can be harmful if people don't consume enough of the fatty acids (the basic components of fat) that are indispensable to well-being. On the other hand, even diets furnishing sufficient amounts of these essential fatty acids can be problematic if they're supplied by foods that undermine health in some other way, or when overall fat intake is out of balance.

The accepted viewpoint of how much fat is enough and how much is too much needs to be rethought in order to define a diet that is both health-enhancing and pleasurable. The conventional advice is to limit total fat intake to 30 percent of calories. Many health advocates feel that a 20 percent ceiling is preferable. For people already experiencing heart disease or those at high risk, there are professionals who suggest confining fat calories to 10 percent. Although with proper attention this 10 percent can probably be accomplished without compromising health, the need for such austerity isn't confirmed. (This meager allotment is also very difficult to stick with over the long term.) Furthermore, some health organizations believe that severe restriction can actually be harmful and counsel a minimum of 15 percent calories from fat.

The most widely promulgated model suggests evenly dividing fats between saturated, monounsaturated, and polyunsaturated fatty acids (a 10-10-10 ratio based on 30 percent total fat). As this Guideline demonstrates, this is neither accurate nor sufficiently informative.

Basic Steps

1. **Rather than focusing on the amount of fat you eat, pay more attention to obtaining the proper balance of individual fatty acids in your diet. This isn't an invitation to overindulge in fatty foods, but when fats are in the right proportion quantity is less of an issue.**
   • Fats can be safely consumed in a range as wide as 10 to 40 percent of total calorie intake, depending on your health and the foods this fat comes from. At both the high and low ends, the specific foods that provide this fat are particu-

larly crucial. This Guideline is devoted to helping you decide what your personal fat percentage should be.

• Fats are made up of many different fatty acids. They are commonly known under the collective headings saturated, monounsaturated, and polyunsaturated. There are, however, distinctions within these categories. As this Guideline explains, individual fatty acids have a variety of significant effects, which is why balance is so important. There is no one formula that works for everyone. However, The Golden Combination, on page 306, outlines ideal proportions. Use this information to devise an overall strategy for yourself, but don't become fixated on numbers.

• The table Foods and Their Fatty Acids, on page 314, will help you determine which foods deserve more attention than others.

2. Give priority to fat-containing plant foods in the whole form in order to obtain fatty acids in a natural proportion and in the context of other nutrients.

• The best way to satisfy the requirement for the polyunsaturated fatty acids that are considered essential is to eat full-fat soy products, wheat germ, and moderate amounts of nuts and seeds.

• If you want additional fats in your diet, the dominant fatty acids in olives, avocados, and almonds are the least controversial.

3. Keep fats from animal sources to a minimum.

• There is no known requirement for any fats that are found exclusively in animal foods.

• If you choose to consume fish for the potential health benefits of the particular fatty acids they offer, check the government fish advisories concerning pesticides, heavy metals, and other environmental contaminants (see "Resources").

4. When you use concentrated fats in the form of oil, for general purposes virgin olive oil is the preferred choice, followed by cold-pressed canola oil and specially bred high-oleic sunflower and safflower oils.

• A variety of specialty oils, such as flaxseed, hemp, and sesame oil, can also be useful for health and culinary purposes. For an ideal balance of polyunsaturated fatty acids, consider hemp oil. To emphasize the omega-3 polyunsaturated fatty acids, try flaxseed oil. For information on these and other oils see Right Fat Foods, on page 307.

• To protect oils from becoming rancid, store them in a dark place or in opaque containers. Refrigeration is preferred for all but olive oil, which keeps well at cool room temperatures. (In a colder environment olive oil thickens; this isn't harmful, but the oil must be returned to room temperature to be usable.) Flaxseed and hemp oils are particularly prone to oxidation; in addition to keeping them refrigerated, they should be consumed within two to three months of opening.

5. Avoid any fat described as partially hydrogenated or hydrogenated.

• The processing technique known as hydrogenation changes the physical construction of fats. The resulting fats, found in margarine, vegetable shortening, and many commercial cooking oils, interfere with critical biological activities.

6. To help you determine if the fat in your diet should be given special attention or might be the cause of health problems, take the Fat Self-Test, below.

• If you suspect an improper ratio of fats in your diet based on medical or nutritional advice or what you read in Chapter 2, "Walking the Dietary Fat Tightrope," consult the table Foods and Their Fatty Acids, on page 314, to discover how you can improve it.

• Don't rely on any one fatty acid to treat a particular disease process without getting proper medical attention and looking at overall dietary habits.

The Next Step

I. To achieve a workable and successful plan, you should have some knowledge of how fats influence health and what foods contain the most suitable fatty acids. These subjects are covered in detail in Chapter 2.

II. Before you go on, take the Fat Self-Test that follows in order to better assess what your needs might be. If you answer yes to any of the questions, your choice of fat-containing foods might be creating problems or need special attention. To learn more about your situation, see the discussion What Happens When Fat Consumption Is Out of Balance, on page 323.

III. To integrate the right fats into the menu, see "In Nikki's Kitchen."

★ FAT SELF-TEST ★

If you answer yes to any of the following questions, your choice of fat-containing foods might be creating problems or need special attention. To learn more about your circumstance, see the discussion What Happens When Fat Consumption Is Out of Balance, on page 323.

1. Are your blood levels of cholesterol (including HDL, LDL, and VLDL) and triglycerides above satisfactory range?
2. Have you been diagnosed with non-insulin-dependent (type II) diabetes?
3. Do you suffer from any inflammatory ailments, such as arthritis, fibromyalgia, polymyalgia, asthma, irritable bowel disease, menstrual cramps, psoriasis, and lupus?
4. Do you have an illness related to impaired immune function, including chronic infections, fatigue syndrome, HIV/AIDS, and the like?
5. Do you or a close relative have a personal history of heart disease, cancer, or osteoporosis?

GOLDEN GUIDELINE #3:
VITAL NUTRIENT HELPERS

The body has a remarkable ability to take carbohydrates, fat, and protein and turn them into the energy it runs on, vital cell components, and a host of regulatory substances. In order for this to happen, these primary nutrients require a crew of assistants. We have dubbed them *nutrient helpers*.

The human body behaves much like a large office. All of the workers take part in getting assignments accomplished efficiently and correctly. The executives generally receive most of the recognition; however, the support team of assistants, secretaries, mail room employees, on down to the maintenance staff is critical to optimum functioning. Although some people's jobs appear to be minor, if they slack off, show up late, or don't come in at all, the entire system runs less smoothly. If this sort of problem isn't recognized soon enough, it inevitably leads to breakdowns.

Nutrient helpers in the diet resemble the less-visible coworkers in the office. That is, when it comes to promoting good nutrition, certain food components get most of the attention. But without adequate participation of some lesser-known yet critical elements, the body doesn't operate at peak levels. If these failings aren't corrected, serious defects will arise.

The helpers we focus on here are vitamins E, C, and beta-carotene; the B vitamins thiamin (B_1), niacin (B_3), pantothenic acid, folate (also known as folic acid), B_6 (pyridoxine), biotin, and choline (considered a candidate for "vitaminhood"); the minerals chromium, zinc, magnesium, selenium, and copper; the sulfur-containing amino acids methionine, cystine, and cysteine; and the phytochemicals known as allyl sulfides. This is by no means an exhaustive list of all the coworkers that perform essential jobs. These were chosen because they're particularly germane to the nutrition goals presented here.

This selection of nutrient helpers is also meant to give an awareness of how many different elements there are in our diets that serve us, and to provide a glimpse at the complex nature of human nutrition. This multilevel interactive web of nutrients illustrates why wholefoods are so important, and why following unbalanced diets or trying to satisfy needs with supplements is fraught with risks.

As you read on, keep in mind these 1995 findings of the U.S. government-funded study, "What We Eat in America":

- Among the women surveyed, zinc, magnesium, copper, B_6, and vitamin E generally didn't meet recommended intake levels.
- Men fell short in zinc, magnesium, and copper.
- Adolescent males and men in most age categories over thirty were low in vitamin E, while men over seventy also lacked vitamin B_6.

In various age and gender groups, other nutrients, including calcium and iron, were also low; however, they aren't subjects of this chapter. Moreover, not all nutrients are included in these surveys, so data about chromium and selenium weren't obtained. Other government reports claim that most Americans consume only marginal levels of chromium.

Basic Steps

1. Incorporate generous amounts of fresh vegetables, legumes, whole grains, fruit, seeds, and nuts—the best food sources of the nutrient helpers—into recipes, meals, and snacks.

• Specific foods that contain notable quantities of individual nutrient helpers are listed in Dietary Sources of Nutrient Helpers, on page 356. (Many are important for other reasons as well, and receive additional attention in other Guidelines.)

2. Pay attention to your special needs regarding nutrient helpers.

• Some people need to pay particular attention to certain nutrient helpers:

People with high or low blood sugar or insulin levels should up their intake of foods providing chromium. They should also consume a variety of foods containing zinc and B vitamins.

People who don't eat meat need to consume other foods offering zinc.

People who have a high dietary intake of calcium or take calcium supplements require more dietary zinc and magnesium.

People who regularly engage in strenuous exercise should give extra consideration to foods furnishing chromium, zinc, and vitamin E.

People who drink alcohol must get plenty of folate in their diet.

To fulfill these needs see Vitamin Helpers, on page 357, and Mineral Helpers, on page 358.

• Foods that furnish vital sulfur-containing amino acids play a variety of helper roles. While these amino acids are essential for everyone, some people have a greater need due to circumstances that place a drain on body stores. In order to transform these amino acids into the desired proteins, the diet must also have available supplies of vitamin B$_6$, choline, and folate. People with special concerns include those who come in contact with chemical carcinogens, anyone taking medications, and people with a high proportion of body fat.

For suitable foods see Amino Acid Helpers, on page 360, and Vitamin Helpers, on page 357.

• A number of commonly used prescription and nonprescription drugs can compromise levels of nutrients that enjoy helper status:

Women who take oral contraceptives should increase consumption of foods containing vitamin B$_6$, folate, and vitamin C, while those using premarin for hormone replacement should emphasize folate.

Large daily doses of aspirin may cause urinary loss of vitamin C.

Frequent use of antacids can destroy thiamin.

Cortisone tablets and prednisone can create increased needs for vitamin B_6, vitamin C, and zinc.

Indocin can deplete thiamin and vitamin C.

Quite a few specialized drugs interfere with folate.

Note: Always read the accompanying literature or ask the pharmacist or your physician about the possibility of nutritional complications if you're taking any medications.

3. Optimize your antioxidant defenses.

• You can build resistance to disease by consuming a variety of foods containing nutrient helpers that serve as antioxidants: the vitamins E, C, and beta-carotene; the mineral selenium; the amino acids methionine and cystine; and phytochemicals such as carotenoids, thiosulfinates, and flavonoids. You'll find suitable foods in Dietary Sources of Nutrient Helpers, on page 356. For more on some of these food constituents, see Golden Guideline #4: More Reasons to Eat Your Vegetables (and Fruit).

• Your need for antioxidants may be greater if you smoke, spend a lot of time outdoors, are a heavy alcohol drinker, are exposed to chemicals, take medication on a regular basis, or live in a relatively polluted environment. Added antioxidant protection can also benefit people with elevated triglycerides or VLDL and LDL cholesterol levels, as they are more susceptible to oxidative damage to lipoproteins in the bloodstream.

4. Enjoy your eggs.

• Eggs can make a valuable contribution of some of the most important nutrient helpers. Unless you have a genetic condition that obstructs cholesterol metabolism, eating four to six eggs a week shouldn't create any problems. Many people can eat more than this without adversely affecting blood cholesterol levels (see page 361).

5. Get the unique benefits of garlic, onions, and mushrooms.

• These foods offer some key health-enhancing and flavoring components (see pages 361–365).

6. Steer clear of dietary schemes that overemphasize or severely restrict any of the three primary nutrients: carbohydrates, fat, and protein.

• The body is designed to utilize all the primary nutrients. It depends on each to perform its particular job. If either carbohydrate, fat, or protein is scarce, another of these nutrients is forced to assume its assignments. This places extra demands on the nutrient helpers and ultimately just about everything runs less efficiently. Likewise, an excess of carbohydrate, fat, or protein puts a strain on various body systems, as discussed in other Golden Guidelines.

11

Goldbecks'
Golden
Guidelines

The Next Step

I. For a deeper understanding of how the body relies on a multiplicity of nutrients, and how this knowledge can enhance well-being, we suggest you read Chapter 3, "Preventing System Breakdowns."

II. If you recognize the importance of the nutrient helpers, knowing the details of why the body needs them may not interest you. In that case, proceed directly to Dietary Sources of Nutrient Helpers, on page 356.

III. To put all this into action, turn to "In Nikki's Kitchen." Dishes that rely on legumes, and especially soy foods, feature vegetables or fruit, and make use of various nuts and seeds and their butters (such as almond butter and tahini) will boost your consumption of nutrient helpers.

GOLDEN GUIDELINE #4:
MORE REASONS TO EAT YOUR VEGETABLES (AND FRUIT)

Vegetables and fruit continue to grow in importance as the key to all good diets. Traditionally, produce has been embraced for its vitamin, mineral, and fiber content. But now newly discovered constituents make vegetables (and fruit) even more powerful health protectors.

You really shouldn't need any other reason to eat vegetables and fruit than for pleasure. It would seem that succulent summer tomatoes, sun-drenched sweet corn, earthy potatoes, tree-ripened peaches, crisp winter apples, and the like are inherently appealing enough to attract us. However, in today's world these gifts of nature must compete with sugared and salty foods that seduce us with their quick energy and jade our tastebuds. If you care about your health though, you'll have to face the not-so-terrible task of eating vegetables and fruit in abundance.

A diet rich in plant foods actively promotes health by:
1. Furnishing the vitamins and minerals that act as catalysts for all the activities that take place within the body.
2. Providing antioxidant nutrients that minimize oxidative activity inside the body.
3. Enhancing the elimination of digestive waste and removal of carcinogens via fiber.
4. Contributing water, which helps fulfill the body's daily liquid requirement.

Basic Steps

1. Eat as much and as many different vegetables as you can.

- Whether you eat your day's ration in bits and pieces or a few large portions, two key concepts apply: abundance and diversity. If over the course of a week you don't consume at least six pounds combined of vegetables and fruit, and mostly the former, you aren't eating enough of these foods.

- While for most people there's no upper limit on vegetables, individuals who are carbohydrate intolerant should be more modest when it comes to eating vegetables with a high G-Force. And when you do eat these sweet or starchy plants, slow down their G-Force by consuming protein-rich foods such as soy products, legumes, and yogurt just before or along with them. (For more about carbohydrate intolerance and G-Force, see Chapter 1.)

- Smokers should make an even greater effort to fulfill this Guideline, particularly with items in the leafy green and deep yellow-orange categories.

2. Fruit is best limited to two to four daily servings.

- Fruit furnishes many of the same beneficial nutrients as vegetables, but because of its high sugar content can create problems for people with varying degrees of carbohydrate intolerance. People who want to limit carbohydrates can reduce or even skip fruit altogether, so long as they compensate with extra vegetables.

- A standard serving is one medium size fruit; $^1/_2$ cup chopped raw, cooked, or canned fruit; or $^3/_4$ cup fruit juice.

3. Give priority to fresh seasonal produce.

- Fresh vegetables (and fruit) have the highest nutritional value. It's a good idea to enjoy them both raw (in salads and as snacks) and cooked. Preferred cooking techniques are baking, grilling, steaming, stir-steaming, stewing, and pressure cooking, as featured in "In Nikki's Kitchen."

- Frozen unseasoned vegetables and unsweetened fruit are also acceptable. (You'll find some of them used in our recipes.)

- Canned vegetables and fruit are almost always highly salted or sweetened, which detracts from their value. Moreover, water-soluble nutrients are lost in the canning liquid. An important exception is canned tomato products, which have considerable culinary value and nutritional worth.

- There are also some dried vegetables (sun-dried tomatoes, seaweeds, mushrooms), dried fruit, and numerous herbs and spices that contribute to the healthiest diet in the world.

4. Whenever possible, choose vegetables and fruit that support the concepts of organic and sustainable agriculture.

- Organically raised vegetables and fruit, particularly when locally grown, are more desirable in many ways. They're free of applied pesticides, herbicides, and fungicides, safer for farm workers, and contribute to a cleaner environment.

Goldbecks'
Golden
Guidelines

The Next Step

I. If you wish to know why fresh produce is the key to every good diet, we suggest you read Chapter 4, "A Foundation of Vegetables (and Fruit)." Even if you're already convinced, you'll probably be surprised by some of what you learn and be in a better position to educate others (for example, those you may feed).

II. If you don't need any more reasons to eat your vegetables (and fruit), but could use some ideas for easily adding then to the daily diet, turn to Nikki's dialogue box on page 368.

III. To find ways to eat plenty of produce and enjoy it, take a look at "In Nikki's Kitchen." You might find you like vegetables (and fruit) more than you expected.

GOLDEN GUIDELINE #5: SUPER SOY FOODS

A growing body of research supports a clear connection between regular consumption of soy foods and a reduced risk of several chronic ailments. But even without such protective health effects, soy's exemplary nutritional profile mandates its inclusion as a prominent part of everyone's diet.

Studies demonstrate that soy in the diet helps protect against cancer in general; breast, prostate, and other hormonally influenced cancers in particular; and heart disease. It has great potential to forestall osteoporosis, and may also modulate blood sugar levels in diabetics, and ease the discomforts of menopause.

While once thought of as exotic, and available mostly as chunks of tofu, in a short time soy foods have come a long way. The soybean now comes in a variety of forms and products that have virtually elevated it to the level of a convenience food, although not all soy-containing foods are necessarily equal in attributes.

In addition, soy foods are an extremely versatile cooking ingredient. The numerous ways of preparing soy can satisfy both conventional and adventurous palates, and make it easier than most people expect to enjoy this remarkable food on a regular basis.

Basic Steps

1. Make soy foods a regular part of your daily diet.
• Substantial evidence indicates that eating soy foods regularly supports health on a broad scale. In order to provide protection against heart attacks and the various cancers that may be reduced by eating soy, a target intake is about 25 grams of protein daily from one or several soy foods (see Mixing and Matching Soy Protein, on page 412).

• Familiarize yourself with today's soy food selections and find ways to include them in everyday meals in an enjoyable manner. Among the most commendable soy foods are tofu, tempeh, soy "milks," soy nuts, soybeans, soy sprouts, soy flour, miso, and products that feature them. All offer important nutrients that can boost your daily intake. (For a description of these foods see pages 415–419.)

The Next Step

During her presentation in 1994 at the First International Symposium on the role of Soy in Preventing and Treating Chronic Disease, Anne Goldberg, of the Lipid Research Center, Washington University School of Medicine, St. Louis, Missouri, spoke strongly in support of the role of soybeans in coronary artery disease prevention. But she was also moved to point out that "the main obstacles to greater use of soy protein in the therapy of hyperlipidemia [elevated cholesterol and triglycerides] include lack of knowledge by physicians and patients of its effects" and the need for "readily available packaged products, recipes, and cookbooks . . . to make incorporation of soy protein into the American diet a reality."

I. If you want to gain this "knowledge" of how soy benefits health, turn to Chapter 5, "In Praise of Soybeans."

II. For some quick ideas on how to use the soy products that are readily available in natural food stores and supermarkets, turn to Nikki's dialogue box on page 425.

III. The need for reliable and enjoyable soy recipes is satisfied with dishes such as Tempeh Breakfast Links, Savory Baked Tofu, Hearty Miso-Vegetable Soup, Tofu Chili, Maple-Pecan Tempeh, Creamy Miso Mustard Dressing, Toasted Soy Spread, Banana–Oat Bran Muffins, Fruit and Tofu Tart, and White Ginger Tea.

GOLDEN GUIDELINE #6:
PROTEIN WITHOUT FEAR: BEANS

The protein in fiber-rich, low fat beans rounds out the menu for people seeking optimal nutrition.

Protein got its name from the Greek word *proteos*, meaning primary or taking first place. Every cell in every living organism, from the tiniest microbe to the biggest animal, is dependent on protein. However, it might be said that people have taken this scientific fact too seriously, to the point where many of us overconsume protein, to our detriment. (The general adult requirement of 45 to 65 grams a day is frequently exceeded by as much as twofold. A modest 4-ounce serving of beef, for example, furnishes 32 grams of protein.)

Some of the problems associated with the consumption of protein from animal products are avoided when beans, also known as legumes, take first place instead. But everyone seeking effective nutrition, from meat eaters to vegetarians, will profit by eating beans, due to their protein-packed/low-fat profile, protective fiber, and diverse vitamin and mineral makeup.

The *American Cancer Society 1996 Dietary Guidelines* urge people to "choose beans as an alternative to meat." Unfortunately, this concept may require a change in attitude. Legumes carry a legacy of being both humble and unexciting. It's true that there was a time when beans were the province of those without means, but this is no longer so. Legumes are for everyone, particularly since in the last two decades they have been made the star of so many imaginative meals.

Basic Steps

1. Bring beans to the table on a regular basis.
• One cup of most cooked beans—a generous-size serving—supplies 14 to 18 grams of protein or about one third to one fourth of people's daily need for protein. This comes with very little fat, and ample amounts of protective fiber and resistant starch. With 12 to 15 grams of fiber, a cup of beans satisfies half of the suggested daily intake.
• Despite a high proportion of carbohydrate, beans have a relatively low G-Force, which means they don't cause spikes in blood sugar or insulin levels.
• Beans confer protection against coronary disease, birth defects, and certain cancers.

2. If your diet is high in protein, and you want to reduce the risk of potential health problems, let beans provide the largest share.
• If you have a typical high protein intake from foods of animal origin, or follow a "high-protein diet," switching to beans may reduce your risk of osteoporosis.
• If you have high blood pressure and eat a lot of animal protein, switching to beans may bring the numbers down.
• If you're prone to kidney stones, try replacing animal protein with beans.

The Next Step

I. Few people have a realistic understanding of how much protein they should be eating. To determine your individual protein needs in order to knowingly consume adequate amounts, see Calculating Your Protein Profile, on page 433.

II. To discover the particular ways in which beans boost health, read chapter 6, "The Beauty of Beans."

III. To begin benefiting from beans, include at least one of the bean dishes from "In Nikki's Kitchen" on your daily menu.

GOLDEN GUIDELINE #7:
PROTEIN WITHOUT FEAR: YOGURT AND YOGURT CHEESE

Foods with a rich creamy texture are highly prized, but often include too much fat, particularly troublesome saturated fat. Yogurt and yogurt cheese, easily made at home by draining yogurt, are versatile foods that furnish a good source of protein that's low fat or fat free, without sacrificing the sensual pleasures of fatty foods.

Plain, unflavored yogurt is one of the most versatile foods in the world kitchen. In addition to popular uses as a quick meal, a snack, on cereal, with fruit, and the like, yogurt can replace sour cream and mayonnaise in spreads, salads, dressings, dips, and baking. Unlike these high-fat items, yogurt offers protein, calcium, and B vitamins in a trim package. On top of this, the bacterial cultures, as well as an unusual fatty acid found in yogurt, point to additional advantages conferred by regular consumption of this adaptable food.

One would think that with all these virtues, yogurt couldn't be made any better. But it can. An amazingly effective way to make yogurt a standard part of your diet is to transform its soft puddinglike consistency into a thick, spreadable cheese. This is effortlessly accomplished by "gravity processing"; that is, allowing its liquid to drain off with the aid of a yogurt cheese funnel or similar device. This simple process results in a magical transformation to a unique food that ranges in texture from rich and creamy to a compact spread, depending on how long you allow it to drain.

Why are we so hot about this cool food? While plain yogurt continues to be a commendable food choice, yogurt cheese has some added attributes that can make your pursuit of the healthiest diet in the world considerably easier:

• Yogurt cheese, which can be made with nonfat or low-fat yogurt, has a texture generally found only in high-fat foods that is associated with an extremely pleasurable effect on the palate.
• Yogurt cheese has a mild flavor that is less tart than the yogurt it came from.
• Yogurt cheese is resistant to heat, making it more practical than yogurt in cooking.
• Yogurt cheese concentrates some of yogurt's nutrients. Consequently, an equal volume delivers extra value.

*Goldbecks'
Golden
Guidelines*

Basic Steps

1. Prepare yogurt cheese on a regular basis so that it's on hand at all times.

• A few simple tools and the force of gravity are all you need. Your refrigerator should always contain one batch ready to use, and one in progress. Directions are on page 244.

2. Use the recipes in this book to gain experience using yogurt cheese.

• In "In Nikki's Kitchen" you'll find ways to use yogurt cheese in everything from soups to desserts. It lends its creaminess to Succulent Stuffed Mushrooms, Chiles Rellenos, White Pita "Pizzas," Brussels Slaw, Creamy Garden Vegetables, Baked Artichoke Cheese, Smothered Eggplant, and Strawberry Frozen Yogurt.

3. Be inventive using yogurt cheese on your own.

• You will quickly discover that yogurt cheese can be used to replace some or all of the mayonnaise, sour cream, and cream cheese in many dishes that are already in your repertoire. Even unskilled cooks will easily find new applications.

• Some simple tips for using yogurt cheese are listed in Nikki's dialogue box on page 444.

4. Assess your need for yogurt in relation to the rest of your diet.

• One of the most important contributions of yogurt and yogurt cheese is calcium. Certain hereditary and dietary factors can raise the need for this mineral. For example, women whose mothers suffer from osteoporosis may be more predisposed to this ailment and their calcium requirement may be higher. Likewise, the more animal foods in your diet, the more attention you should pay to upping your consumption of calcium-containing foods. A high intake of alcohol and caffeine can also boost calcium needs.

• Other conditions where calcium might be helpful include hypertension, kidney stones, and possibly colon cancer.

5. Don't forget about plain yogurt. It, too, is a great food.

• If you're concerned about animal fat, yogurt comes in low-fat and no-fat options. However, before you make a determination, you should read about some potential benefits of the fat in yogurt on page 445.

• Be sure to buy a yogurt that hasn't been pasteurized after culturing and states on the label that it contains live and active (or viable) cultures. Otherwise the friendly flora, whose health benefits are discussed on page 442, will be lacking.

• Make an attempt to purchase a brand that doesn't contain the growth hormone BST. As this information isn't noted on the label, organic yogurt is the safest bet, or query companies directly.

The Next Step

I. To discover why yogurt and yogurt cheese are so important, read Chapter 7, "Yogurt: Beyond Milk."

II. To find simple ways to incorporate yogurt cheese into your daily food plan, see Nikki's dialogue box on page 444.

III. For recipes that take advantage of the versatile nature of yogurt and yogurt cheese, such as Mushroom Pâté, Chunky Red Chili Mashed Potatoes, Stewed Red Cabbage, Cauliflower Gratin, Baked Potatoes with Whipped Artichoke Filling, Curried Tomato and Cucumber Salad, Black Bean Hummus, Cold Cucumber-Yogurt Soup, Lemon-Tahini Dressing, Creamy Walnut Pesto, Applesauce-Date Cake, and Whipped Yogurt "Cream," turn to "In Nikki's Kitchen."

GOLDEN GUIDELINE #8: LIQUIDS OF LIFE

About two-thirds of the human body is composed of water. Because we continuously use water in various body processes and lose water through perspiration and waste elimination, replenishing the supply is a necessity. While individual circumstances dictate how much fluid each of us needs to consume daily, a minimum of 50 ounces is a standard recommendation. This demand can be fulfilled entirely with water—both by itself and within foods. There are also health benefits to be obtained from leaf tea, modest juice consumption, and possibly limited amounts of alcohol.

Finding something suitable to drink is a surprisingly complex job. Among other things, people question the cleanliness of their water, worry about the caffeine in many popular beverages, and have been given misleading information about the value of juice. In addition, it's hard to know what to believe regarding publicity that makes tea seem like a cure for whatever ails us, and we have all heard conflicting information about the suitability of alcohol.

Water is the world's most abundant drink and it should be a significant part of the nourishing elements that we take in every day. But water isn't always as pure as it should be, and in today's marketplace it isn't necessarily the beverage with the most appeal. There are ways to improve both of these situations, but for many people it may require some adjustment.

On a worldwide basis, tea is the most widely consumed beverage aside from water. Animal studies have produced a particularly strong argument in favor of tea drinking, whether green or black, regular or decaffeinated. (One can't help but be amused at the thought of lab animals enjoying high tea.) The evidence as far as humans go, however, is still equivocal and incomplete. (Note that the positive findings on tea apply only to leaf teas, not herbal teas, which are botanically and chemically unrelated. Herbal teas are made from a vast assortment of plants that can have many physiological functions ranging from healing to harmful.)

Most people believe that fruit juice is a healthful beverage. Indeed, pure (100 percent) fruit juices furnish a variety of essential nutrients and adjunctive food factors, such as phytochemicals. However, they're also a concentrated source of simple carbohydrates. As a result, not only does fruit juice make a considerable contribution in terms of calories, but as you will read in Chapter 1, its native sugars can disturb blood sugar levels, disrupt our innate appetite-controlling mechanisms, and interfere with many people's ability to manage their weight. While juice is certainly preferable to soft drinks, which are equally sweet but lack nutrients, most people are best off eating fruit, not drinking it. (For more on fruit juice, see Juicy Prospects, on page 370.)

Regarding vegetable juices, carrot juice, too, is amply endowed with carbohydrates. Perhaps the sole commonly consumed exception is tomato-based juices. Unfortunately, the value of canned tomato juices is usually diminished by high sodium content. (Unsalted versions are available.) Of course, a homemade vegetable broth or soup could help satisfy your liquid needs. Note that you will find juices used in some of our recipes. In this form, their impact is diluted.

Where alcohol is concerned, reports that wine drinking may hold the answer to why the French have a low incidence of heart disease have prompted many people to take up social drinking or conclude that red wine ought to be their beverage of choice. Even though there is a respectable body of research supporting the heart-protective influence of alcohol in general, and wine in particular, the dangers of excess alcohol consumption are profound. There is a fine line between the optimal amount and too much. Furthermore, most of alcohol's protective effects can be derived from other foods. This means if you don't already drink, there's no reason to start. On the other hand, there appears to be no reason to condemn a prudent intake of alcohol.

Basic Steps

1. Consume the equivalent of at least 50 ounces (six 8-ounce glasses) of liquid a day, with water the preferred choice.

- To determine more individualized fluid needs, see How Much Water Should You Drink?, on page 460.
- The liquid within food counts. Serve water-based foods such as soups, stews, sauces, and gravies. In addition, you can get essential water from vegetables, fruit, and cooked grains and legumes.

2. Encourage water drinking by making it readily accessible.
- Keep containers of water in the refrigerator. Set water out on the table at mealtime. Drink the water that's poured for you in restaurants.
- Use bottled still or sparkling water if this is more appealing than tap water.
- Give everyone in your household a personal water bottle to carry with them.
- Dilute juices by one-half or more with sparkling or still water for a tasty thirst-quencher with substantially fewer calories and a lower G-Force.
- Water from private wells and municipal water sources should be tested every six months to one year. If called for, install an appropriate water filter or a home water cooler.

3. Make one of your beverages (leaf) tea.
- Leaf teas (as distinguished from herbal teas) contain high levels of phytochemicals to which health-protective roles have been ascribed. Since the potential of tea to reduce the risk of cancer and heart disease hasn't yet been attributed to any one component, and the composition of teas differs by type, drinking all kinds of tea—green, oolong, and black—is suggested.
- Avoid presweetened teas. Downing a bottle of sweetened ice tea (or making it from a mix) is not much better than guzzling soda or sweetened punch.
- Avoid drinking tea that's boiling hot, as it can be a dangerous irritant.

4. If you want to take advantage of the potential health benefits of alcohol, limit yourself to just one drink a day for women, two for men, and be sure to maintain good nutrition.
- One drink equals 12 ounces of beer, 4 to 5 ounces of wine, or 1.5 ounces of distilled spirits (see page 469).
- Imbibe slowly and in the company of food and water.
- Any positive effects of alcohol are negated by binge drinking. What you don't drink one day can't be added to the next day's allotment.
- Any protection against heart disease may be offset by an increased risk of cancer, which has been associated with just a few drinks a week for some women, and starts to rise for all genders above two drinks a day.
- Be attentive to maintaining your nutritional status. Alcohol can interfere with certain nutrients and increase the need for others. Vitamins C, E, A, B_6, B_{12}, riboflavin, folate, zinc, and the amino acid methionine are all intertwined in some fashion with alcohol. If you drink alcohol, be sure to eat foods rich in all these nutrients (for details see Golden Guidelines #3 and #4 and parallel chapters).
- If you drink alcohol, increase your water intake to compensate for its diuretic effect.

Goldbecks' Golden Guidelines

• The combined effects of smoking and drinking are greater than either alone. If you smoke, don't drink alcohol.

• Alcohol is never recommended for children, adolescents, or pregnant women.

• Consult your doctor and pharmacist about any contraindications regarding alcohol for all medications you take.

The Next Step

I. If you don't need more information about the importance of suitable liquids in your diet, make sure to take action so that your daily needs are met.

II. For a thorough understanding of why liquids are so crucial, and why some may be better for you than others, read Chapter 8, "Drink Up."

III. If you drink alcohol, be sure to read the section Alcohol: To Drink or Not to Drink, on page 468.

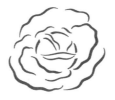

PART II

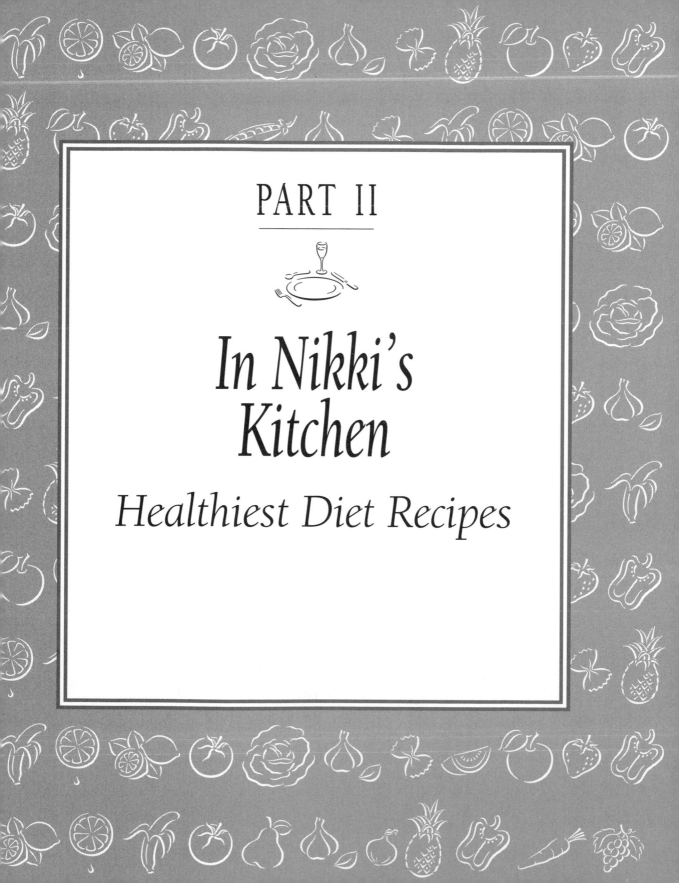

In Nikki's Kitchen

Healthiest Diet Recipes

The Healthiest Breakfasts in the World

The healthiest diet in the world starts with breakfast. This is the first opportunity to begin changing the pattern of your meals. Everyone should eat something worthwhile in the morning. Moreover, if you get up early you can divide breakfast into two snack-type meals before lunch.

People have different opinions about what foods qualify as breakfast fare. In one of our earlier books, *The Good Breakfast Book,* we note that "most foods that are good for you are good for you at any time of day." Nonetheless, below we offer some breakfast tips, menus, and a selection of recipes whose form will be familiar. In addition to the recipes that appear here, you'll find several suitable breakfast items in other recipe sections, such as Yogurt Cheese in "Gold Star Basics" and a variety of muffins and biscuits in "Simple Baking." Take a look at "Drinks," as well, for beverage ideas.

Breakfast Tips

Here are some basic tips you can use regardless of whether you eat your morning meal at home or out:

• Carbohydrate-dominant foods such as bagels, rolls, and pastries are typical of many breakfasts. Be sure to complement your carbohydrates with protein. As often as possible, make soy- and yogurt-based proteins the breakfast choice.

• Choose cereals, breadstuffs, crackers, pancakes, and the like made from whole grains. Top cereal with ground flaxseed and wheat germ, ingredients that should also be included when making your own baked goods.

• Eat cereal with yogurt or soy milk.

• Top pancakes with yogurt cheese (or yogurt) and fruit instead of drowning them in butter and sweet syrup.

• Try to include some vegetables at breakfast: a slice of tomato, cucumber, sprouts, and/or lettuce added to the filling on a bagel or sandwich; mushroom, peppers, onions, leftover vegetables, and the like in tofu scrambles or omelets. A baked potato (white or sweet, made in advance) topped with yogurt cheese is an easy breakfast addition.

- Include fresh fruit on cereal, pancakes, or nut butter sandwiches.
- Make soy part of your breakfast fare. Along with using soy milk on cereal and in shakes, add soy flour to muffins, biscuits, and pancakes, and try the Soybean Pancakes and tofu and tempeh breakfast recipes below. (For more tofu and tempeh of this type, see *The Good Breakfast Book*.)
- Drink tea or water.

Nikki's Select Breakfast Menus

I.
Scrambled Eggs with Cheese* on whole-grain toast

II.
Mexican Scramble* with corn tortillas and sliced avocado

III.
Ultimate Oatmeal* with fresh berries or sliced banana

IV.
Appleberry-Corn Muffins† with Yogurt Cheese† or almond butter

V.
Orange Griddlecakes* with Tempeh Breakfast Links*

VI.
Yogurt with fresh fruit

VII.
All-in-One Breakfast Shake*

*Recipes below.
†Recipes in other sections.

Breakfast Recipe Notes

Of course, just as breakfast needn't be limited to traditional foods, the recipes in this section don't have to be reserved for the morning. For example, Vegetable Tofu Scramble and Mexican Scramble make excellent dinners. And, for a light evening meal, griddlecakes can fill the bill.

All-in-One Breakfast Shake

~

Cereal, soy, and fruit in one easy-to-fix and easy-to-enjoy package. You can add variety with your choice of juice, and by altering the fruit with the season, replacing the banana with a very ripe pear, a large peach, or ³/4 cup sweet berries.

1¹/4 cups soy milk
1 medium banana
¹/2 cup orange, apple, or
   pineapple juice

¹/4 cup oats
2 tablespoons wheat germ
2 to 4 ice cubes, optional
nutmeg, optional

Combine everything except the ice cubes and nutmeg in blender. Process at high speed until smooth. (For a frothier shake, add ice cubes and process until completely melted.) Pour into serving glasses. Sprinkle with nutmeg, if desired.

YIELD: 2 LARGE 12-OUNCE SERVINGS

Ultimate Oatmeal

~

Ultimate Oatmeal provides an excellent example of how easy it is to integrate the Golden Guidelines into familiar recipes. To reflect the principles set forth in Golden Guideline #1: Carbohydrate Compatibility, breakfast oats are enhanced with extra oat bran, wheat germ, and flaxseed. The recipe is purposely proportioned to produce a thick porridge that can handle a generous amount of soy milk. (If a thinner cereal is preferred, add additional freshly boiled water at the end as needed.) At serving time, garnish each bowl according to personal taste with sunflower seeds, chopped walnuts, and cinnamon.

¹/3 cup oats
2 tablespoons oat bran
1¹/4 cups water
pinch salt for pot, optional

1 tablespoon flaxseed meal
  (page 239)
1 tablespoon wheat germ

Combine the oats, oat bran, water, and salt, if using, in a pot. Place over medium heat. Bring to a boil, reduce the heat, and simmer gently for 5 minutes. Stir once or twice during cooking. Remove from the heat and stir in the flaxseed meal and wheat germ. Cover and let sit for a few minutes before serving.

YIELD: 1 SERVING

*In
Nikki's
Kitchen*

Scrambled Eggs with Cheese

A single egg goes farther when you combine it with Yogurt Cheese. Although this dish is flavorful and creamy without any embellishment, those who like their eggs more elaborate can add chopped scallions, chives, mushrooms, leftover cooked vegetables, and assorted herbs according to taste. The technique used in this recipe of beating the egg in the hot pan requires a bit more skill than the conventional (alternative) approach, in which the egg is beaten first in a bowl and then poured into the hot pan. I like this method because there's less cleanup. However, you do need to move quickly. If not, the egg may set too rapidly and you'll end up with unblended whites, rather than consistently yellow eggs. For 2 or 3 servings, multiply the ingredients proportionally and prepare in a 10- or 12-inch omelet pan. For more than this, cook in separate batches.

1 egg
1 tablespoon Yogurt Cheese
 (page 244)

salt and pepper

Heat an 8-inch seasoned omelet pan. If not well seasoned, wipe with oil.

When hot, break the egg directly into the pan and quickly beat with a fork until yolk and white are integrated. Cook over low to moderate heat, stirring with a spoon or lifting the cooked portion with a spatula as it sets. When the egg is almost cooked to your liking, drop the Yogurt Cheese in several dollops on top. Fold the cooked portion of egg over the cheese and cook briefly, until the Yogurt Cheese is creamy.

Season to taste with salt and pepper.

YIELD: 1 SERVING

Vegetable-Tofu Scramble

Many people find scrambled tofu a marvelous replacement for eggs. The addition of turmeric is more for color than taste; it truly gives the tofu the appearance of eggs. Serve on a plate with brown rice or potatoes, or turn into a great sandwich stuffed into a whole wheat pita, rolled into a tortilla, or piled on toast.

1/4 cup chopped onion
1/4 cup diced green pepper
1 cup mixed vegetables of choice,
  cut into small pieces: asparagus,
  broccoli, celery, carrots,
  cauliflower, corn kernels, green
  beans, mushrooms, red cabbage,
  snow peas, zucchini

1 tablespoon water
1 teaspoon soy sauce
8 ounces firm tofu
1/4 teaspoon turmeric
salt and pepper

Combine the vegetables, water, and soy sauce in a skillet and place over medium heat. When hot, turn the heat low, cover, and cook, stirring occasionally, for 10 to 15 minutes or until the firmest vegetables are fork tender.

Add the tofu to the skillet and mash into rough chunks with a potato masher. Sprinkle the entire dish with the turmeric. Raise the heat a little and continue to cook and stir for a few minutes, until the tofu is hot.

Season to taste with salt and pepper.

YIELD: **2** SERVINGS

VARIATION: For *Mexican Scramble*, add 1 tablespoon minced hot pepper (jalapeño, serrano, hot chile, according to taste preferences) along with the vegetables. Just before adding the tofu, season the vegetables with 1/2 teaspoon oregano, 1/4 teaspoon cumin, and 1 teaspoon chili powder and cook briefly. Omit the turmeric. Top each serving with 2 tablespoons warm salsa. Accompany with tortillas, sliced avocado, and additional salsa for individual seasoning.

Soybean Pancakes

High in protein, flourless, and surprisingly delicate.

1 cup cooked soybeans   1/4 cup soy milk
2 eggs

Combine all ingredients in a blender or food processor and puree until smooth. Pour the batter onto a preheated, nonstick or lightly oiled grill or skillet, allowing 1/4 cup batter per pancake. When bubbles form on the surface and the bottom is lightly browned, turn and cook until the other side is set.

YIELD: **10** PANCAKES; **2** SERVINGS

Orange Griddlecakes

~

Serve these sweet, cakelike pancakes topped with yogurt cheese and sliced bananas, peaches, or berries. A good choice for a brunch or even a light dinner. Recipe can be multiplied as needed.

3/4 cup whole wheat flour
2 tablespoons wheat germ
2 tablespoons soy flour
2 tablespoons flaxseed meal
  (page 239)

1 teaspoon baking powder
1/2 teaspoon baking soda
1/4 teaspoon salt
1 1/4 cups orange juice
1 teaspoon canola oil

Combine the dry ingredients in a mixing bowl. Add the juice and oil. Stir gently until the dry ingredients are completely moistened.

Pour the batter by 1/4 cupfuls onto a hot oiled or nonstick griddle. Cook until the bottom is golden. Turn and cook the other side.

YIELD: 8 PANCAKES; 2 SERVINGS

Mixed Grain Griddlecakes

~

Try these hearty pancakes with one of the delicious pancake toppings that follow.

1/2 cup cornmeal
1/4 cup whole wheat flour
2 tablespoons wheat germ
2 tablespoons soy flour
2 tablespoons flaxseed meal
  (page 239)

2 1/2 teaspoons baking powder
1/4 teaspoon salt
1 1/4 cups soy milk
1 teaspoon maple syrup
1 teaspoon canola oil
1 banana, sliced, optional

Combine the dry ingredients in a mixing bowl. Add the milk, maple syrup, and oil. Stir until the dry ingredients are completely moistened. Let stand a few minutes, until the batter absorbs liquid and thickens. Stir in the fruit, if desired.

Pour the batter by generous 1/4 cupfuls onto a hot oiled or nonstick griddle. Cook until the bottom is golden. Turn and cook the other side.

YIELD: 6 PANCAKES; 2 SERVINGS

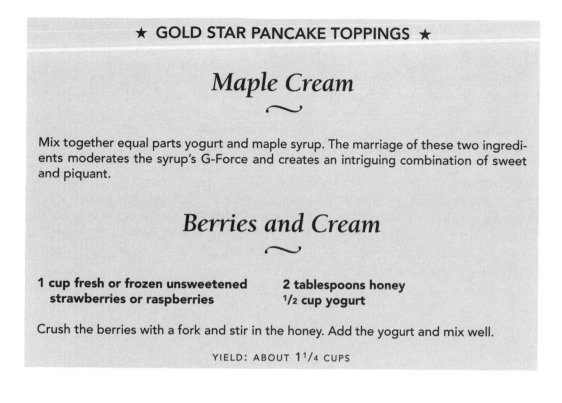

Maple Cream

Mix together equal parts yogurt and maple syrup. The marriage of these two ingredients moderates the syrup's G-Force and creates an intriguing combination of sweet and piquant.

Berries and Cream

1 cup fresh or frozen unsweetened strawberries or raspberries

2 tablespoons honey
¹/₂ cup yogurt

Crush the berries with a fork and stir in the honey. Add the yogurt and mix well.

YIELD: ABOUT 1¹/₄ CUPS

Tempeh Strips

These tasty strips are good with pancakes, alongside eggs, or on a sandwich. They can also be served on top of a grain—brown rice, millet, quinoa, kasha.

8 ounces tempeh
1 tablespoon soy sauce

2 tablespoons water
canola or olive oil

Cut the tempeh into strips ¹/₈ inch thick. Combine the soy sauce and water. Heat enough oil in a skillet to coat the bottom. When hot, add the tempeh strips and brown lightly on both sides. Sprinkle the soy sauce mixture over the browned tempeh, cover, and cook 1 to 2 minutes, until most of the liquid is absorbed. Remove the lid and cook to evaporate any remaining moisture.

YIELD: 24 STRIPS; 4 SERVINGS

Tempeh Breakfast Links

Fat, juicy tempeh links can be used in the same way as the crisper Tempeh Strips above, with pancakes, eggs, or a grain.

8 ounces tempeh	**¹/₄ cup water**
1 tablespoon soy sauce	

Cut the tempeh into 12 ¹/₄-inch "fingers." Combine the soy sauce and water. Heat a heavy skillet, preferably cast iron. Put the tempeh and about half of the diluted soy sauce into the skillet and cook until the tempeh starts to color on the bottom. Turn the tempeh over, add the remaining liquid, cover, and cook for 5 minutes. Remove the cover and cook until the liquid is gone and the tempeh is nicely colored on both sides.

YIELD: 12 LINKS; 3 TO 4 SERVINGS

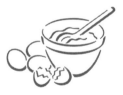

*The
Healthiest
Diet in
the World*

The Healthiest Lunches
in the World

Whether your midday meal is eaten at home or you pack a lunch to go, it can easily meet the criteria in the Golden Guidelines. You might want to divide your lunch into two parts to gain the benefits of the small-meal pattern. Sandwiches are typically split in halves, while salads, soups, yogurt, and the like can easily be consumed at intervals.

Some sample menus and recipes are provided below. They feature dishes that are quickly prepared or conveniently made ahead. For packed lunches, a thermos makes it possible to carry homemade soups and chili.

Additional lunch ideas can be found throughout the recipe section. For example, in "Appetizers and Hors d'oeuvres" you'll discover spreads such as Mushroom Pâté, Tofu Pâté, Deviled Tofu, Bean Guacamole, Black Bean Hummus, Roasted Red Pepper–Chickpea Dip, and Tomato Cream Cheese for filling sandwiches. "Spreads" includes valuable ideas for seasoning sandwiches. Depending on your time schedule, the recipes in "Soup," "Main Dishes," and "Accompaniments" can be made expressly for lunch, or you can plan ahead to have leftovers to reheat or eat cold. In "Salads and Salad Dressings" you'll find dressings to enhance your enjoyment of huge salads at lunchtime; you might even want to bring a jar with you for box lunches or dining out.

Lunch Tips

While it's easiest to heed the Golden Guidelines if you eat lunch at home or bring it with you, there are plenty of ways to comply when eating out. The suggestions below provide some tips.

• Choose salad as either your main dish or accompaniment. Ask for beans or tofu to be added, if available. Request the dressing on the side so you can monitor the amount. Better still, ask for oil (preferably olive) and vinegar (something mild like balsamic or cider) and make your own dressing. Best yet, bring some homemade dressing with you.

• Whenever available, opt for whole grains in the form of brown rice, millet, buckwheat, and such. Choose whole-grain bread, crackers, and pasta.

• Sandwiches should always include vegetables (or fruit). Whenever suitable, add chopped celery, sweet red or green pepper, cucumber, or other vegetables to sandwich fillings. Cover the filling with lettuce, tomato, sprouts, and the like. Make your "peanut (almond or cashew) butter and" sandwiches with sliced pear, apple, banana, or berries.

• Always include raw vegetable sticks—celery, carrots, cucumber, zucchini—in the lunch bag, as well as a piece of fresh or dried fruit.

• Minimize added fat. Sandwiches can easily be made without butter or mayonnaise. Simple replacements include mustard and ketchup (or preferably, our Better Than Ketchup) and, of course, yogurt cheese. Other flavorful choices are found in "Spreads." One of the tastiest ways to moisten and flavor bread is with mashed cloves of roasted garlic (see page 242).

• Yogurt (with added vegetables or fruit) is a good choice at almost any meal.

• When ordering pizza, have it topped with onions, peppers, mushrooms, broccoli, artichokes, or other available vegetables. Do the same with pasta, as in "primavera."

• Add beans to the lunch menu by choosing soups (lentil, split pea, minestrone) and bean-topped salads. When dining out, frequent restaurants that feature bean-based cuisines, including Middle Eastern, Mexican, and Indian (where you'll also find yogurt).

• For more soy foods, order tofu dishes in Chinese and Japanese restaurants and seek out Indonesian, Thai, and natural foods restaurants for both tofu and tempeh.

• Drink water and/or unsweetened tea.

Nikki's Select Lunch Menus

I.
Quick Corn Chowder* and Tofu "Tuna"* sandwich

II.
Quick Vegetable-Bean Soup* and Vegetable-Cheese Spread* on crackers

III.
Baked Italian Tempeh* sandwich with raw carrot, cucumber, and celery sticks

IV.
Garden Chili† with Baked Tortilla Crisps†

V.

Chef's salad of greens, vegetables, Quick Grilled Tofu, and
Lemon-Tahini Dressing†*

VI.

Quick White Pita "Pizza"† and salad with Creamy Italian Dressing†

VII.

*Black Bean Hummus† in whole wheat pita with lettuce, avocado,
salsa, and sprouts*

*Recipe below.
†Recipe in other sections.

Lunch Recipe Notes

This reminder probably isn't necessary, but don't neglect some of these lunch dishes for other meals as well. Tempeh burgers make a great quick dinner, the tofu salads are equally good at breakfast or a cold salad smorgasbord in the evening, and Quick Grilled Tofu and Savory Baked Tofu are excellent in sandwiches, on top of salads, or as snacks anytime.

Vegetable-Cheese Spread

Yogurt Cheese is an ideal base for many tasty sandwich spreads. The version below can be altered by adding sliced radishes, chopped celery, water chestnuts, sun-dried tomatoes, fresh dill, or other herbs or flavorings to taste. If you have a chance to prepare it ahead, chilling imparts a slightly firmer consistency.

1 cup Yogurt Cheese (page 244)	2 scallions, finely chopped
1/4 cup finely chopped red or green pepper	1 small carrot, shredded
	1/2 teaspoon salt

Combine all ingredients. If possible, chill for several hours (or longer) to stiffen.

YIELD: 1 CUP; ENOUGH FOR 4 SANDWICHES

Tofu Sandwich Salad

~

Serve on sandwiches, crackers, or as part of a salad plate. Excellent stuffed into whole wheat pita with lettuce, sliced tomato, cucumber, raw onion, and sprouts.

8 ounces firm or extra firm tofu
1 tablespoon lemon juice
2 teaspoons prepared mustard
1 1/2 tablespoons light miso
1/2 teaspoon paprika

1/2 cup chopped celery or green or
 red pepper
2 tablespoons chopped mild onion
 or scallions, optional

Method 1: Mash the tofu with a fork or potato masher. Mix in the remaining ingredients. Knead gently with your hands to form an evenly blended, cohesive mass.

Method 2: Combine all ingredients in a food processor. Process using a start/stop motion until the vegetables are finely chopped; stop before the mixture turns into a puree.

YIELD: 1 1/2 CUPS; ENOUGH FOR 4 SANDWICHES OR 3 TO 4 SERVINGS ON A PLATE

Tofu "Tuna"

~

Another choice for sandwiches, crackers, and salad plates. A bit more substantial in texture than Tofu Sandwich Salad.

3/4 pound firm or extra firm tofu
 (2 cups mashed)
3 tablespoons tahini
wedge of lemon

2 teaspoons soy sauce or to taste
1/3 cup shredded carrot
1/3 cup chopped celery, red or green
 pepper, or cucumber

Mash the tofu well using a potato masher or fork. Mix in the tahini. Squeeze in the lemon juice and add soy sauce to taste. Fold in the vegetables. Use at once or chill.

YIELD: 2 1/4 CUPS; 4 SERVINGS

*The
Healthiest
Diet in
the World*

Quick Grilled Tofu

～

Tofu slices can be quickly grilled and used for sandwiches or cut in strips and placed on top of main-dish salads. While nothing more than a quick seasoning with soy sauce is needed, you can add a few drops of hot sesame oil or hot pepper sauce to the soy sauce for a more sprightly taste, or rub the surfaces with chili powder, curry powder, or other seasoning mix of choice. If you don't have access to a grill, a wire cake rack set over a gas burner is an easy substitute. As an alternative to grilling, tofu can be broiled; however, the flavor isn't really the same.

tofu	**soy sauce**

Cut the tofu into 1/2-inch-thick slices, allowing 2 to 3 per serving. Season on both sides by sprinkling with soy sauce and spreading gently with your fingers to disperse.

Place the tofu on a grill or set on a wire cake rack over a gas burner. Cook for a few minutes, until the bottom is grilled to taste. Turn and repeat.

YIELD: PREPARE IN ANY QUANTITY NEEDED

Savory Baked Tofu

～

These firm, well-seasoned tofu slices are terrific in sandwiches, on a plate with cooked grains or potatoes, or simply eaten out of hand. Serve right from the oven, at room temperature, or chilled.

1/4 cup soy sauce	1 tablespoon lemon juice
1/4 cup water	1 pound firm or extra firm tofu,
1 large clove garlic, split	sliced 1/4 inch thick
1 teaspoon grated fresh ginger or	
1/4 teaspoon dried ground ginger	

Preheat the oven to 350°F.

In a 9 × 13-inch baking dish, or other shallow casserole big enough to hold the tofu in a single layer, combine all ingredients except the tofu. Lay the tofu slices in a single layer in the pan. Let sit at least 5 minutes, then turn so both sides are coated with the soy mixture. If you have time you can do this ahead and marinate for a while.

Bake, uncovered, for 30 minutes, until the tofu is dry and nicely browned.

YIELD: ABOUT 16 SLICES; 4 SERVINGS

Baked Italian Tofu

⌒

This recipe produces a thick coating around the tofu to make a flavorful filling for sandwiches. It takes 30 minutes to prepare and can be eaten hot from the oven, reheated, or at room temperature.

1 pound firm or extra firm tofu	1 teaspoon oregano
1 cup canned crushed tomatoes	1 teaspoon dried basil
1 tablespoon balsamic vinegar	1/4 teaspoon salt
2 large cloves garlic, minced	

Preheat the oven to 375°F.

Cut the tofu into 12 to 16 slices, each about 1/4 inch thick. Combine the remaining ingredients.

Spread half of the sauce over the bottom of a 9 × 13-inch baking dish or similar shallow pan that can hold the tofu snugly in a single layer; divide into 2 pans if necessary. Lay the tofu slices in the tomato sauce. Spoon the remaining sauce over the tofu, spreading it so that all surfaces are well coated.

Bake, uncovered, for 30 minutes.

YIELD: **4 SERVINGS**

VARIATION: For *Baked Italian Tempeh*, replace the tofu with tempeh and cut into 1/4-inch-thick patties.

Baked Mexican Tofu

⌒

Here the tofu is embedded in a rich spicy coating. Roll into tortillas or use as a sandwich filling. As with Baked Italian Tofu, the tofu can be eaten hot from the oven, reheated, or at room temperature.

1 pound firm or extra firm tofu	1/4 teaspoon cayenne
1 1/2 cups canned crushed tomatoes	2 teaspoons chili powder
1 tablespoon wine vinegar	1 teaspoon cumin
1 large clove garlic, minced	1/2 teaspoon salt

Preheat the oven to 375°F.

Cut the tofu into 12 to 16 slices, each about 1/4 inch thick. Combine the remaining ingredients.

Spread half of the sauce over the bottom of a 9 × 13-inch baking dish or similar shallow pan that can hold the tofu snugly in a single layer; divide into 2 pans if necessary. Lay the tofu slices in the sauce. Spoon the remaining sauce over the tofu, spreading it so that all surfaces are well coated.

Bake, uncovered, for 30 minutes.

YIELD: 4 SERVINGS

VARIATION: For *Baked Mexican Tempeh*, substitute tempeh for tofu. Cut into 1/4-inch-thick patties or strips.

Tempeh Burgers

~

Place on whole wheat hamburger rolls or toasted whole wheat English muffins and load on the sprouts, sliced fresh tomato, onion, and Better Than Ketchup to taste.

8 ounces tempeh	**1/3 cup water**
2 tablespoons soy sauce	

Cut the tempeh into burger-size squares. You can leave them the thickness of the tempeh or slice each through the middle to make 2 thinner patties.

Combine the soy sauce and water. Heat a heavy skillet, preferably cast iron. Put the tempeh and about half of the diluted soy sauce into the skillet, cover, and cook for 5 minutes, until the tempeh starts to color on the bottom. Turn the tempeh over, add the remaining liquid, cover, and cook for 5 minutes. Remove the cover and cook until the liquid is gone and the tempeh is nicely colored on both sides.

YIELD: 2 SERVINGS

Quick Corn Chowder

~

Takes just minutes to prepare and heat.

2 cups corn kernels (fresh or frozen)
4 cups soy milk
2 slices whole wheat or other
   whole-grain bread (remove crusts
   if tough)

1 thin slice onion
2 teaspoons salt

Combine all ingredients in a blender or food processor. Process at high speed for 20 seconds, until chunky. Pour into a pot and warm through over moderate heat without boiling.

YIELD: 4 TO 6 SERVINGS

Quick Vegetable-Bean Soup

~

Thirty minutes from start to table.

1 small onion, chopped
2 carrots, cut into coins
2 stalks celery, sliced
2 cloves garlic, sliced
4 cups water mixed with any bean
   cooking or canning liquid

2 cups cooked or canned beans
2 tablespoons tomato paste or
   1/4 cup canned crushed tomatoes
lots of fresh parsley
1 tablespoon miso

Combine the onion, carrots, celery, and garlic in a 2- to 3-quart soup pot, cover, and stew over moderate heat for 10 minutes. Add 2 cups water, bring to a boil, cover, and cook for 10 minutes. Add the beans, tomato paste or crushed tomatoes, parsley, and remaining 2 cups water combined with any bean cooking or canning liquid. Simmer 2 minutes. In a small bowl, dilute the miso with a little of the hot soup. Return to the pot, remove from the heat, cover, and let sit 5 minutes before serving.

YIELD: 2 QUARTS; 4 TO 6 SERVINGS

Miso Soup

~

This light soup is meant to accompany a sandwich or salad. To turn it into a heartier lunch entrée, add up to 1 cup frozen corn or peas, or precooked carrots, squash, or other vegetables of choice during the last few minutes of cooking (long enough to warm through). Cooked brown rice or whole-grain pasta can also be added. Garnish each bowl with sliced raw scallion, chopped parsley, and toasted nori seaweed.

1/2 cup chopped onion or sliced scallion
2-inch strip kombu seaweed
6 cups water

8 ounces soft, regular, or firm tofu, cut into cubes
3 tablespoons light or dark miso

Combine the onion, kombu, and water in a soup pot and bring to a boil. Add the tofu and simmer 5 minutes. If adding other vegetables or grains, now is the time.

Reduce the heat to very low. In a separate vessel, stir a little of the hot broth into the miso and mix until smooth. Stir back into the soup. Cook gently without boiling for 1 to 2 minutes longer.

YIELD: 4 SERVINGS

In Nikki's Kitchen

Golden Guideline Snacks

There are benefits derived from eating several small meals or meals interspersed with healthful snacks, rather than three big meals or fewer each day (see Golden Guideline #1: Carbohydrate Compatibility). To get you started, incorporate the following ideas at intervals over the course of a day. Recipes (where needed) are found in the upcoming sections.

- When you cook, plan leftovers for snacking.
- When you eat, rather than forcing yourself to finish everything on the plate, put some aside for a "minimeal" later on.
- Munch on raw vegetables with bean or yogurt cheese dips, such as our Black Bean Hummus, Roasted Red Pepper–Chickpea Dip, and Superior Spinach Dip.
- Scoop up Black Bean Salsa with lettuce leaves or whole wheat pita bread.
- Put together a Quick White Pita "Pizza."
- Fix or reheat a bowl of quick soup.
- Grab a handful of soy nuts.
- Whip up a Banana-Soy (or other fruit) Shake.
- Enjoy a cup of yogurt and sliced cucumber or fresh fruit.
- Spread celery stalks or slices of fresh fruit with almond butter.
- Eat a homemade muffin or slice of whole-grain bread with yogurt cheese.

When devising similar snacks on your own, remember to include some protein at each of these "sittings." Soy products, legumes, yogurt, and yogurt cheese are the primary means. Unsalted seeds, nuts, and nut butter can also be used, but be modest when it comes to quantity. Two tablespoons of nut butter or 1/4 cup of nuts and seeds is adequate; you can extend this by making a trail mix containing the nuts and seeds, mixed with a more ample volume of whole-grain ready-to-eat cereal. A small amount of raisins, currants, or other cut-up dried fruit can be added for sweetness.

One of our favorite protein-packed snacks is presented below.

Tofu Jerky

Tofu Jerky makes a flavorful snack that's easily prepared in a food dehydrator or oven. When stored in an airtight container, it keeps for months. The basic recipe can be spiced up by adding hot sauce or a good pinch of cayenne pepper if you want it hot. Chili powder makes a chili jerky; oregano and basil create pizza jerky.

1 pound firm or extra firm tofu	1 tablespoon grated fresh ginger
1/4 cup soy sauce	1 clove garlic, minced
1/4 cup water	1 teaspoon honey, molasses, or
2 tablespoons lemon juice	maple syrup

Slice the tofu into 1/8-inch-thick pieces. Combine the remaining ingredients and place in a shallow pan (or 2) large enough to hold the tofu in a single layer. Lay the tofu slices in the soy sauce marinade and turn to coat both sides. Let marinate in the refrigerator for several hours. (It can stay there all day or overnight.) Turn a few times for maximum penetration.

Remove the tofu from the marinade. If drying in a dehydrator, place on trays and set temperature to about 140°. For oven drying, set temperature to 200°F., place the tofu pieces on a wire rack (such as a cake cooking rack or grilling rack with fairly narrow spacing), place on a baking sheet, and insert in the oven.

Dry the tofu until it is very chewy, but not yet crisp. Average timing is 4 to 6 hours, but this varies somewhat with the tofu, oven, or dehydrator, and even the ambient room conditions.

Store in airtight containers.

YIELD: **12** TO **16** PIECES

*In
Nikki's
Kitchen*

The Healthiest Dinners in the World

As you explore the rest of "In Nikki's Kitchen," you'll discover numerous menu suggestions accompanying individual recipes. To give you a preview of the menus, below are seven dinners that follow the principles of the Golden Guidelines and illustrate how varied and tempting the healthiest diet in the world can be.

Dinner Tips

Whether your dinners feature selections from "In Nikki's Kitchen" or not, there are a few routines you can develop at dinnertime to help fulfill the Golden Guidelines:

• Set out a plate of raw vegetables for nibbling before the meal. It can include carrot and celery sticks, cucumber slices, pepper strips, broccoli and cauliflorets, fennel wedges, jicama, and the like. For added value and appeal, accompany with a dip or dressing such as Black Bean Hummus, Tofu-Mustard Dip, Superior Spinach Dip, Piquant Mustard-Tomato Dressing, Creamy Tofu Russian Dressing, or Lemon-Tahini Dressing.

• Dress up dinner plates with a seasonal raw vegetable garnish of cherry tomatoes, spicy radishes, celery hearts, alfalfa sprouts, sprigs of dill, fresh basil leaves, or similar decorative elements.

• Add a green salad, preferably containing more than one leafy green.

• Toss leftover beans and/or cooked vegetables into green salads.

• Garnish salads with toasted pine nuts, pumpkin seeds, sunflower seeds, or walnuts.

• Enhance salads with homemade dressings that feature tofu, miso, and yogurt to increase your intake of these essential foods.

• Likewise, to fill in gaps of various guideline components, keep a supply of homemade spreads in the refrigerator and use them on whole-grain crackers for instant hors d'oeuvres or on your dinner bread. For example, Soy Butter and Toasted Soy Spread can help balance your intake of fatty acids and increase your consumption of soy products; boost your intake of nutrient helpers with such offerings as Mushroom Pâté and Onion Butter; to add more beans, set out Black Bean Hummus or Chickpea Pesto; yogurt cheese intake can be fostered with choices such as Herb Cheese or Vegetable-Cheese Spreads.

• Set out a pitcher of water and/or unsweetened tea.

Note: Before you begin cooking, you may want to take a look at "The Golden Pantry" in order to stock the kitchen with foods that support the Golden Guidelines. As a final reminder, we believe people should use organic products as much as possible. This is especially important when it comes to foods you consume on a regular basis. Furthermore, you'll note that a number of recipes call for orange or lemon peel; for these applications, we urge you to seek out organic specimens.

Nikki's Select Dinner Menus

I.
Cauliflower Gratin
Tomato Couscous
Sesame Green Beans
Warm Mushroom Salad

II.
Bean Guacamole with Baked Tortilla Crisps
Quick Mixed Vegetables in Tomato Juice, Mexican Style
Millet Polenta

III.
Mildly Sweet-and-Sour Tofu and Vegetables
Mustard Brussels Sprouts
Brown Rice or Buckwheat Soba

IV.
Maple-Pecan Tempeh
Louisiana Sweet Potatoes
Country Greens

V.
Cold Cucumber-Yogurt Soup
White Beans with Swiss Chard
Moroccan Carrot Slaw
Whole-Grain bread with Tahini-Garlic Spread

VI.
Cowboy Beans
Golden Biscuits
Creamy Miso-Mustard Coleslaw

VII.
Creamy Stuffed Italian Artichoke Bottoms
Portobello Pasta
Fennel & Orange Salad

The
Healthiest
Diet in
the World

Appetizers and Hors d'oeuvres

Appetizers and hors d'oeuvres include recipes you can both put out before the meal for snacking and serve as a first course at the table. Some of these dishes—for example, Cold Tofu with Sesame Sauce, Tofu-Stuffed Artichokes, and Tomato Gratin—make excellent entrées as well. Others, such as Bean Bruschetta and the various Pita "Pizzas," also make suitable accompaniments to many main courses.

Bean Guacamole

A new twist on the popular Mexican avocado dip, with added protein, less fat, and fewer calories. Suitably served with Baked Tortilla Crisps.

1 cup cooked white beans (navy, great northern, cannellini)
1 large ripe avocado
1/4 cup chopped Italian plum tomato (1 medium)

2 tablespoons lemon juice
2 tablespoons finely chopped cilantro or flat-leaf parsley
hot pepper sauce
salt

Mash the beans completely with a potato masher. Add the avocado to the beans and mash until evenly combined. Stir in the tomato, lemon juice, and cilantro or parsley and mix well. Add the hot pepper sauce and salt to taste.

YIELD: 4 TO 6 SERVINGS

Most U.S.-grown avocados come from California and are the Hass variety, characterized by a thick, pebbly skin that turns black when ripe. Hass avocados have a rich, buttery texture and subtly sweet, nutty flavor. They're the foundation for guacamole, and their creaminess makes them an agreeable stand-in for butter. The less common Florida specimens are considerably larger and have bright green, smooth skins. Florida avocados contain about half the fat of California varieties and more water. This is reflected in their blander taste and firmer flesh. Unlike California avocados that are easily mashed, Florida avocados are more suitable for service that calls for slicing or dicing.

Baked Tortilla Crisps

An easy way to make fat-free corn or whole wheat tortilla chips for hors d'oeuvres, dips, or snacking, or crisp tacos to use as the base for a Mexican bean or tofu entrée.

**6 to 8 6-inch corn or whole wheat
   tortillas or 4 larger tortillas**

Preheat the oven to 500°F.
   Run cold water quickly over each tortilla. Let drain briefly.
   To prepare as chips for dipping, stack the tortillas and cut 6-inch tortillas into 6 wedges, larger tortillas into 8 wedges. Spread in a single layer on a baking sheet. To prepare for tacos, place the tortillas directly on the oven rack.
   Bake for 5 minutes. Turn and bake for 2 to 3 minutes longer, until crisp. If the tortilla wedges stick to the baking sheet, gently loosen with a spatula.

YIELD: 4 SERVINGS

Black Bean Hummus

A marriage of cuisines, blending the traditional ingredients of the Mideast chickpea dip called hummus with the popular black beans of South America and spicing it up with hot sauce. This very convenient appetizer can be prepared with fresh cooked or canned beans, served right away, or made ahead and refrigerated. Serve at room temperature for best flavor, with raw vegetables, Baked Tortilla Crisps, or whole wheat pita for dipping.

2 cups cooked black beans
1/4 cup bean cooking liquid, if needed
2 tablespoons lemon juice
2 cloves garlic, finely minced
1/2 teaspoon hot pepper sauce or to taste

2 tablespoons tahini
2 tablespoons Yogurt Cheese (page 244)
salt

Drain the beans, conserving the cooking liquid. Do not rinse.

Puree the beans in a blender or food processor, adding bean liquid as needed to make a smooth puree. (The need for added liquid will depend on how soft the beans are and the amount of liquid that clings to them.)

Transfer the bean puree to a shallow bowl. Using a fork, beat in lemon juice, garlic, and hot pepper sauce. Then beat in tahini and Yogurt Cheese.

Add salt to taste if the beans were unsalted. Adjust the hot sauce according to taste.

YIELD: 2 CUPS; 4 TO 6 SERVINGS

*In
Nikki's
Kitchen*

Roasted Red Pepper–Chickpea Dip

~

For dipping, provide whole wheat pita triangles, endive leaves, or small inner leaves of lettuce, strips of red and green pepper, and raw or lightly steamed cauliflower and broccoli florets. This dip can be made with fresh cooked or canned chickpeas and prepared as long as a day in advance and refrigerated.

1 medium red pepper (4 to
  6 ounces)
2 cups cooked chickpeas
about 1/4 cup bean cooking liquid
2 cloves garlic

1/2 teaspoon salt (omit if beans are
  salted)
2 tablespoons wine vinegar
1/4 cup Yogurt Cheese (page 244)

Place the red pepper on a baking sheet and broil 4 to 6 inches beneath heat for about 15 minutes, until the skin is blistered. Turn several times to cook evenly. Alternatively, hold the pepper over a flame using tongs and brown on all sides. When the skin is completely blistered, wrap the pepper in a clean cloth to steam for a few minutes. When cool, peel off the skin using a small paring knife, cut open, and remove the seeds and any thick ribs.

Puree the chickpeas in a blender or food processor, adding liquid as needed to make a smooth, creamy puree. Add the roasted pepper, garlic, salt, wine vinegar, and Yogurt Cheese. Process again until smooth.

Transfer to a shallow serving bowl. If possible, let sit for 30 minutes (or longer) to blend the flavors.

YIELD: 2 CUPS; 4 TO 6 SERVINGS

Tofu-Mustard Dip

~

When soft tofu is pureed it forms the basis of a vegetable dip as creamy as any built around sour cream or mayonnaise. If soft tofu isn't available, regular or firm tofu can be used in this recipe, but in that case you'll need to add a few tablespoons of soy milk (or other suitable liquid such as vegetable broth or bean cooking liquid) to make the consistency suitable for dipping. The amount needed will vary according to the density of the tofu.

8 ounces soft tofu
2 tablespoons lemon juice
1 1/2 tablespoons prepared mustard
1 1/2 tablespoons light miso
1 tablespoon soy sauce

1/2 teaspoon paprika
2 large cloves roasted garlic or
  1 large clove raw garlic
1 cup peeled diced cucumber

In a blender or food processor fitted with the steel chopping blade, combine all ingredients. Process until the mixture is a smooth puree.

YIELD: JUST UNDER 2 CUPS; 6 TO 8 SERVINGS

Superior Spinach Dip

1 package (10 ounces) frozen
  spinach, thawed
1 1/2 cups Yogurt Cheese (page 244)
1/4 cup chopped fresh dill
1/4 cup chopped parsley

1/4 teaspoon hot pepper sauce
1 tablespoon lemon juice
1/2 teaspoon salt
2 tablespoons minced scallion

Drain the spinach and squeeze out as much liquid as possible. Chop finely. Combine the Yogurt Cheese, dill, parsley, hot pepper sauce, lemon juice, and salt. Mix well. Stir in the spinach and scallion until evenly blended. Serve at once or chill until serving time.

YIELD: 2 CUPS; 6 TO 8 SERVINGS

NOTE: If the dip seems stiff, loosen by adding plain yogurt.

*In
Nikki's
Kitchen*

Tomato Cream Cheese

⁓

A rich tomato flavor. Spread on thin slices of whole-grain toast. Will keep for about 5 days in the refrigerator.

3 tablespoons chopped, rehydrated
  dried tomatoes (see Note)
1/2 cup Yogurt Cheese (page 244)

1 tablespoon tomato paste
1 teaspoon dried basil

Combine all ingredients in a small bowl and stir until uniformly mixed. Chill for several hours before serving.

YIELD: ABOUT 1/2 CUP

NOTE: To rehydrate dried tomatoes, run quickly under cold water. Let sit for about 5 minutes to soften before chopping. Tomatoes can still be a bit firm, as they will continue to soften in the cheese.

> ## ★ TOMATO TIP #1 ★
>
> When using only part of a can of tomato paste, spoon the remainder into an ice cube tray and freeze. When firm, transfer the tomato paste cubes to plastic bags. Use frozen or let sit a few minutes at room temperature to soften, depending on what best suits your needs.

Tofu Pâté

⁓

Serve on crackers for hors d'oeuvres. Prepare ahead of time so the pâté has time to chill.

1 tablespoon soy sauce
1/2 cup finely chopped onion
1/4 cup shredded carrot
1/4 cup parsley
1/4 cup walnuts

6 ounces firm or extra firm tofu
  (1 cup diced)
about 2 tablespoons water
salt

Combine the soy sauce, onion, and carrot in a skillet and cook, stirring frequently, for 3 to 5 minutes, until tender. Let cool.

Combine the parsley and walnuts in a food processor or blender. Process until the parsley is finely minced. Add the tofu and process until smooth. Add water, if needed, to reach a spreadable consistency.

Transfer the tofu to a bowl and stir in the cooked vegetables. Season with salt to taste. Chill well before serving.

YIELD: ABOUT 1¹/₄ CUPS; 4 TO 6 SERVINGS

Deviled Tofu

Serve on cucumber rounds, sweet red or green pepper wedges, or whole-grain rye crackers. Can be eaten just after preparation or held in the refrigerator.

8 ounces regular or firm tofu
2 teaspoons prepared mustard
¹/₂ teaspoon soy sauce
¹/₈ teaspoon turmeric

¹/₄ cup minced green pepper
¹/₄ cup minced onion
salt
¹/₈ teaspoon paprika

Mash the tofu with a fork until crumbly. Add the remaining ingredients, except the paprika, and mix well. Spread on cucumber rounds, pepper wedges, or crackers and sprinkle paprika on top.

YIELD: 1¹/₂ CUPS; 4 TO 6 SERVINGS

Mushroom Pâté

~

This savory pâté combines common white cultivated mushrooms with the more intense "wild" varieties such as portobello, cremini, and/or shiitake. The best flavor balance is achieved when the mild cultivated mushrooms make up about half the mix. Mushroom Pâté should be prepared at least several hours ahead and will keep several days in the refrigerator. Serve on thin slices of toasted whole-grain bread or mound on a serving plate and garnish with parsley sprigs and cherry tomato wedges.

3/4 pound mixed cultivated white
  and wild mushrooms, coarsely
  chopped (4 cups)
1/2 cup chopped shallots
2 cloves garlic, chopped
3 tablespoons cooking sherry
2 teaspoons soy sauce

1/2 cup pumpkin seeds
1/4 cup sliced hazelnuts or almonds
1/3 cup Yogurt Cheese (page 244)
1/4 teaspoon salt
1/4 teaspoon hot pepper sauce or
  to taste

Combine the mushrooms, shallots, garlic, sherry, and soy sauce in a skillet. Cook, stirring frequently, until the mushrooms release their juices and are tender. This will take about 8 to 10 minutes. Cook 3 to 5 minutes longer, until most of the liquid evaporates.

While the mushrooms cook, grind the pumpkin seeds and nuts to a fine meal in a blender or food processor. Transfer to a mixing bowl.

Transfer the cooked mushroom mixture to a blender or food processor and puree to a coarse texture. Scrape into the bowl with the ground seeds and nuts.

Incorporate the mushrooms into the seeds and nuts, along with the Yogurt Cheese, salt, and hot pepper sauce.

Chill several hours. Adjust the salt and hot pepper sauce to taste before serving. Keeps several days in the refrigerator.

YIELD: 2 CUPS; 8 OR MORE SERVINGS

Rolled Eggplant Stuffed with Mushroom Pâté

~

Bite-size hors d'oeuvres for elegant entertaining. Make at least several hours or as long as a day in advance.

1 medium eggplant, about 6 inches
  long and 3/4 pound

olive oil
1 cup Mushroom Pâté (above)

Preheat the broiler.

Peel the eggplant and cut lengthwise into slices about 1/4 inch thick. Use the 6 largest slices for this recipe. (Reserve any remaining eggplant for another use; see Note.) Generously oil a baking sheet with olive oil, place the eggplant slices on the oil, then turn them over so both sides are lightly coated with oil. Broil about 6 inches below the heat for about 5 minutes on each side, or until tender and lightly browned.

Arrange 3 scant tablespoons Mushroom Pâté in a lengthwise strip down the center of each eggplant slice. Roll, jelly-roll style, along the long edge to cover filling. Chill.

Using a very sharp knife, cut into 1-inch segments to serve.

YIELD: ABOUT **30** PIECES

NOTE: Any remaining eggplant slices can be broiled at the same time, cut into strips, tossed with a favorite salad dressing (for example, Tomato-Basil, Orange-Parsley, or Yogonaise), and served as a side dish.

Pesto-Stuffed Mushrooms

Serve on a platter as a party hors d'oeuvre or at the table as a first course.

3/4 **to 1 cup Chickpea Pesto (page 196) or Creamy Walnut Pesto (page 196)**

12 to 16 medium to large mushrooms or about 24 small mushrooms

Preheat the oven to 350°F.

Prepare the pesto of choice. Remove the mushroom stems and reserve for another use; clean the mushroom caps. Fill the caps with a spoonful of pesto. Depending on their size, they will hold a little more or less than a tablespoonful, or if you choose small mushrooms for platter service, each will hold a generous teaspoonful of filling.

Place the mushrooms, filling up, in a baking dish. Bake for 15 minutes, or until the mushrooms are tender. Very large mushrooms may take 5 minutes longer (or about 20 minutes) to cook.

YIELD: **4** TO **6** SERVINGS

In Nikki's Kitchen

Succulent Stuffed Mushrooms

~

Allow 2 to 4 of these stuffed mushrooms per person, depending on the size of mushrooms, mode of service (sit-down appetizers or casual hors d'oeuvres), the rest of the menu, and the eaters' appetites.

1/2 cup Yogurt Cheese (page 244)
1 1/2 teaspoons mixed herbs:
  oregano, parsley, basil, sage,
  thyme, or your favorite
  seasoning mix

8 medium to large mushrooms

Preheat the oven to 350°F.
  Combine the Yogurt Cheese with the herbs and mix well.
  Remove the stems from the mushrooms and reserve for another use. Clean the caps. Fill each cap with seasoned Yogurt Cheese.
  Place the mushrooms on a baking sheet and bake for 15 to 20 minutes, until tender. Remove from the oven and let cool briefly before serving.

YIELD: 2 TO 4 SERVINGS

Creamy Stuffed Italian Artichoke Bottoms

~

The tangy flavor and creamy texture of the Yogurt Cheese filling is a striking contrast to the firm artichoke base. As these are quite rich, 2 bottoms are generally enough for a serving. However, you may wish to provide extra depending on the rest of the menu and people's appetites.

1/2 cup Yogurt Cheese (page 244)
1/2 teaspoon oregano
3 tablespoons minced parsley
1 clove garlic, finely minced
1/4 cup shredded and finely chopped
  zucchini or thawed, pressed,
  chopped frozen spinach

2 tablespoons grated Parmesan
  cheese
8 canned artichoke bottoms

Preheat the oven to 350°F.
  Combine the Yogurt Cheese with the remaining ingredients except the artichokes. Before adding the zucchini or spinach, press out as much of the moisture as possible.
  Drain the artichokes and pat dry. Mound a spoonful of seasoned Yogurt

Cheese onto each artichoke bottom. Sprinkle with a little additional Parmesan cheese, if desired.

Place on a baking pan and bake for 12 to 15 minutes, until the filling is hot.

YIELD: **4** SERVINGS

VARIATION: For *Creamy Stuffed Greek Artichoke Bottoms*, replace the parsley with dill and the Parmesan cheese with feta.

Baked Artichoke Cheese

⌒

Bite-size vegetable-cheese squares make an unusual and convenient hors d'oeuvre for entertaining. Everything can be put together well in advance and baked just before serving. (If more than 1 hour ahead, refrigerate.) Moreover, service can be hot, warm, or at room temperature; leftovers can even be chilled and eaten cold as a snack or sandwich filling.

1 can (14 ounces) artichoke hearts in water
1¼ cups Yogurt Cheese (page 244)
½ cup grated cheese (parmesan, provolone, cheddar, jack, feta, or other natural cheese alone or mixed)

2 tablespoons chopped sun-dried tomatoes
2 tablespoons coarsely chopped walnuts
⅛ teaspoon hot pepper sauce
¼ cup chopped fresh dill or parsley

Preheat the oven to 350°F.

Drain the artichokes; chop into small pieces. Combine with the remaining ingredients. Transfer to a 9-inch square or shallow 1-quart baking dish. Bake for 30 minutes, until firm and lightly browned on top. Let sit at room temperature for a few minutes to set before cutting. Cut into 2-inch squares and arrange on a platter to serve.

YIELD: **16** 2-INCH PIECES

*In
Nikki's
Kitchen*

Tomato Gratin

This flavorful tomato–Yogurt Cheese casserole goes well with most cuisines. Best made with ripe, summer tomatoes. Note that these are modest appetizer-size servings. For 4 to 6 hearty eaters or to feature at a meal, you can double the recipe in a shallow 2-quart or 9 × 13-inch baking dish.

3/4 cup Yogurt Cheese (page 244)
3 tablespoons chopped green or
  black olives
3 tablespoons chopped capers
3 large or 4 medium tomatoes
  (1 1/2 pounds)
freshly ground pepper

2 cloves garlic, finely chopped
1 tablespoon chopped fresh basil
2 tablespoons chopped parsley
2 tablespoons pumpkin seeds
1 tablespoon wheat germ
1 teaspoon olive oil

Preheat the oven to 350°F.

Combine the Yogurt Cheese, olives, and capers. Slice the tomatoes into 1/4-inch-thick rounds. Place half the tomato slices in overlapping layers in a shallow 9-inch baking dish or glass pie plate. Season generously with the pepper and sprinkle with half the garlic, basil, and parsley. Top with half the Yogurt Cheese mixture, using a spoon to drop in dollops evenly over the tomato slices. Repeat the layers.

Grind the pumpkin seeds to a meal in a blender or food processor. Combine with the wheat germ and sprinkle evenly over the top of the assembled dish. Drizzle with the olive oil. Bake for 30 minutes. Serve warm, but not piping hot.

YIELD: **4 SERVINGS**

Tofu-Stuffed Artichokes

Depending on the size of the rest of the meal, you may want to cut the artichokes in half for appetizers. To serve Tofu-Stuffed Artichokes as the entrée, set on top of cooked rice or other grain of choice. In either case, serve with Agliata as a dipping sauce (page 204) or wedges of fresh lemon.

4 medium to large artichokes
1¹/2 cups mashed tofu (12 ounces)
¹/3 cup dry whole-grain bread
  crumbs
2 tablespoons flaxseed meal
  (page 239)
¹/4 cup sunflower seeds, ground
  (6 tablespoons sunflower meal)

2 tablespoons wheat germ
2 cloves garlic, minced
¹/4 cup chopped parsley
1 teaspoon oregano
¹/2 teaspoon salt

To prepare the artichokes for stuffing, cut off the sharp tips, spread the inner leaves, remove the small leaves attached to the heart, and scrape out the hairy "choke." Cut off any stem so the artichoke sits firmly upright. (If there's enough stem to eat, peel, slice in half lengthwise, and cook along with the artichoke.) Rinse the artichokes under cold water and invert to drain.

To make the filling, combine the remaining ingredients in a bowl, mixing well until thoroughly blended. Knead gently by hand until the mixture holds together. Stuff about ¹/4 cup filling into the hollow at the center of each artichoke. Pack any remaining filling between the leaves.

Place the artichokes upright in a vegetable steamer set over boiling water. Surround with any prepared leftover stems. Steam the artichokes 35 to 45 minutes, until tender. Or pressure-cook 13 to 15 minutes.

YIELD: 4 TO 8 SERVINGS

*In
Nikki's
Kitchen*

Cold Tofu with Sesame Sauce

~

Cold tofu in a rich piquant sauce will be familiar to anyone who has eaten the popular Chinese dish cold noodles with sesame paste. It's easy to assemble and there's no cooking involved. In addition to appetizer service, this recipe can be offered as an entrée, joined by brown rice, buckwheat soba, or a favorite grain; a cooked vegetable (steamed broccoli, cooked greens, Stir-Steamed Sesame Cabbage, Sesame Green Beans, Asian Sesame-Ginger Carrots); and Fennel & Orange Salad, mixed seasonal greens, or refreshing cold cucumber slices.

6 tablespoons tahini
2 tablespoons almond butter
1/4 cup white or rice wine vinegar
1/4 cup soy sauce, divided
2 to 3 tablespoons hot water or
  black or green tea

1 teaspoon spicy sesame oil
  (see Note)
1 teaspoon shredded ginger
1 pound soft tofu
2 scallions, thinly sliced, including
  dark-green portion

In a shallow bowl, combine the tahini and almond butter. Using a fork, beat in the vinegar, followed by 2 tablespoons soy sauce and 2 tablespoons hot water or tea. The mixture should be the consistency of rich cream. If too thick, beat in additional hot water or tea until the desired consistency is reached. Beat in the sesame oil. Pour the sauce into a shallow serving bowl large enough to hold the tofu in a single layer. Drizzle the remaining 2 tablespoons soy sauce over the sesame sauce. Scatter the ginger on top.

Cut the tofu into bite-size cubes. Arrange in a single layer in the sesame sauce. Cover with the scallions. Serve at room temperature.

YIELD: 6 APPETIZER SERVINGS OR 4 SERVINGS AS THE PROTEIN PORTION OF A MEAL

NOTE: Toasted sesame oil with a pinch of cayenne (to taste) can be substituted for spicy sesame oil.

*The
Healthiest
Diet in
the World*

Alan's Curry Tofu Cubes with Dipping Sauce

~

These tasty tofu cubes, which are prepared in the pressure cooker, are incredibly easy and versatile. The seasonings can be varied (Alan suggests Herbamare) and the cubes themselves can be served on top of salads, along with pasta or a cooked grain bathed in a favorite gravy or tomato sauce, or mixed with almost any cooked vegetable. They also make especially good hors d'oeuvres with a dipping sauce such as Agliata, Spicy Orange-Nut Sauce, Tomato-Almond Pesto, or a tomato salsa.

1 pound firm or extra firm tofu   **1 tablespoon curry powder**

Pat the surface of the block of tofu dry and cut into $3/4$-inch cubes. Toss in a bowl with seasonings to coat.

Place the tofu cubes in the steamer basket of a pressure cooker set above boiling water. Close the cooker and bring to pressure. Pressure-cook 8 minutes. Release the pressure using the pressure release valve. (On older models, run under cold water to bring the pressure down.)

YIELD: 4 SERVINGS

Skewered Tempeh with Orange-Nut Crust

~

These mini kebabs are a nice appetizer to pass around at a party or set out on an hors d'oeuvres buffet. Any extra sauce can be served on the side for dipping, or as a dipping sauce for vegetables.

24 ounces tempeh   **$1^{1}/_2$ cups Spicy Orange-Nut Sauce (page 198)**

Preheat the broiler.

Cut the tempeh into 1-inch cubes. Thread on 8 skewers. Set the skewers so the ends rest on opposite edges of a shallow baking pan with the tempeh hanging above the surface.

Coat the top of the tempeh generously with the sauce. Broil for about 5 minutes, or until golden. Turn the skewers and spread the sauce over the uncooked side of the tempeh. Broil for another 5 minutes, or until the coating forms a crust.

YIELD: 8 SKEWERS; 4 TO 8 SERVINGS

Bean Bruschetta

~

Bean Bruschetta is an excellent way to add more beans to the menu. Serve as an hors d'oeuvre, as an accompaniment to grain or vegetable entrées, for lunch with vegetable soup or a big salad, or even as a snack. The beans (home-cooked or canned) and greens can be used warm or at room temperature, making the components of this dish easy to prepare ahead or at the last minute. The recipe is also easily multiplied for serving a crowd.

4 cups cut-up greens, such as Swiss chard, arugula, escarole, spinach, beet greens (about 1/2 pound)
2 teaspoons red wine vinegar
1 cup cooked white beans
2 cloves garlic, minced
2 teaspoons olive, flaxseed, or hemp oil

salt and pepper
4 slices whole-grain bread or 2 whole wheat pitas separated into rounds
2 tomato heels (ends), if available

Combine the greens with the wine vinegar in a heavy skillet, preferably cast iron. Cook, stirring frequently, for about 5 minutes, until wilted. When cool enough to handle, finely chop.

Mash the beans with a potato masher. Add the minced garlic and oil of choice. Season to taste with salt and pepper.

Grill the bread on both sides over a gas burner or toast until golden. If the tomato heels are available, rub on one side of the hot bread to moisten.

Cover the moistened side of each bread slice with 1/4 cup of the mashed beans and top with 2 tablespoons cooked greens.

YIELD: 4 SERVINGS

★ TOMATO TIP #2 ★

Rubbing the ends, or heels, of a tomato on freshly toasted or grilled bread is an excellent way to keep the bread moist and add flavor.

Quick White Pita "Pizzas"

Cut into triangles for hors d'oeuvres or as part of an antipasto first course. You can also serve 2 rounds per person as an entrée or one as an individual "pizza" to accompany a meal.

2 2-ounce whole wheat pita breads　　**Vegetable Topping (see below)**
3/4 cup Yogurt Cheese (page 244)

Preheat the oven to 400°F.

Use a fork to perforate the circumference of the breads. Separate each into 2 rounds.

Spread each pita round with 3 tablespoons Yogurt Cheese. Top with the Vegetable Topping of choice.

Place on a baking sheet and bake for 15 minutes, until lightly browned at the edges. Let sit for a few minutes to set the filling before serving.

YIELD: **4** TO **6** APPETIZER SERVINGS; **2** TO **4** SERVINGS AS AN ENTRÉE OR ACCOMPANIMENT

VEGETABLE TOPPINGS: These are some of our favorite variations. Use them as is or for inspiration.

Greens: Top each round with 1/2 cup shredded raw greens, such as spinach, romaine or leaf lettuce, arugula, endive, radicchio, or a combination. Season with 1/8 teaspoon crushed hot red pepper flakes. Top with 1 tablespoon pine nuts, grated parmesan cheese, or crumbed feta.

Mushroom: Top each round with 1/3 cup thinly sliced raw mushrooms and 1 tablespoon frozen green peas. Scatter a clove of slivered garlic on top. Season with 1/8 teaspoon oregano or mixed Italian seasonings.

Artichoke: Follow directions for mushroom topping, replacing mushrooms with 1/3 cup thinly sliced canned or cooked artichoke hearts.

Sweet Red Pepper: Follow directions for mushroom topping, replacing mushrooms with 1/3 cup thin strips of red pepper. Instead of green peas, use capers.

White Pita "Pizzas"

～

As with the quicker pita pizzas above, cut into triangles for hors d'oeuvres or part of an antipasto, or serve whole as individual pizzas. If you have any roasted garlic on hand, squeeze a few cloves on top just before serving.

2 2-ounce whole wheat pita breads
Vegetable Filling (see below)
3/4 cup Yogurt Cheese (page 244)

1/4 to 1/2 cup crumbled feta or
grated Parmesan cheese, optional

Preheat the oven to 400°F.

Use a fork to perforate the circumference of the breads. Separate each into 2 rounds.

Mix prepared (and cooled) Vegetable Filling of choice with Yogurt Cheese until evenly blended. Cheese eaters can add crumbled feta or parmesan if desired. Spread to completely cover each pita round.

Place on a baking sheet and bake for 15 minutes, until lightly browned at the edges. Let sit for a few minutes to set the filling before serving.

YIELD: **4** TO **6** APPETIZER SERVINGS; **2** TO **4** SERVINGS AS AN ENTRÉE OR ACCOMPANIMENT

VEGETABLE FILLINGS

Cooked Greens: Combine 1/2 pound (5 to 6 cups loosely packed) greens of choice (spinach, beet greens, Swiss chard, or a mixture including some radicchio, arugula, and endive, if desired) in a heavy skillet with 1 tablespoon balsamic vinegar. Cover and cook until tender, about 10 minutes. Chop coarsely. If desired, add 1/4 cup minced fresh dill. Cool to lukewarm before mixing with the cheese(s).

Broccoli: Chop broccoli florets into very small pieces to make 2 cups. Combine with 1 tablespoon balsamic vinegar and 2 tablespoons water in a heavy skillet. Cover and cook until tender, about 8 to 10 minutes. Season with 1 teaspoon dried oregano. Cool to lukewarm before mixing with the cheese(s).

Pepper and Onion: Slice 1 large or 2 medium Spanish, Vidalia, or red onions in half lengthwise. Cut each half crosswise into thin half-rings. You should have about 2 cups. Chop sweet green or red pepper to make 1/2 cup. Combine the vegetables with 1 tablespoon balsamic vinegar in a heavy skillet. Cover and cook over low heat, stirring occasionally, for 20 minutes, until the onions are tender. Cool to lukewarm before mixing with the cheese(s). Season lightly with salt if not using Parmesan or feta cheese and liberally with fresh pepper.

NOTE: Instead of using pita bread, "pizzas" can be made using slices of whole-grain bread, toasting one side first, piling the filling on the untoasted side, then baking as directed.

Soups

Soup is more of an art than a science. There are so many variables when it comes to ingredients, proportions, and textures that cooks should feel free to improvise. Although long-simmered vegetable broth makes an indisputably rich soup base, not everyone has the time to prepare homemade stock. This shouldn't be a deterrent, for as the recipes in this section demonstrate, a delicious soup can be made without this effort.

Since soups generally improve with reheating, it's a good idea to make more than you need for one meal. By planning ahead in this manner, you can easily enjoy a bowl of soup for lunch or a snack without any extra work.

Russian Vegetable Soup

Serve this soup with plenty of Yogurt Cream (page 244) to spoon into each soup bowl.

3 cups water
1 cup tomato pulp or puree
1 onion, diced
1 cup peeled and shredded or finely chopped carrots
1 cup peeled and shredded or finely chopped beets

1 cup shredded or finely chopped potatoes
2 cups thinly shredded cabbage
2 teaspoons salt
1 tablespoon lemon juice

Combine the water and tomato in a soup pot and bring to a boil. Add the vegetables, season with salt, cover, and simmer about 30 minutes, until the vegetables are tender. When cooking is completed, add the lemon juice.

YIELD: 1¹/2 QUARTS; 4 TO 6 SERVINGS

★ HOW TO MAKE A QUICK SOUP ★

A quickly made soup may lack the depth of flavor that characterizes a long-simmered soup, but when time is a factor a very satisfactory soup can be made in the manner described here in just 30 minutes. Such soup doesn't require a precise recipe and can be conveniently made with common vegetables that are likely to be on hand.

For each quart or so of soup:

Chop up a large onion (and/or leek, if available) and put it in a soup pot with a spoonful of olive oil. Cover and steep over medium heat.

Meanwhile, prepare additional vegetables, as listed below, and add in order as they're ready. Include:

a clove or two of chopped garlic (optional)
a sliced celery stalk (with leaves, if available)
2 carrots (diced or cut into coins)
some chopped green leafy vegetables (kale, Swiss chard, beet greens, cabbage, romaine, or such)

Other possible additions include:
diced potatoes
cut-up string beans
broccoli or cauliflorets
turnips
parsnips

When all the vegetables have cooked in the covered pot for a few minutes to release their juices, add about a cup of water, or enough to cover, and a generous pinch of salt. Bring to a boil, cover the pot, and simmer for 10 to 15 minutes, until the vegetables start to soften.

At this point you can add 1 to 2 cups cooked dried beans (along with some of their cooking liquid) or if you don't have any beans, toss in some diced tofu. You can also add a cup or so of cooked rice, barley, millet, or other precooked grain that's around, or even some uncooked whole wheat couscous or pasta.

Next add 1 to 2 cups tomato juice and 2 to 3 cups cold water, according to how tomatoey you want the soup to be, how much vegetable has been used, and how thin or thick you want it to end up being.

Replace the cover and cook about 10 minutes longer, or until everything is tender. During the last minute you can add some frozen peas or corn if more vegetables are desired.

When soup is really hot its flavor is difficult to judge. Therefore, it's best to let people adjust the seasoning to taste by providing salt and pepper at the table. A generous dollop of yogurt cheese in each bowl makes the soup richer.

Hearty Miso-Vegetable Soup

As with most soups, the vegetables can be altered according to what's in season, what's in the pantry, or the whim of the cook. Using the ingredients below, this soothing soup will be ready in just 30 minutes. Adding sesame oil makes it more robust, and by choosing hot sesame oil you can add some zing.

1 large onion, quartered and thinly sliced

2 large carrots, thinly sliced

2 medium potatoes, diced

6 cups of water

2 to 3 cups chopped greens (chard, beet greens, cabbage, even romaine lettuce can be used)

1 cup corn kernels (fresh or frozen)

$^1/_2$ cup minced fresh dill or parsley, optional

$^1/_3$ cup light miso

$^1/_4$ cup sliced scallions

1 teaspoon toasted plain or spicy sesame oil, optional

In a 3- to 5-quart soup pot, combine the onion, carrots, and potatoes. Cover, place over moderate heat, and let the vegetables sweat for 5 minutes. Stir. If the onions haven't wilted, replace the cover and sweat a few minutes longer.

Add the water and bring to a boil. When boiling, add the greens, corn, and dill if using. Cover, and simmer gently for 10 to 15 minutes, until the vegetables are tender.

Place the miso in a small bowl and stir in some hot soup broth to melt. Stir back into soup.

Cover, remove from the heat, and let rest 5 to 10 minutes before serving.

Garnish each bowl with some sliced scallions and season with a little sesame oil, if desired.

YIELD: ABOUT 2 QUARTS; 6 SERVINGS

NOTE: If reheating leftovers, try not to boil. The enzymes in miso like to be treated gently.

In Nikki's Kitchen

Country Mushroom Soup

This delicate mushroom soup provides an admirable first course in just a half hour.

3/4 pound mushrooms, quartered (about 4 cups)
1 clove garlic, sliced
1/4 teaspoon nutmeg
2 tablespoons chopped parsley
2 1/2 cups vegetable broth or water flavored with a few spoonfuls of canned crushed tomatoes, tomato puree, or tomato paste

2/3 cup fresh whole-grain bread torn into pieces
1/2 teaspoon salt (omit if broth is salted)
freshly ground pepper
1 1/2 cups soy milk

Put the mushrooms in a 2-quart soup pot, cover, set over medium heat, and cook for 10 minutes, until the mushroom liquid runs freely. Stir in the garlic, nutmeg, and parsley; cook briefly.

Add the broth or tomato-flavored water, bread, salt, and a generous amount of pepper. Bring to a boil, cover, and simmer over low heat for 10 minutes.

Transfer the soup to a blender or food processor fitted with the steel chopping blade; coarsely chop. The soup should be chunky, with tiny pieces of mushrooms, rather than smooth.

Return the soup to the pot and stir in the soy milk. Cook over gentle heat, stirring frequently, until hot. Do not boil; this could curdle the milk, which would detract from the appearance, although not the flavor. Adjust salt and pepper to taste before serving.

YIELD: ABOUT 5 1/2 CUPS; 4 SERVINGS

Mushroom-Barley Soup

Pressure cooking makes an exceptionally creamy Mushroom-Barley Soup. If you don't have a pressure cooker, follow the second set of directions for conventional stove-top cooking. With either version, letting the soup rest awhile before serving enhances the richness.

3/4 pound mushrooms, coarsely chopped (4 cups)
1 cup chopped onion
2 tablespoons soy sauce

1 cup hulled barley
6 cups water
1 teaspoon salt or to taste
freshly ground pepper

For pressure cooking, combine the mushrooms, onion, soy sauce, barley, and water in a pressure cooker. Cover the pot and bring up to pressure over high heat. Reduce the heat to just maintain the pressure and cook for 50 minutes. Remove from the heat and let sit 10 minutes before releasing the pressure and opening the pot.

For conventional stove-top cooking, combine the ingredients in a 5-quart pot. Bring to a boil, cover, and reduce the heat so the soup simmers gently. Cook for 1½ to 2 hours, until tender.

When the soup is done cooking, add salt and pepper to taste.

YIELD: 2 QUARTS; 6 SERVINGS

Pan-Asian Tomato-Rice Soup

A very tasty first course, with a multicultural mix of ingredients. If you want to serve this soup as a main dish, double the recipe for 6 servings. To dress the soup up, float a few thin rounds of toast in each bowl.

½ cup drained canned tomatoes
1 tablespoon curry powder
6 cloves garlic, cut into pieces
1 cup liquid from canned tomatoes, divided
3 cups water

½ teaspoon salt
½ pound firm or extra firm tofu, cut into cubes
1½ cups cooked brown rice
1 tablespoon miso
2 tablespoons chopped cilantro

In a 3- to 5-quart soup pot, combine the tomatoes and curry powder. Cook over moderate heat for 2 minutes while mashing the tomatoes with the back of a spoon. Add the garlic and ½ cup tomato liquid. Bring to a boil, cover, and simmer over low heat for 10 minutes. Transfer to a blender or food processor and puree.

Return the puree to the pot and add the remaining ½ cup tomato liquid, the water, and salt. Bring to a boil, add the tofu, cover, and simmer gently for 10 minutes. Add the rice and simmer, uncovered, for 5 to 10 minutes, or until the rice is hot.

In a small bowl, combine a little hot soup with the miso and stir until melted. Add back to the soup, mix well, cover, remove from the heat, and let stand for 5 minutes. Adjust the salt to taste and scatter the cilantro on top.

YIELD: 1 QUART; 4 APPETIZER SERVINGS

Carrot Soup with Tomato-Ginger Cream

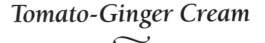

Tomatoes, carrots, and orange make a surprisingly good soup that's even more delectable with swirls of Tomato-Ginger Cream. In hot weather, prepare in advance and serve chilled with dollops of Tomato-Ginger Cream floating on top.

2 cups tomato juice
6 medium carrots, sliced into coins
1 shallot, sliced, or 1/4 cup chopped
   sweet Vidalia or red onion
3/4 cup orange juice

1 teaspoon slivered orange rind
1 cup water
1 teaspoon honey, if needed
Tomato-Ginger Cream (see below)

Bring the tomato juice to a boil in a medium saucepan. Add the carrots and shallot or onion, reduce the heat so the liquid is barely simmering, cover, and cook for 15 minutes.

Add the orange juice, orange rind, and water. Cover and simmer 15 minutes, until the carrot is tender.

Puree in a food mill, blender, or food processor until evenly blended but still somewhat rough textured. If done in a blender, it may be necessary to divide into 2 batches.

Return the soup to the pot; taste. If a bit sharp or acidic, add honey to taste. Simmer, uncovered, for 5 minutes. Ladle the hot soup into serving bowls. Top each with a generous spoonful of Tomato-Ginger Cream and swirl into soup. Serve any remaining cream at the table.

YIELD: ABOUT 5 CUPS; 4 TO 6 SERVINGS

Tomato-Ginger Cream

6 tablespoons Yogurt Cheese
  (page 244)
2 tablespoons tomato juice
1 teaspoon orange juice

1 teaspoon grated fresh ginger or
  1/4 teaspoon dried ground ginger

At any time during the cooking of the soup, combine the Tomato-Ginger Cream ingredients, beating with a fork until smooth.

Carrot Bisque

This is another carrot soup that's excellent either hot or cold. If soup needs to be reheated, avoid boiling.

3 cups carrot coins (6 medium carrots)
1/2 cup chopped onion
1/2 cup sliced celery (include a few leaves if available)
1 tablespoon chopped fresh ginger
1/2 teaspoon salt

1/4 teaspoon cinnamon
1 bay leaf
3 cups water
1 tablespoon soy sauce
2 tablespoons almond butter
1 cup soy milk
freshly ground pepper

Combine the carrots, onion, celery, ginger, salt, cinnamon, bay leaf, and water in a 2- to 3-quart soup pot. Bring to a boil. Cover and simmer over medium-low heat for 15 minutes, or until the carrots are tender. Let cool slightly.

Transfer about half of the soup to a blender or food processor. Add the soy sauce and almond butter. Puree until smooth. If there's room in the machine, add the remaining soup. Otherwise, puree what's left separately. Combine all of the carrot puree with the soy milk in the soup pot. Place over moderate heat and warm through without boiling. Season generously with freshly ground pepper to taste.

YIELD: 6 CUPS; 4 TO 6 SERVINGS

In Nikki's Kitchen

Minestrone

Minestrone is the classic Italian vegetable soup. The vegetables can be varied according to what's available. Green beans, fresh green peas, turnips, or fennel are among those that can be added or substituted for the vegetables included here.

1 tablespoon olive oil
2 cloves garlic, chopped
1 small onion, chopped
3 cups tomato juice
4 cups water
2 carrots, diced
1 stalk celery, diced
1/2 pound potatoes, diced
1 teaspoon salt
1 tablespoon chopped parsley

1 tablespoon chopped fresh basil or
    1 teaspoon dried basil
1 small zucchini, diced
1/2 cup whole wheat elbow
    macaroni, small shells, or broken
    spaghetti
2 cups cooked red or white
    kidney beans
2 1/2 cups shredded greens (spinach,
    Swiss chard, chicory, romaine)

Combine the oil, garlic, and onion in a 5-quart soup pot and cook for a few minutes, until softened. Add the tomato juice, water, carrots, celery, potatoes, salt, parsley, and basil. Bring to a boil, cover, and simmer for 20 minutes.

Add the remaining ingredients, cover, and simmer 20 to 30 minutes longer, until the vegetables are quite tender.

YIELD: ABOUT 2 QUARTS; 6 TO 8 SERVINGS

Mom's Thick Split Pea Soup

Split pea soup is a time-honored favorite at our house, handed down from Nikki's mother. It reheats well and can also be frozen successfully.

2 cups dried split peas
8 cups water
2 medium onions, chopped
4 carrots, chopped

4 to 6 leafy celery tops, chopped
1 large bay leaf
1 1/2 teaspoons salt
freshly ground pepper

Combine the split peas and water in a 3- to 5-quart soup pot and bring to a boil. Prepare the vegetables and add as ready, along with the bay leaf and salt.

When boiling, cover and cook over low heat for 1 to 1 1/2 hours, until the peas are very soft. Mash with a fork or puree in a food mill. Simmer uncovered for a few minutes to thicken. Season generously with freshly ground pepper.

YIELD: ABOUT 2 QUARTS; 8 SERVINGS

Greek Lentil Soup

This is another soup that we serve quite often, sometimes varying it by adding some cooked brown rice or small whole wheat shells or macaroni, and always topping it with generous amounts of yogurt.

1 tablespoon olive oil	1 bay leaf
2 medium onions, chopped	1½ teaspoons salt
2 stalks celery, chopped	4 cups shredded spinach or other
2 cups dried lentils	dark leafy greens
8½ cups water	2 to 3 tablespoons lemon juice
2 tablespoons tomato paste	

Heat the oil in a 5-quart soup pot and sauté the onions for about 3 minutes, until limp. Add the celery, lentils, water, tomato paste, and bay leaf. Bring to a boil, cover, and simmer over low heat about 45 minutes, until the lentils are just tender.

Add the salt and greens, cover, and cook for 15 minutes, or until the beans are completely tender. The consistency should be fairly thick, but if the soup appears to be too dry, add a little water during this phase. When fully cooked, add the lemon juice to taste.

YIELD: ABOUT 2 QUARTS; 6 TO 8 SERVINGS

73

Black Bean Soup

⌒

This bean soup hails from South America. We often serve it as an entrée, setting out brown rice, yogurt, chopped green pepper, and chopped raw onion on the side for everyone to add to their bowl. We complete the menu with a tossed green salad and either warm corn tortillas or a crusty whole-grain bread.

1 cup black beans	1 teaspoon oregano
3¹/₂ cups water	1 teaspoon salt
1 bay leaf	2 tablespoons wine vinegar
1 clove, garlic, chopped	¹/₂ teaspoon hot pepper sauce or
1 small onion, chopped	to taste
¹/₂ medium green pepper, chopped	

Combine the beans and water in a 2- to 3-quart soup pot and let soak for 8 hours, or bring to a boil for 2 minutes, remove from the heat, cover, and let soak for 1 to 2 hours.

Add the bay leaf, garlic, onion, green pepper, and oregano to the beans. Bring to a boil, cover, and simmer over low heat for 1 hour, or until the beans are tender.

Add the salt, vinegar, and hot pepper sauce and cook 5 minutes longer. Taste for seasoning and adjust if necessary. Remove about half of the beans from the pot and puree. Stir back into the soup and cook for a few minutes, until slightly thickened. If the soup is too thick, add up to ¹/₂ cup water.

YIELD: ABOUT 1¹/2 QUARTS; 4 SERVINGS

Leek and White Bean Soup

⌒

This is a rich potage with a southern French/Italian flair. To complete the dish, float rounds of toasted whole-grain bread thickly spread with roasted garlic in each bowl. You might also offer additional cloves of roasted garlic on the side.

2 cups dried white beans	2 tablespoons chopped fresh sage or
9 cups water	¹/4 cup chopped parsley
1 pound leeks	freshly ground pepper
1 teaspoon salt	

Combine the beans and water in a 3- to 5-quart soup pot and let soak for 8 hours, or bring to a boil for 2 minutes, remove from the heat, cover, and let soak for 1 to 2 hours. Return the beans to a boil, cook for 5 minutes, cover, and simmer gently over low heat for 20 minutes, until partially tender.

While the beans cook, prepare the leeks by trimming off the dark green portion and the root, cutting in half lengthwise, and running under cold water to remove any dirt lodged between the layers. Then cut across into thin slices. You should have between 2$^1/_2$ and 3 cups.

Add the leeks and salt to the partially cooked beans, replace the cover, and continue to cook for 30 minutes, or until the beans are very tender.

Using a potato masher, mash the beans to a pulpy consistency. Simmer 5 minutes. Season with fresh sage or parsley and freshly ground pepper, and adjust salt to taste.

YIELD: 2 QUARTS; 4 TO 6 SERVINGS

Cold Cucumber-Yogurt Soup

A warm-weather favorite.

$^1/_2$ cup fine bulgur or whole wheat
  couscous
1 cup boiling water
$^1/_4$ cup chopped onion
$^1/_4$ cup fresh dill
2 medium cucumbers, peeled and
  cut into chunks (about 3 cups)

2 cups yogurt
salt and pepper
$^1/_3$ cup coarsely chopped walnuts
6 lemon wedges

Place the bulgur or couscous in a bowl and cover with the boiling water. Let soak for 15 to 20 minutes, until softened and the liquid is absorbed.

While the grain soaks, combine the onion, dill, and cucumbers in a blender or food processor. Process to a thick puree. Transfer to a bowl.

Add the yogurt to the cucumber puree and mix well. Stir in the soaked grain. Season to taste with salt and pepper. Refrigerate until ready to serve.

Ladle the soup into individuals bowls. Garnish with the chopped walnuts and set a lemon wedge on the rim of each bowl; squeeze the lemon juice into the soup before eating.

YIELD: 4$^1/_2$ CUPS; 6 SERVINGS

NOTE: Bulgur, also known as cracked wheat, comes in several textures. If the fine bulgur called for in this recipe isn't available, reduce coarse varieties to a fine grind in a blender or food processor, or use whole wheat couscous instead.

Main Dishes

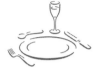

Cauliflower Gratin

This easily prepared casserole takes just 30 minutes, but for added convenience, it can be assembled in advance and refrigerated until baking time. Complete the menu with a grain, a cooked green bean or carrot accompaniment, and a tossed salad.

1 medium to large cauliflower
  (about 2 pounds)
1¹/₂ cups Yogurt Cheese (page 244)
1¹/₂ tablespoons prepared mustard
¹/₃ cup dry whole-grain bread or
  cracker crumbs

2 tablespoons wheat germ
¹/₄ teaspoon salt
¹/₄ teaspoon nutmeg

Preheat the oven to 375°F.

Break the cauliflower into florets and steam 5 to 8 minutes, until just tender. When done, arrange the florets in a shallow 2-quart baking dish so that they're snuggled together.

Combine the Yogurt Cheese and mustard. Smear over the cauliflower using a rubber spatula or flat knife. Combine the crumbs, wheat germ, and seasonings. Sprinkle evenly over the coated cauliflower. Bake for 20 minutes.

YIELD: **6** SERVINGS

Mushroom Ragout

This creamy mushroom mélange can be served on toast or over baked potatoes, kasha, rice, or bow-tie noodles.

¹/₂ pound cultivated white mushrooms	¹/₄ cup cooking sherry or dry wine
¹/₂ pound mixed wild mushrooms of choice (portobello, cremini, shiitake, or chanterelles)	2 teaspoons soy sauce
	¹/₂ cup Yogurt Cheese (page 244)
	¹/₂ teaspoon salt
¹/₂ cup thinly sliced shallots	freshly ground pepper

Clean the mushrooms and slice the caps and stems into bite-size pieces. You should have about 3 cups.

Combine the mushrooms, shallots, sherry, and soy sauce in a skillet. Cook, stirring frequently, for 8 to 10 minutes, or until the mushrooms release their juices and are tender. Remove from the heat and stir in the Yogurt Cheese and salt. Return to low heat and cook, stirring continuously, for 1 to 2 minutes, until creamy and warm. Do not boil.

Season with freshly ground pepper to taste and spoon over toast, potato, or grain of choice.

YIELD: 4 TO 6 SERVINGS

Chiles Rellenos

~

In selecting chiles for this dish, which literally means "stuffed chiles," poblano and Anaheim are most authentic, but can't be found everywhere. In addition, their flavor isn't predictable—they may range from mild to hot. Italian frying peppers, which are offered as an alternative, have a mild, slightly bitter taste and are more widely available. Serve the stuffed peppers and their sauce on brown rice, quinoa, Millet Polenta, 3-Grain Polenta Bread, or a bed of black beans. Cucumber-Tomato Salsa and a green salad are good accompaniments.

8 4- to 6-inch poblano or Anaheim chiles or Italian frying peppers
1½ cups Yogurt Cheese (page 244)
1½ cups corn kernels (fresh or frozen)
⅓ cup thinly sliced scallions
4 cups Quick Spicy Mexican Tomato Sauce (page 201) or other tomato sauce

Arrange the peppers on a baking sheet. Broil until the skins are lightly charred, turning to cook all sides. This will take about 15 minutes. When done, wrap the peppers in a clean dish towel to steam for 5 to 10 minutes. Remove the skins. (For more details on preparing Roasted Peppers, see page 242.)

Cut a slit in the side of each pepper. Carefully remove any seeds. Pat the inside of the peppers with a paper towel to absorb moisture.

In a bowl combine the Yogurt Cheese, corn, and scallions. Spoon the mixture into the peppers. If the surface of the peppers gets messy during filling, wipe with a damp cloth when finished.

Pour the tomato sauce into a skillet large enough to hold the peppers in a single layer. Arrange the peppers slit side up in the sauce; the sauce should generously surround the peppers but not reach as high as the slit. Bring the sauce to a boil over medium heat. Lower the heat so that the sauce gently simmers. Partially cover, leaving the lid slightly ajar to allow steam to escape. Cook for 20 minutes.

YIELD: 4 SERVINGS

The Healthiest Diet in the World

Russian Vegetable Pie

The creamy filling of this savory pie is packed with vegetables and lavishly infused with dill. The rich taste belies the fact that it's fat free. If you've always shied away from making a pie crust, the ease of this one will change that. As an added bonus, the filling can be prepared at the last minute or well in advance and chilled until baking.

Filling:

1 small onion, thinly sliced (about ¹/₂ cup)

1 medium carrot, shredded (about ¹/₄ cup)

1 cup thinly sliced mushrooms

¹/₄ cup slivered green pepper

2 cups coarsely shredded cabbage

¹/₄ cup dill

¹/₄ teaspoon salt

1 cup Yogurt Cheese (page 244)

Crust:

²/₃ cup whole wheat flour

¹/₃ cup cornmeal

2 tablespoons wheat germ

1 teaspoon baking powder

¹/₄ teaspoon baking soda

2 tablespoons olive oil

¹/₃ cup nonfat yogurt

1¹/₂ teaspoons prepared mustard

To make the filling, combine the vegetables, including the dill, in a heavy skillet. Cover and steep over medium heat, stirring occasionally, for 15 minutes, until tender. Season with salt. Cool to lukewarm.

Preheat the oven to 425°F.

To prepare the crust, combine the dry ingredients in a mixing bowl. Stir in the olive oil and mix with a pastry blender, wire whip, or fork until completely incorporated and crumbly. Stir in the yogurt and mix until the ingredients are well blended, kneading gently in the bowl with your hands at the end to form a ball of dough.

Oil a 9-inch pie pan. Press the dough over the bottom and up the sides of the pan to make a pie shell. Prick the surface liberally with a fork. Bake for 10 minutes. Remove from the oven and lower the heat to 375°F.

Complete the filling by combining the cooled vegetables with the Yogurt Cheese. Stir until evenly combined. Spread the mustard lightly over the bottom of the partially baked crust. Add the vegetable-cheese filling.

Bake 20 minutes, until the filling is firm and the edges of the crust are golden brown. Remove from the oven and let sit for at least 10 minutes before cutting. Serve warm or at room temperature.

YIELD: **8** APPETIZER SERVINGS; **4** SERVINGS AS AN ENTRÉE

Baked Stuffed Onions

Baking onions brings out their natural sugar and provides a sweet receptacle for this delicate grain filling. If you don't have access to fresh mint, prepare the grain with mint tea and use fresh parsley in the filling. For an extra minty taste, use both the mint tea and the fresh mint. You can turn this into an elegant meal by starting out with Roasted Red Pepper–Chickpea Dip or Superior Spinach Dip, serving Zucchini "Pasta" along with the Baked Stuffed Onions, and finishing up with a tossed green salad and whole-grain French bread.

4 medium red onions or Vidalia
onions
1 cup cracked wheat (bulgur)
2 cups boiling water or mint tea
2 tablespoons toasted pine nuts or
pumpkin seeds (page 241)

2 tablespoons minced fresh mint or
1/4 cup minced parsley
1/2 teaspoon salt
1/4 cup balsamic vinegar

Preheat the oven to 375°F.

Remove the outer papery layer from the onions. Cut in half crosswise. Remove the centers from each onion half, leaving 2 to 3 layers of rings and the bottom intact to form a small bowl. A grapefruit spoon is a good tool for this job. If there is a hole in the bottom, place a piece of the scooped-out onion over it to cover.

Chop enough of the scooped-out onion to make 1 cup. Reserve the rest for another use. Place the chopped onion in a bowl with the cracked wheat. Cover with the hot water or mint tea. Let sit 10 minutes. Drain off any liquid that hasn't been absorbed. Stir in the pine nuts or pumpkin seeds, mint or parsley, and salt. Pack into the onion bowls, pressing with your hands and mounding to fill tightly.

Place the onions side by side in a baking pan that holds them snugly. Cover and bake for 30 minutes. Remove the cover and continue baking for about 15 minutes, or until the onions are tender.

Remove the onions from the pan and place on a serving dish. Add the balsamic vinegar to the baking pan, place on the stove, and cook for 2 to 3 minutes, stirring to mix any pan juices or dislodged filling with the vinegar. When slightly thickened and syrupy, remove from the heat and spoon on top of each onion. If the pan doesn't come clean, stir in a little water and spoon this, too, over the onions.

YIELD: 4 SERVINGS

Baked Potatoes with
Whipped Artichoke Filling

⌒

Serve 2 halves per person as the focal point of the meal. One half makes a good accompaniment.

4 medium baking potatoes
4 large cloves garlic
1/2 cup Yogurt Cheese (page 244)
6 canned artichoke hearts, drained
  and chopped

salt and pepper
paprika

Preheat the oven to 400°F.

Scrub the potatoes and prick in several places with a fork. Place the potatoes and unpeeled garlic cloves on a baking sheet. Bake the garlic for 15 to 20 minutes, until soft but barely colored. Remove from the oven and continue baking the potatoes until completely tender. This will take from 45 minutes to 1 hour.

Remove the potatoes from the oven and reduce temperature to 350°F.

Holding the potatoes in a clean cloth or oven mitt, cut in half lengthwise and carefully scoop the insides into a mixing bowl, leaving the skins intact. Hold the baked garlic cloves at the root end and squeeze the insides into the bowl with the potatoes. Using a potato masher, mash until no lumps remain. Add the Yogurt Cheese and whip with a fork until creamy. Fold in the artichoke pieces. Season to taste with salt and pepper. Pack the whipped artichoke-potato filling into the potato shells. Sprinkle the surface of the potatoes liberally with paprika. If desired, the potatoes can be prepared to this point and rebaked later. If held more than 1 hour, refrigerate and increase baking time by 5 to 10 minutes to compensate.

Return the potatoes to the oven for about 10 minutes, until piping hot.

YIELD: 8 SERVINGS AS AN ACCOMPANIMENT; 4 SERVINGS AS AN ENTRÉE

*In
Nikki's
Kitchen*

Zucchini "Pasta"

~

Crisp zucchini cut in linguinelike strips makes a delightful pasta alternative. Prepared here with a lightly cooked zucchini-tomato sauce, this dish is crunchy, colorful, and appealing both visually and to the taste buds. It is nicely complemented by a bean salad.

Sauce:

2 tablespoons cooking sherry or
   red wine
1 medium zucchini, diced small
2 large cloves garlic, minced
4 plum tomatoes, diced

2 tablespoons minced parsley
2 tablespoons minced fresh basil
2 tablespoons capers
freshly ground pepper

"Pasta":

4 medium zucchini (about
   10 ounces each)

1/4 to 1/2 cup crumbled feta cheese
   or grated Parmesan

To prepare the sauce, heat the sherry or wine in a large skillet. Add the zucchini and garlic and cook for 5 minutes, stirring occasionally. Add the tomatoes, parsley, basil, and capers and cook 2 to 3 minutes more, until heated through. Season generously with pepper.

To prepare the "pasta," bring a large pot of salted water to a boil. Trim the ends from the zucchini and cut each lengthwise into halves. Place the zucchini halves cut side down on a cutting board and slice them lengthwise into thin strips.

Add the zucchini to the boiling water and cook for 3 minutes. Do not overcook. Drain well. Combine with the sauce and serve, topping each portion with 1 to 2 tablespoons cheese.

YIELD: 4 SERVINGS

Quick Mixed Vegetables in Tomato Juice

~

The basic design of this recipe can be used to turn any combination of vegetables into an Indian, Italian, or Mexican feast. Be sure to include legumes in the mixture for protein. A generous topping of yogurt or yogurt cheese provides additional protein, but this can also be supplied by another component of the meal. For example, the Indian version of this dish can be served with Channa Dahl, rice, and Curried Tomato and Cucumber Salad; for an Italian dinner, Quick

White Pita "Pizzas" or Bean Bruschetta are a natural complement; Quick Mixed Vegetables in Tomato Juice, Mexican Style work well with rice, black beans, and corn tortillas.

2 tablespoons dry wine or cooking sherry
1/2 cup coarsely chopped onion
1/2 cup diced green pepper
2 tablespoons minced hot chile pepper, optional
1 1/2 pounds combined vegetables of choice (green beans, broccoli or cauliflorets, cabbage, carrots, corn, zucchini, crookneck or other summer squash, asparagus, snow peas, mushrooms, potatoes, cooked chickpeas, kidney beans, white beans, or other legumes), cut into bite-size pieces (6 to 8 cups)

1 cup tomato juice
3 cloves garlic, chopped

Indian:

1 dried red chile pepper* or 1/4 teaspoon crushed red pepper flakes*
1/2 teaspoon turmeric*

2 teaspoons grated ginger†
1 teaspoon cumin†
1/4 cup chopped cilantro‡

Italian:

2 tablespoons fresh or 1 teaspoon dried basil†
1 teaspoon oregano†

1 tablespoon balsamic vinegar‡
1/4 cup chopped fresh parsley‡

Mexican:

1 dried red chile pepper* or 1/4 teaspoon crushed red pepper flakes*
2 teaspoons chili powder*
1 teaspoon cumin†

Combine the wine, onion, peppers, vegetables of choice, and seasonings marked * in a saucepan. Cook over medium-high heat, stirring, for 2 minutes.

Add the seasonings marked †, along with the tomato juice and garlic. Stir to blend. Reduce the heat, cover, and cook for 12 to 15 minutes, until the vegetables are tender. Cooking time will vary somewhat depending on the vegetables, size of pieces, and personal taste. Stir occasionally to promote even cooking.

Remove from the heat and stir in the seasonings marked ‡.

YIELD: 4 TO 6 SERVINGS

Creamy Garden Vegetables, Greek or Italian Style

~

This creamy vegetable sauce can be made Greek style—with dill and feta cheese—or Italian style—with parsley, basil, oregano, and Parmesan. For the Italian version, be sure to use high-quality, freshly grated, flavorful Parmesan, romano, or similar grating cheese in order to get the proper taste. Serve over a bed of brown rice, Millet Polenta, or whole-grain pasta. To complete the meal, add Bean Bruschetta or a simple side dish of cooked beans, plus a green salad.

1 small onion, cut into thin crescents
2 cups coarsely chopped mushrooms
4 cups vegetables of choice, cut into thin strips 1 to 2 inches long or comfortable bite-size pieces, including asparagus, broccoli stalks, carrots, cauliflorets, celery, corn kernels, fennel, green beans, leeks, shredded greens, sweet red or green pepper, snow peas, zucchini, yellow crookneck squash

1/4 cup minced fresh dill weed or
1/4 cup Italian flat-leaf parsley plus
2 tablespoons chopped fresh basil or 1/2 teaspoon dried basil and
1 teaspoon dried oregano
2 tablespoons cooking sherry
1 cup Yogurt Cheese (page 244)
1/3 cup crumbled feta cheese or grated Parmesan cheese
freshly ground pepper

Combine the onion, mushrooms, vegetables, herbs, and cooking sherry in a heavy skillet. Cover and cook over moderate heat for 10 minutes, or until the vegetables are just tender and the mushroom liquid runs freely.

Remove from the heat and stir in the Yogurt Cheese. Return to low heat and cook, stirring continuously, until the Yogurt Cheese melts and the sauce is creamy. Do not boil. Add the feta or Parmesan. Remove from the heat. Season generously with freshly ground pepper.

YIELD: **4 SERVINGS**

The Healthiest Diet in the World

Broiled Tofu with Parsley Dressing

Serve 2 slices of this very quick and flavorful recipe per person as an entrée, along with a grain, cooked vegetable, and salad. You can also serve it as an hors d'oeuvre by cutting each slice into cubes or strips after cooking.

1 pound firm or extra firm tofu
2 teaspoons soy sauce
2 tablespoons water
1 cup lightly packed parsley leaves
   or a combination of parsley
   and dill
2 large cloves garlic, sliced

1 teaspoon paprika
1/8 teaspoon crushed red pepper
   flakes, optional
2 tablespoons lemon juice
2 tablespoons wine vinegar

Slice the tofu into 8 pieces, about 1/2 inch thick each. Pat dry.

In a shallow baking pan large enough to hold the tofu in a single layer, combine the soy sauce and water. Dip each tofu slice in the diluted soy sauce, turning so both sides are seasoned. Arrange the tofu slices in a single layer in the liquid remaining in the pan.

In a food processor, combine the herbs and garlic; mince. Add the paprika, red pepper flakes, if desired, lemon juice, and vinegar. Process until evenly blended. Spread thickly on top of each tofu slice.

Broil 4 to 6 inches below heat for 5 to 8 minutes, until lightly browned on top.

YIELD: **8** SLICES; **4** SERVINGS

*In
Nikki's
Kitchen*

Baked Tofu Sticks

These Baked Tofu Sticks are flavorful and fun to eat. Serve with lemon wedges and Better Than Ketchup or Salsa Cruda for dipping. For a complete meal, begin with grapefruit and accompany the Baked Tofu Sticks with corn on the cob and Creamy Miso-Mustard Coleslaw or a green salad.

2 pounds firm tofu	1/4 cup finely chopped walnuts
2 eggs	1 teaspoon salt
1/2 cup cornmeal	1 teaspoon paprika
1/2 cup wheat germ	generous pinch cayenne

Preheat the oven to 400°F.

Cut the tofu into sticks 3/4 inch thick and about 3 inches long. You should have 24 sticks. Pat dry with paper towels.

Crack the eggs into a shallow bowl and beat lightly with a fork.

Combine the cornmeal, wheat germ, walnuts, salt, paprika, and cayenne on a plate. Mix well. Dip the tofu in the egg. Roll in the dry mixture to coat. Transfer to a wire rack and let sit while preparing the remaining tofu. The recipe can be prepared well in advance up to this point and refrigerated. In fact, this will give the coating a chance to set.

Place on an oiled baking sheet. Bake 15 to 20 minutes, until the coating is golden.

YIELD: **6** SERVINGS

Simmered Soft Tofu with Vegetables

This delicate tofu-vegetable combination can stand on its own or as a topping for whole wheat linguine, brown rice, or other cooked grain.

1/4 cup soy sauce	1 pound soft tofu
2/3 cup water	1/3 cup minced parsley
1 small onion, diced	1/4 cup sliced scallions
1/2 cup diced red pepper	
1 hot pepper, minced, optional	
3 cups snow peas or green beans cut into 1-inch pieces or 3 cups frozen green peas	

Combine the soy sauce and water. Pour 1/4 cup of this mixture into a large skillet. Add the onion and peppers. Bring to a simmer, cover, and cook over medium heat for 5 minutes.

Add the snow peas or green beans to the skillet along with the remaining soy sauce mixture. Cover and cook 8 to 10 minutes longer, until the vegetable is just tender. If using frozen green peas, proceed immediately to the next step.

Drain the tofu if necessary and pat dry. Break into generous bite-size chunks using a spoon. Add to the skillet along with the frozen green peas (if using), parsley, and scallions. Simmer, uncovered, for 5 to 8 minutes, until the tofu is hot.

YIELD: 4 SERVINGS

NOTE: For a more robust dish, add 1/2 cup sliced portobello mushrooms or soaked dried porcini mushrooms to the skillet along with the snow peas or green beans.

Mildly Sweet-and-Sour Tofu and Vegetables

Serve with brown rice or rice pasta. For extra flavor, drizzle a little toasted sesame oil on the grain.

1 cup orange juice
1/4 cup canned crushed tomatoes
2 tablespoons soy sauce
1 small onion, cut into crescents
1/2 red pepper, cut into strips
1 tablespoon minced fresh ginger
4 cups vegetables cut into slim
  pieces (carrots, cauliflower,
  broccoli, fennel, green beans, snow
  peas, turnips, or your choice)

1 pound firm or extra firm tofu, cut
  into strips
1/2 cup frozen green peas, optional
1/4 cup white or rice wine vinegar
1 1/2 teaspoons prepared mustard

Combine the orange juice, crushed tomatoes, and soy sauce. Pour 1/4 cup of this mixture into a large skillet. Add the onion, red pepper, and ginger. Cover and cook for 5 minutes.

Add the vegetables and tofu to the skillet, along with the remaining orange juice mixture. Bring to a boil, cover, and simmer gently for 10 to 15 minutes, or until the vegetables are just tender.

Add the green peas, if desired (depending on the vegetables you have chosen they might be nice for color), vinegar, and mustard. Mix well. Simmer uncovered for 5 minutes. Taste for seasoning, adding more mustard if necessary; this will vary according to personal preference and the strength of the mustard.

YIELD: 4 SERVINGS

Smothered Tofu with Peas

~

Slow-cooked onions form a sweet gravy that smothers the tofu. The peas provide an appealing color contrast, but aren't mandatory for taste. Fresh, high-quality paprika makes a big difference in the flavor of this dish, where it's the predominant seasoning. A bit more cayenne than is indicated will provide a lift if the paprika is too bland. Serve with your favorite grain, pasta, or crusty whole-grain bread and round out the menu with a cooked vegetable and salad.

3 large Vidalia, Maui, Bermuda, or
   Spanish onions, halved and thinly
   sliced
2 tablespoons soy sauce
3/4 cup water, divided

1 pound firm or extra firm tofu
1 tablespoon paprika
generous pinch cayenne
1 cup green peas (fresh or frozen)

Combine the onions, soy sauce, and 1/4 cup water in a heavy skillet. Cover and cook over medium-low heat, stirring occasionally, for 15 minutes. The onions should be soft.

While the onions cook, cut the tofu into bite-size cubes. After 15 minutes, add the tofu to the onions, along with the paprika, cayenne, and another 1/4 cup water. Mix well, cover, and continue to cook for 15 minutes, stirring occasionally, until the onions are very soft and almost saucelike in consistency.

When you uncover the pot to stir, gradually add the remaining 1/4 cup water to produce a rich gravy. If using fresh peas, add after 5 minutes, allowing 10 minutes for them to cook. If using frozen peas, wait until cooking is almost complete before adding.

YIELD: 4 SERVINGS

Creamed Tofu with Peas

~

A homey meal when served over cooked grain (brown rice, wild rice, kasha, millet, quinoa) or spooned over whole-grain English muffins or toast.

8 ounces frozen tofu
boiling water
8 ounces firm tofu
3 tablespoons cornstarch

1/4 cup soy sauce
3 cups soy milk
1 teaspoon poultry seasoning
1 cup green peas (fresh or frozen)

Unwrap the frozen tofu and place in a bowl. Pour on boiling water to cover and let stand while preparing the gravy. Cut the fresh tofu into 1/2-inch cubes.

Combine the cornstarch with the soy sauce in a saucepan and stir smooth. Gradually stir in the soy milk. Place over moderate heat and cook, stirring constantly, until the sauce thickens and just comes to a gentle boil.

Squeeze the moisture from the frozen tofu, return to the bowl, and sprinkle lightly with additional soy sauce. Squeeze to distribute the flavoring evenly, then tear the tofu into bite-size pieces.

Stir the poultry seasoning into the gravy. Add the fresh cubed tofu, thawed seasoned frozen tofu, and peas. Simmer gently, stirring continuously, for about 2 minutes.

YIELD: 4 SERVINGS

VARIATION: Replace the peas with fresh or frozen corn kernels or tiny broccoli florets.

★ FREEZING TOFU ★

Another aspect of tofu's versatility is that it can be frozen for long-term keeping. In addition, freezing dramatically changes the texture—so much that it's like an entirely different food in terms of use. Where fresh tofu is soft and dense, frozen tofu is chewy with an open, coarse texture. Some people liken it to chicken; in fact, it can be torn into small pieces and used instead of poultry in chicken salads and many other recipes that call for poultry (see Tofu à la King below). Freezing also increases tofu's spongelike ability to absorb flavors. Firm tofu is the preferred choice for freezing.

To freeze, slice the tofu into 1/2-inch-thick pieces, each weighing about 2 ounces. Wrap each in freezer paper or foil. This individual packaging keeps tofu pieces from sticking together and makes it easy to remove them as needed and defrost them quickly. As an alternative, tofu pieces can be packaged in a single bundle by laying them out next to one another and building layers, if need be, with a piece of freezer paper between them. Freeze and use within six months.

Defrost frozen tofu before using by removing the freezer packaging and placing the tofu in a bowl. Submerge in boiling water and let stand about 10 minutes, or until the water is cool enough to touch. Remove the tofu and repeat the process if still partially frozen. When completely thawed, press the tofu firmly between your palms to expel all moisture. It's now ready to use.

Tofu à la King

The traditional way to serve à la king is over biscuits, and Golden Biscuits are perfect for this. Other options are to spoon this rich flavorful sauce over whole-grain toast or brown rice.

3/4 pound frozen tofu
boiling water
1 cup cold water
2 tablespoons soy sauce
4 tablespoons cooking sherry, divided
1 medium onion, chopped

1/2 cup chopped red pepper
2 cups diced mushrooms
1/4 cup whole wheat flour
1 1/2 cups soy milk
1/2 teaspoon salt
hot pepper sauce
1/4 cup chopped parsley

Unwrap the tofu, place in a bowl, cover with boiling water, and let thaw while preparing the remaining ingredients. When defrosted, drain and squeeze each piece between your palms to remove the moisture. Combine the cold water and soy sauce and marinate the tofu while cooking the sauce.

In a 1 1/2-quart saucepan, combine 2 tablespoons sherry, the onion, red pepper, and mushrooms. Cover and cook about 8 minutes, until the mushrooms are soft and have released their liquid. Stir in the flour, then gradually stir in the milk.

Cook over moderate heat, stirring continuously, until thick and beginning to boil. This will take about 5 to 8 minutes.

Remove the tofu from the soy marinade, press once again to expel moisture, and tear into bite-size pieces. Add to the sauce along with the remaining 2 tablespoons sherry, the salt, and a dash of hot pepper sauce. (If the sauce seems too thick, gradually stir in a little more soy milk.) Continue to cook and stir for a few minutes to heat through. Adjust seasoning to taste.

Spoon over biscuits, toast, or rice and garnish with parsley.

YIELD: **4** SERVINGS

Rosanne's Watercress Tofu

~

While any style of tofu can be used, we prefer tender soft tofu in this dish. If watercress isn't available, substitute fresh spinach, arugula, or a combination of these greens. The addition of sesame oil isn't imperative; however, we particularly enjoy the flavor it imparts. As an alternative, the oil can be omitted and offered at the table as a condiment for individual seasoning; moreover, for those who like their food spicy, hot chile pepper–infused sesame oil can be similarly employed. Excellent served over brown rice mixed with up to one-third kamut or barley.

2 good-size bunches watercress
  (total 12 ounces)
1/2 cup thinly sliced scallions
2 tablespoons soy sauce
1 pound tofu, cut into
  bite-size cubes

2 tablespoons chopped fresh ginger
1/4 cup sunflower seeds
3/4 cup water
1 teaspoon toasted sesame oil,
  optional but recommended

Trim the tough stems of the watercress. You should have about 8 cups loosely packed tops.

Preferably in a wok or otherwise in a large skillet, combine the scallions with 1 tablespoon soy sauce and cook, stirring continuously, for a few minutes. Add the remaining tablespoon soy sauce, the tofu, ginger, and sunflower seeds. Continue to cook and stir for about 5 minutes, gradually adding water as the pan becomes dry.

Add any remaining water and the watercress. Continue cooking and stirring for 5 to 10 minutes, until the greens wilt and become tender. Season with sesame oil.

YIELD: 4 SERVINGS

Eggplant Rollatini

Rolled filled eggplant slices are similar to manicotti or cannelloni, with the vegetable serving the same purpose as the pasta does in these familiar Italian dishes. These delicate rollatini are deceptively filling. The entrée can be complemented with pasta or rice, but if a low-carbohydrate meal is preferred, a generous tossed salad is sufficient. The entire dish can be assembled in advance and refrigerated for later baking. It also reheats well, but isn't recommended for freezing.

2 medium eggplants (about 1 to
  1½ pounds each)
olive oil
1 pound firm tofu
2 tablespoons lemon juice
2 tablespoons tahini
2 tablespoons light miso

1 clove garlic, minced
1 10-ounce package frozen chopped
  spinach, thawed, or 1 cup finely
  chopped, pressed fresh spinach
4 cups Puttanesca Sauce (page 202)
  or other tomato sauce

Preheat the broiler.

Peel the eggplants and cut lengthwise into slices about ¼ inch thick, making 16 slices. (Any extra can be used in other recipes, as explained in Rolled Eggplant Stuffed with Mushroom Pâté, page 54.) Generously oil a baking sheet with olive oil, place the eggplant slices on the oil, then turn them over so both sides are lightly coated with oil. Broil 6 inches below the heat for about 5 minutes on each side, or until lightly browned. You may have to do this in 2 batches.

To prepare the filling, puree the tofu in a food processor or mash thoroughly with a potato masher. Mix in the lemon juice, tahini, and miso. Add the garlic. Squeeze the spinach to remove all moisture and stir into the tofu until evenly combined.

Preheat the oven to 350°F.

Place a sausagelike strip of filling across the center of each eggplant slice, using about 2 tablespoons. Roll the eggplant over the filling. Pour half the sauce into a 9 × 13-inch baking pan and spread to cover the bottom. Place the filled eggplant rolls side by side in the sauce. Pour the remaining sauce over all. Cover and bake for 20 minutes. Remove the cover and bake for 10 minutes longer, until easily pierced with a fork.

YIELD: 4 AMPLE SERVINGS

Tofu Chili

This quickly made chili can be served on corn bread or with rice and tortillas.

1 pound frozen tofu
boiling water

1³/₄ cups Quick Spicy Mexican
Tomato Sauce (page 201)

Unwrap the tofu, place in a bowl, and pour on boiling water to cover. Let sit for 5 to 10 minutes, until the water is cool enough to touch. Remove the tofu and squeeze to remove moisture. If any pieces aren't defrosted, repeat the process.

Using your hands, tear the tofu into bite-size pieces. Combine with the sauce in a pot and simmer for 5 minutes, until heated through.

YIELD: 4 SERVINGS

In
Nikki's
Kitchen

Fajitas

❤

Fajitas are a popular Mexican dish that you eat by scooping up the vegetable mixture with pieces of tortilla and then putting diced avocado and yogurt to taste on top. The version below is made using frozen tofu; it can be varied with strips of tempeh instead. Because marinating is involved, preparation should begin at least an hour before cooking. For the rest of the meal, serve brown rice (perhaps cooked in diluted tomato juice, or if reheated with added tomato juice) and Cucumber-Tomato Salsa or just some cucumber wedges for contrast.

1 pound frozen tofu
boiling water
1/2 cup fresh lime juice (2 to 3 limes)
2 tablespoons soy sauce
2 cloves garlic, minced
2 teaspoons chili powder
2 hot peppers, minced
2 medium onions, sliced into thin crescents

1 large red or green pepper, cut into strips
2 medium zucchini (8 to 10 ounces each), cut into sticks 2 inches long and 1/4 inch thick
8 corn tortillas or 4 large whole wheat tortillas
1 avocado, peeled and diced
yogurt, optional

Unwrap the tofu, place in a bowl, and cover with boiling water. Let stand until the water is cool enough to touch and the tofu is defrosted. Repeat this step if necessary to completely defrost. Remove the tofu and squeeze to extract any moisture. Cut into thin strips.

In a large container or bowl, combine the lime juice, soy sauce, garlic, chili powder, and hot peppers. Add the tofu strips and marinate 1 hour at room temperature, or longer in the refrigerator.

Place a 15-inch skillet or wok over high heat. Add the onions, sweet pepper, zucchini, marinated tofu, and any remaining marinade. Cook, stirring often, for about 10 minutes, until the vegetables are cooked but still crisp.

To prepare the tortillas, cook one at a time by warming briefly over a burner; transfer to a cloth napkin and wrap to keep warm and pliable. Continue to pile up tortillas until they're all cooked. Or stack the tortillas together, wrap in foil, and heat in an oven at 350 to 400°F. for about 10 minutes, until steamy.

Serve the avocado and yogurt on the side so the tofu-vegetable mixture can be scooped into the tortillas and garnished to taste.

YIELD: 4 SERVINGS

*The
Healthiest
Diet in
the World*

Individual Tofu Loaves

Cloak these Individual Tofu Loaves with a generous blanket of sauce. We think they make an especially good match with Sweet Onion Gravy, Creamy Mushroom Gravy, or Tahini-Mushroom Gravy. You can also serve them with a rich tomato sauce.

1 pound firm or extra firm tofu	**$^1/_2$ teaspoon ground ginger**
$^1/_4$ cup oat bran	**$^1/_4$ cup chopped walnuts**
2 teaspoons poultry seasoning	**2 tablespoons miso**

Preheat the oven to 375°F.

Pat the tofu dry, cut into chunks, and place in a mixing bowl. Mash with a fork or potato masher. Add the remaining ingredients. Knead with clean hands until the mixture is well blended and holds together when compressed.

Shape into 4 mounds and place on an oiled baking sheet. Bake for 20 minutes, until the surface is browned.

YIELD: **4** SERVINGS

VARIATION: For *Tofu Burgers*, shape mixture into 8 flat patties instead of 4 mounds. Bake as above. Serve on whole wheat buns with your favorite accompaniments: ketchup, sliced onion, tomato, sprouts, lettuce, or a spicy salsa.

Soy Balls

~

The character of these Soy Balls is determined largely by the sauce they're combined with. This could be an Italian- or Mexican-style tomato sauce or something creamy, such as Creamy Mushroom Gravy. Serve over pasta, brown rice, barley, kasha, or on whole-grain bread for a hot sandwich. Round out the menu with a cooked vegetable (broccoli, brussels sprouts, Blackened Green Beans, carrots) and salad.

1 pound firm tofu	1 teaspoon oregano
1/2 cup wheat germ	1 tablespoon soy sauce
1 large clove garlic, minced	2 to 3 cups sauce of choice
3 tablespoons minced fresh onion	

Preheat the oven to 375°F.

Pat the tofu dry, cut into chunks, and place in a mixing bowl. Mash with a fork or potato masher. Add the remaining ingredients, except the sauce. Using your hands, knead the mixture in the bowl until it's evenly combined and holds together when compressed. Using generous tablespoonfuls, shape into 16 1 1/2-inch balls.

Place the Soy Balls on an oiled baking sheet. Bake for 20 minutes, until firm and golden. Just before serving, heat the sauce, add the Soy Balls, and warm through.

YIELD: 16 BALLS; 4 SERVINGS

Stuffed Peppers

~

These stuffed peppers are a good vehicle for using up leftover cooked grain.

3 cups tomato juice	2 cups cooked grain (kasha, millet,
2 cloves garlic, minced	barley, oat groats, short-grain
2 carrots, chopped	brown rice)
1 small hot pepper, optional	1/4 cup chopped onion
4 green peppers	1 tablespoon soy sauce
1 pound regular or firm tofu	

In a large skillet or broad pot that will hold the pepper halves in a single layer, combine the tomato juice, garlic, carrots, and hot pepper, if using. Bring to a boil.

Cut the peppers in half lengthwise through the stem. Remove the seeds and any tough ribs.

Mash the tofu using a potato masher or fork. Combine in a bowl with the grain, onion, and soy sauce and mix well. Pack into the pepper halves.

Place the peppers, filling up, in the sauce, reduce the heat to a gentle simmer, spoon a little sauce over each pepper, cover, and cook for 30 minutes, until the peppers are just tender and the carrots in the sauce are soft.

Remove the peppers from the pot and using a potato masher mash the carrots into the sauce to a coarse consistency. (If desired, the sauce can be transferred to a blender and pureed.) Spoon the sauce over the peppers to serve. If not serving immediately, return the peppers to the sauce and reheat briefly before eating.

YIELD: 4 SERVINGS

Tofu-Stuffed Sweet Red Peppers

Place two stuffed pepper halves on rice and top with rich, garlic-laden Agliata sauce as an entrée. The peppers can also be served as appetizers by placing half a pepper on a bed of fresh salad greens for each serving and topping with Agliata.

4 large red peppers (1/2 pound each)
1 1/2 pounds regular or firm tofu
2/3 cup dry whole-grain bread crumbs
1/4 cup flaxseed meal (page 239)
1/2 cup sunflower seeds, ground (3/4 cup sunflower "meal")

1/4 cup wheat germ
3 large cloves garlic, minced
1/2 cup chopped parsley
2 teaspoons oregano
1 teaspoon salt

To prepare the red peppers for stuffing, cut in half lengthwise through the stem. Remove the seeds and any thick ribs. Rinse under cold water and invert to drain.

To make the filling, mash the tofu with a potato masher or fork and combine in a bowl with the remaining ingredients. Mix well to thoroughly blend, then knead gently by hand until the mixture holds together. Pack about 1/2 cup filling into each pepper half.

Place the pepper halves, filling up, in a vegetable steamer set over boiling water. Steam for 20 minutes, until the pepper shell is just tender.

YIELD: 8 APPETIZER SERVINGS; 4 SERVINGS AS AN ENTRÉE

In Nikki's Kitchen

Maple-Pecan Tempeh

~

Tempeh cutlets with a sweet nutty topping provide the focal point of a "Southern" meal that includes Louisiana Sweet Potatoes (or plain baked or mashed sweet potatoes) and cooked greens.

1 pound tempeh
about 3 tablespoons prepared
  mustard
about 1/3 cup cornmeal

3 tablespoons soy sauce
3 tablespoons maple syrup
1/4 cup chopped pecans
water

Cut the tempeh into 8 "cutlets," each one about 1/4 inch thick. Spread a thin coating of mustard on both sides of the tempeh cutlets. Dredge with the cornmeal.

Wipe a large heavy skillet with oil to coat and heat. Cook the tempeh 3 to 5 minutes on each side, until browned.

Combine the soy sauce, maple syrup, and pecans. Spoon evenly over the tempeh.

Turn the heat to low. Pour about 1/4 cup water into the bottom of the skillet; stand back—the water will sputter. Cover the pan and cook 5 minutes.

YIELD: 4 SERVINGS

Baked Corn-Tempeh Hash

~

Hash is generally regarded as a "family" dish, and this one is quite tasty. For more elegant service, stuff inside tomatoes or peppers, as described in the Note.

1 medium green pepper, chopped
1 medium onion, chopped
1/2 pound tempeh, crumbled or
  coarsely chopped (2 cups)
2 tablespoons cooking sherry or
  dry wine
2 medium tomatoes, diced, or
  2 cups drained canned tomatoes

1/4 teaspoon nutmeg
1/4 teaspoon cayenne
1/2 teaspoon salt
1/2 cup crumbled whole-grain bread
1/2 cup soy milk
1 cup corn kernels (fresh or frozen)

Preheat the oven to 350°F.

Combine the green pepper, onion, tempeh, and cooking sherry or wine in a skillet. Cover and cook over moderate heat for 8 to 10 minutes, until the onion has softened. Add the tomatoes, nutmeg, cayenne, and salt. Cook over medium-high heat, stirring frequently, for about 5 minutes, until the tomato softens. Remove from the heat.

While the tempeh cooks, combine the crumbled bread and soy milk in a small bowl. When the tempeh mixture is done cooking, mash the bread and add to the skillet along with any unabsorbed soy milk and the corn. Mix well.

Transfer the hash mixture to an oiled 9-inch or shallow 1-quart casserole. Bake for 30 minutes. The hash should be piping hot, but still a bit moist. Baking for too long or at too high temperatures will dry out the hash. If this seems to be occurring, pour a little soy milk over the surface as the hash bakes.

YIELD: 4 SERVINGS

NOTE: For more elegant service, stuff into 8 medium-size hollowed-out tomatoes or blanched peppers (remove the tops and steam for 5 minutes) or a combination of the two. Plan on 2 stuffed vegetables per serving. Bake as above, placing the tomatoes in an oiled baking dish and the peppers in a baking dish surrounded by hot water to a depth of 1 inch.

Picadillo

Picadillo is a classic Latin American dish—a cross between hash and a thick, rich sauce, somewhat like Sloppy Joes. While the recipe tends to vary depending on the country of origin and the cook, there's a characteristic mix of seasonings that creates a surprising interplay of sweet, salty, aromatic, and astringent tastes. Serve with brown rice or Sunflower-Rice Patties, Glazed Plantains, and tossed salad. Or simply eat by rolling up into warm corn or whole wheat tortillas.

1 small onion, chopped
1 medium green pepper, chopped
2 cloves garlic, minced
1 pound soy tempeh, cut into thin strips
1 tablespoon soy sauce
3 tablespoons water
1 teaspoon cumin
1 teaspoon cinnamon
1 1/2 cups canned crushed tomatoes or tomato sauce
1/4 cup currants or chopped raisins
2 tablespoons capers
1 tablespoon molasses
1 tablespoon cider vinegar
2 tablespoons chopped olives

In a 3- or 4-quart pot, combine the onion, green pepper, garlic, tempeh, soy sauce, and water. Cover and cook over low heat, stirring occasionally, for 10 minutes. Add the remaining ingredients except for the olives. Cover and continue to cook for 10 to 15 minutes, until quite hot. Stir in the olives at the end.

YIELD: 4 SERVINGS

Tempeh-Mushroom Stew

Serve this classic stew with a grapefruit appetizer, a large salad, and crusty bread.

2 pounds thin-skinned potatoes
  (6 medium)
1 large onion, cut into crescents
1/2 pound mushrooms, sliced
  (3 cups)
1 pound asparagus or green beans,
  trimmed and broken into pieces
  (4 cups)
12 ounces tempeh, cut into
  1-inch cubes

2/3 cup water
1 tablespoon soy sauce
2 cups soy milk
1 teaspoon dried thyme
2 tablespoons lemon juice
3 tablespoons capers
salt and pepper
nutmeg

Cut the potatoes into quarters if small to medium, or sixths if medium to large. Steam the potatoes for 15 to 20 minutes, until tender.

While the potatoes are steaming, combine the onion, mushrooms, and asparagus or green beans in a 3- to 5-quart pot. Cover and place over medium heat. Cook, stirring occasionally, for about 10 minutes, until the onion is translucent and the mushrooms begin to release their liquid.

Add the tempeh, water, and soy sauce to the mushroom mixture. Cover and cook about 10 minutes, until the vegetable is tender.

When the potatoes are cooked, remove one-third and combine in a blender with the soy milk. Puree until smooth. (Skins can be left on the potatoes or not according to preference.)

Cut the remaining potatoes into 1-inch pieces. Add to the mushroom mixture along with the potato puree and thyme. Heat through, stirring gently, for 5 to 8 minutes, until the sauce is thick. If the sauce is too thick, add additional soy milk to reach the desired consistency.

Remove from the heat and stir in the lemon juice and capers. Season to taste with salt and pepper, then grate some fresh nutmeg on top.

YIELD: 4 TO 6 SERVINGS

Asian Grill

Marinated tofu and tempeh are both excellent grilled. This recipe provides enough marinade for 1 pound of tofu or tempeh, or 4 servings. If you want to include some vegetables as well, double the recipe and you'll have enough for 6 to 8 mushroom caps and some broccoli, eggplant, cauliflower, or sweet potato slices. Of course, you can make Asian Grill in larger quantities for feeding a crowd. (For another tasty barbecue marinade, see Spicy Marinade in "Sauces and Toppings.")

^{1}/$_3$ cup fresh lime or lemon juice
^{1}/$_3$ cup soy sauce
2 cloves garlic, minced
1-inch segment ginger, peeled and
  grated

1 teaspoon minced orange rind
1 tablespoon molasses or
  2 tablespoons fruit juice–sweetened
  orange marmalade
1 pound tempeh or tofu

Combine the marinade ingredients in a pan (or 2) large enough to hold the food in a single layer. Slice the tofu or tempeh about ^{1}/$_3$ inch thick, or into 12 squares. (For vegetables, divide broccoli into thin trees and cauliflower into manageable florets; slice eggplant into ^{1}/$_4$-inch-thick rounds; clean mushrooms caps; cut onions into thick rounds or wedges; cut sweet potatoes into ^{1}/$_4$-inch-thick slices.)

Marinate 1 to 2 hours at room temperature or longer in the refrigerator.

Grill over hot coals, brushing on any remaining marinade while cooking.

YIELD: ^{2}/$_3$ CUP MARINADE; ENOUGH FOR 1 POUND OF TOFU OR TEMPEH

*In
Nikki's
Kitchen*

Barbecued Tofu

~

Cook outdoors or on a stove-top grill. With lots of vegetables, a grain, and a green salad this is a generous meal; but if the rest of the menu is sparse, you may want to double the recipe, giving you plenty of food for 6 (or 4 with leftovers).

1 pound firm or extra firm tofu	1½ teaspoons lemon juice
¼ cup soy sauce	1 tablespoon chopped garlic
¼ cup orange juice	½ teaspoon oregano
2 tablespoons tomato paste	freshly ground pepper
1½ teaspoons olive oil	

Slice the tofu ½ inch thick. You should have at least 12 pieces.

Combine the remaining ingredients, adding a generous amount of freshly ground pepper. Mix thoroughly. Transfer to a pan large enough to hold the tofu in a single layer.

Lay the tofu slices in the sauce, turn so both sides are coated, and let sit for several hours in the refrigerator if possible to marinate. Turn once or twice while marinating so the tofu is well coated with the sauce.

Cook over hot coals for about 8 to 10 minutes per side, or until the surface is firm and lightly charred. Use any remaining sauce to baste the tofu while cooking.

YIELD: 4 MODEST SERVINGS

Tempeh Kebabs

~

Depending on what else is on the menu, and whether the kebabs contain just tempeh or vegetables as well, plan on 1 to 2 skewers per person.

12 ounces tempeh	vegetables of choice, optional: onion
½ cup water	wedges, chunks of sweet red or
2 tablespoons soy sauce	green pepper, tomato crescents,
	whole mushrooms

Cut the tempeh into 16 cubes. Combine the water and soy sauce in a bowl. Add the tempeh cubes and let soak for 15 minutes or long enough to absorb the liquid.

Thread 4 cubes of tempeh on each of 4 skewers, alternating with pieces of vegetables, if desired. Grill for about 5 minutes on each side, or until the tempeh is nicely browned.

YIELD: 2 TO 4 SERVINGS

Shish Kebab in a Bag

~

These individual packets of tempeh and vegetables are designed to cook directly in hot coals, making them ideal for cookouts, campfires, or even fireplace cooking. They can be assembled ahead and held in a cooler or refrigerator.

12 ounces tempeh
1/2 cup water
2 tablespoons soy sauce
1 small eggplant (about 1 pound)
2 small tomatoes or 4 plum
   tomatoes
1 green pepper

1 small onion
2 medium potatoes (about
   3/4 pound)
4 nice-size mushrooms
1 teaspoon oregano
1 lemon, cut into 8 wedges

Cut the tempeh into 1-inch cubes. Combine the water and soy sauce in a bowl and add the tempeh cubes. Let marinate while preparing the remaining ingredients. Cut the eggplant and tomatoes into small chunks. Cut the green pepper into strips. Cut the onion into thin rings. Thinly slice the potatoes and mushrooms.

Prepare four 12-inch squares of heavy-duty aluminum foil or double layers of regular foil. Divide the vegetables and tempeh evenly and place in the center of each sheet. Fold up the edges to form a bowl around the vegetables.

Season each packet with 1/4 teaspoon oregano, the juice from 1 lemon wedge, and any leftover soy marinade. Enclose completely in foil, folding the edges several times to seal.

Place the packets directly on the coals of a grill or in the embers of a campfire or fireplace. Cook for 20 minutes. Lift the packets carefully from the heat with long-handled tongs or a spatula. Open one to test for doneness. If the vegetables are tender, they're ready to eat. If not, close and cook as needed.

Distribute the packets and let everyone eat directly from the foil dish, or transfer the contents to plates. Be sure to let the food cool a bit before tasting, as it will be very hot. Serve the remaining lemon wedges on the side along with salt and pepper for individual seasoning.

YIELD: 4 SERVINGS

103

*In
Nikki's
Kitchen*

Thai Salad

A cold salad makes a good warm-weather meal. This one is very pretty and offers a lot of room for creativity. For example, instead of garnishing with sprouts and peas, you can arrange fresh steamed green beans around the circumference of each salad, creating the appearance of a nest. Another option is to surround the salad with freshly steamed broccoli buds. Rice cakes make a good accompaniment. For a more substantial meal, begin with Carrot Soup with Tomato-Ginger Cream or Carrot Bisque, either of which can be served hot or cold.

3/4 pound firm tofu
1/2 cup fresh lime juice
1/4 cup soy sauce
2 teaspoons grated ginger
2 cloves garlic, crushed
3/4 teaspoon crushed red pepper
  flakes
1/4 cup chopped fresh cilantro
1/4 cup sliced scallion or diced
  sweet onion
1/2 cup diced red or green pepper
1 medium cucumber, peeled and
  thinly sliced

6 cups salad greens torn into bite-
  size pieces
1/2 cup sprouts (bean, sunflower,
  radish, alfalfa)
1/2 cup fresh green peas or sliced
  edible pod peas, optional
radishes, optional
1/4 cup unsalted dry-roasted
  peanuts, chopped
toasted sesame oil, optional

Cut the tofu into thin strips. In a medium bowl, combine the lime juice, soy sauce, ginger, garlic, and red pepper flakes. Add the tofu strips and gently mix. Add the cilantro, scallion or onion, red or green pepper, and cucumber. Mix again. Don't worry if the tofu falls apart somewhat. Cover and refrigerate until serving time.

Arrange the greens on 4 serving plates. Top with the marinated tofu and vegetables. Pour any dressing remaining in the bowl on top of the salads. Surround with the sprouts, peas, and/or radishes, if desired. Sprinkle 1 tablespoon chopped peanuts on top of each salad.

Provide the toasted sesame oil at the table for those who wish to sprinkle a little on their salad to temper the intense lime flavor.

YIELD: 4 SERVINGS

Indonesian Tempeh Salad

To add color to this generous main-dish salad, garnish with a few red pepper strips, radishes, or tomato wedges. Accompany with lightly toasted rice cakes. Depending on the season, you could start the meal with hot or cold Carrot Soup with Tomato-Ginger Cream. Or, to go along with the salad, try corn on the cob or Grilled or Oven-Roasted Sweet Potatoes.

1/4 cup pumpkin seeds

1/4 cup peanuts

1 large Vidalia or other sweet onion, sliced into half-rings

2 large cloves garlic

3 tablespoons soy sauce

2 tablespoons lemon juice

1 tablespoon molasses

1/2 teaspoon cayenne or to taste

1/3 cup water

12 ounces tempeh

6 cups mixed salad greens

1 cucumber, peeled and sliced

1 lemon, cut into wedges

Toast the pumpkin seeds in a dry skillet until they pop. Watch carefully and shake the pan during cooking to prevent burning.

Transfer the seeds to a blender or food processor. Add the peanuts, 1 slice of onion, garlic, soy sauce, lemon juice, molasses, cayenne, and water. Puree until evenly blended but not quite smooth.

Slice the tempeh into strips 1/8 inch thick.

Transfer the sauce to a large skillet and heat. Add the remaining onion and tempeh strips and mix to coat with sauce. Cover and cook over moderate heat for 5 minutes. Uncover, mix again, replace the cover, and cook 5 minutes longer.

Pile 1 1/2 cups greens onto each of 4 plates. Surround with the cucumber rings. Mound the cooked tempeh and onions on top of the greens. Use a spoon to scrape any sauce that clings to the pan onto the salads. Garnish with lemon wedges for individual seasoning at the table.

YIELD: 4 SERVINGS

In Nikki's Kitchen

White Beans and Carrots with Creamy Walnut Pesto

~

Pesto sauce is a versatile flavoring agent that shouldn't be regarded as solely for pasta. Unlike the classic version, which is imbued with oil, the only fat in this pesto recipe comes from the walnuts. The creaminess is provided by yogurt cheese and mellow light miso.

1 cup carrot coins
4 cups cooked white beans or black-eyed peas

3/4 cup Creamy Walnut Pesto (page 196)

Steam the carrots or cook in a small amount of boiling water for 5 to 8 minutes, until just tender. Combine with the beans and heat through. Just before serving, and while the beans are still hot, stir in Creamy Walnut Pesto and mix gently until the beans and carrots are completely covered with the sauce.

YIELD: 4 SERVINGS

Braised Fennel with White Beans

~

Fennel has a delicate licorice flavor that goes especially well with white beans. Either home-cooked or canned beans can be used in this dish. If using canned beans, reserve some of the canning liquid if possible for cooking the vegetables, diluting it with water as necessary. And remember to omit the salt if beans are presalted. For the rest of the meal, consider grilled portobello mushrooms, White Pita "Pizzas" with Cooked Greens, or crusty bread with a yogurt cheese spread.

1 large or 2 medium bulbs fennel (1 pound)
1/2 cup bean cooking liquid or water
1 1/2 cups diced red or new potatoes
1 large clove garlic, minced
1/4 teaspoon crushed red pepper flakes

1/2 teaspoon salt (omit if beans are salted)
1 cup diced fresh plum tomatoes or drained canned tomatoes
1 tablespoon lemon juice
2 cups cooked white beans, drained
2 tablespoons chopped black olives

Trim the stem and feathery leaves from the fennel. Discard the stalk. Mince the leaves to make 1 tablespoon. (Reserve the remaining leaves for another use.) Cut the fennel bulb in half lengthwise. Remove the core and discard. Slice the fennel into thin wedges. You should have about 4 cups.

Bring the bean cooking liquid to a boil in a medium saucepan. Add the fennel leaves, fennel wedges, potatoes, garlic, red pepper flakes, and salt. Cover and cook over gentle heat until the potatoes are tender but still hold their shape, about 10 minutes.

Add the tomatoes and lemon juice. Mix well. Stir in the beans and olives. Cook, uncovered, for 2 to 3 minutes, until heated through.

YIELD: **4** GENEROUS SERVINGS

White Beans with Swiss Chard

These white beans in a bed of tender greens have a noticeable bite. Those who like their food mild can reduce or omit the cayenne. This dish tastes best eaten lukewarm or at room temperature. A suggested menu includes Smothered Eggplant, whole wheat pita bread, and some olives, raw carrot sticks, red pepper wedges, and similarly simple accompaniments. Or try it with baked or grilled winter squash. If a grain is desired, barley makes a hearty choice, or choose millet for something lighter.

1 cup dried white cannellini or great northern beans	1/4 teaspoon cayenne
3 cups water	3/4 pound plum tomatoes, chopped (about 2 cups)
5 cloves garlic, minced	1 pound Swiss chard, coarsely chopped
1 large onion, chopped	
2 stalks celery, thinly sliced	1/2 cup dry red wine
2 carrots, diced	1 teaspoon salt

Combine the beans and water in a pot. Bring to a boil, cook 2 minutes, remove from the heat, cover, and let soak 1 hour or longer. Return to a boil for 5 minutes, cover, and simmer gently for 20 minutes.

Meanwhile, in a separate 5-quart pot, combine the garlic, onion, celery, and carrots. Cover and stew over moderate heat for about 10 minutes, until the onion is translucent. Add the cayenne and tomatoes. Cook over medium-high heat, mashing with a spoon until the tomatoes start to soften. Add the Swiss chard, stirring to wilt. When wilted, add the wine, salt, and partially cooked beans along with any cooking liquid. Cover and simmer gently for about 45 minutes, or until the beans are quite tender.

Remove from the heat and let sit at least 10 minutes before serving. Serve lukewarm or at room temperature.

YIELD: **4** TO **6** SERVINGS

In Nikki's Kitchen

Cabbage with White Beans

For this dish you can use either home-cooked or canned beans and their liquid. If the bean liquid is insufficient, you can use water or vegetable broth. Serve with a flavorful grain, such as Kasha with Stewed Onions.

3/4 pound cabbage cut into 1/4-inch-thick strips (4 to 5 cups)
3 cloves garlic, sliced
1 1/2 cups bean cooking liquid, vegetable broth, or water

3 cups cooked white cannellini beans
1 generous tablespoon caraway seeds
salt and pepper

Combine the cabbage, garlic, and bean cooking liquid in a pot, cover, and stew for 10 minutes over moderate heat, until tender. Add the beans and caraway seeds and cook uncovered for about 10 minutes, stirring occasionally, until a rich gravy forms. Season to taste with salt and pepper.

YIELD: **4** SERVINGS

Unstuffed Cabbage

Similar to stuffed cabbage, but much less work. While home-cooked dried beans are preferred, canned can be substituted for a very easy last-minute meal. Best served warm but not piping hot. For maximum appeal, top each serving with generous amounts of yogurt cheese. Accompany with brown rice, quinoa, millet, or cracked wheat.

2 cups tomato juice
2 cloves garlic, minced
1 tablespoon minced fresh ginger
2-inch piece cinnamon stick
2 tablespoons lemon juice
1 tablespoon molasses

1/3 cup chopped dried prunes (5 large to 8 medium pitted prunes)
1 1/2 pounds cabbage, cut into 1/2-inch-wide strips (about 8 cups)
3 cups cooked white cannellini beans, well drained

Combine the tomato juice, seasonings, lemon juice, molasses, and prunes in a pot and bring to a boil. Add the cabbage, cover, and simmer over gentle heat for 10 minutes, until the cabbage is tender. Add the beans. (If using canned beans, rinse in a strainer to remove all traces of canning liquid.) Simmer uncovered for 3 to 5 minutes to heat through. Remove the cinnamon stick.

YIELD: **4** SERVINGS

White Bean Ratatouille

This casserole of beans and vegetables is typical of the fare in the south of France. Although there are a lot of directions, the recipe is really very easy to execute and produces a generous amount. Leftovers can be kept in the refrigerator for about a week and make a good sandwich filling on whole wheat Italian or other crusty whole-grain bread.

1 cup dried great northern, navy, or pea beans
$2^1/2$ cups water
$^3/4$ teaspoon salt, divided
3 cloves garlic, minced
1 pound eggplant
2 stalks celery, sliced into $^1/4$-inch pieces
1 medium green pepper (about 5 ounces), cut into small strips

2 medium yellow crookneck squash (5 to 6 ounces each), sliced into $^1/4$-inch-thick rounds
1 medium onion, thinly sliced
2 cups chopped Italian plum tomatoes (12 ounces)
2 tablespoons capers
2 tablespoons wine vinegar
freshly ground pepper

Combine the beans and water in a pot. Bring to a boil, cook 2 minutes, remove from the heat, and let soak 1 hour or longer. Return to a boil for 5 minutes, cover, and simmer gently for 30 to 40 minutes, until just tender. Drain the beans, reserving any liquid as a cooking medium for another time. Transfer the beans to an oiled 9 × 13-inch baking dish or 3-quart casserole. Stir in $^1/4$ teaspoon salt and scatter one-third of the garlic on top.

While the beans cook, prepare the remaining ingredients. During assembly, preheat the oven to 400°F. Peel the eggplant and cut into $^1/2$-inch cubes. Place in a strainer or colander, sprinkle with $^1/4$ teaspoon salt, and let sit while preparing the remaining vegetables.

For assembly, layer the vegetables and garlic over the beans as follows: celery, eggplant, one-third of the garlic, green pepper, squash, onion, tomatoes, capers, remaining $^1/4$ teaspoon salt, and the remaining garlic. Drizzle the vinegar over all. Cover and bake for 1 hour, or until the vegetables are tender.

Remove the cover and cool for 10 minutes. Adjust salt, if needed, and season with freshly ground pepper to taste. Serve lukewarm or at room temperature.

YIELD: 6 SERVINGS

In Nikki's Kitchen

Black-eyed Peas, Corn, and Greens

~

This colorful dish has a nice bite. Choose the type of hot pepper or adjust the amount of crushed red pepper flakes according to how spicy you like your food to be.

1½ cups dried black-eyed peas
3 cups water
1 hot pepper, chopped, or ½
    teaspoon crushed red pepper flakes
½ teaspoon salt
1 good-size onion, chopped (use
    Vidalia, Maui, or another sweet
    variety when available)

1 pound kale or collard greens,
    coarsely chopped
2 cups corn kernels (fresh or frozen)
3 tablespoons wine vinegar
2 tomatoes, diced

Combine the black-eyed peas and water in a large pot. Bring to a boil for 2 minutes, cover, remove from the heat, and let soak for 1 hour or longer.

Return the beans to a boil for 5 minutes, cover, and cook over low heat at a gentle simmer for 20 minutes, until partially done. Add the hot pepper and salt. Continue cooking for another 15 to 20 minutes, or until the beans are tender.

When the beans are tender, add the onion, greens, and corn. Raise the heat and cook until the greens wilt. Cover, lower the heat, and cook for 10 to 15 minutes, or until the greens are tender. Season with the vinegar, mix well, and remove from the heat.

Place in a serving bowl and garnish with the diced tomatoes.

YIELD: **4** TO **6** SERVINGS

★ THE BEST ANTIOXIDANT VEGETABLES ★

In a U.S. Department of Agriculture study of the relative antioxidant capability of vegetables, the top eight, starting with the most potent, are: kale, garlic, spinach, brussels sprouts, alfalfa sprouts, broccoli flowers, beets, and red bell pepper. The antioxidant rating of kale was three times that of the red pepper.

*The
Healthiest
Diet in
the World*

Lentils with Vegetables, French Style

⌒

A good choice for a buffet, since the recipe makes a lot and the dish should be eaten at room temperature. Don't attempt to make this when you're in a rush, since a fair amount of chopping is involved. Leftovers can be diluted with liquid from canned tomatoes or tomato juice and water for an excellent soup.

1 cup dried lentils
2 1/2 cups water
2 medium red potatoes (3/4 pound), cut into 1/2-inch cubes
1 teaspoon salt, divided
1 cup diced onion
1 medium zucchini (10 ounces), quartered lengthwise then cut across into 1/4-inch strips

1 1/2 cups diced plum tomatoes
2 stalks celery, cut on the diagonal into 1/4-inch slices
1 green pepper, diced
3 cloves garlic, minced
3 to 4 tablespoons lemon juice
1/4 cup minced parsley
freshly ground pepper

Place the lentils in a medium saucepan with the water. Bring to a boil, reduce the heat, cover, and simmer 15 minutes. Add the potatoes and 1/2 teaspoon salt. Replace the cover and cook 15 to 20 minutes longer, until the potatoes are tender but still hold their shape.

Meanwhile, combine the onion, zucchini, tomatoes, celery, green pepper, and garlic in a large skillet. Cook over medium heat, stirring frequently, until the vegetables are crisp-tender, 8 to 10 minutes. Don't overcook. Season with the remaining 1/2 teaspoon salt.

In a large serving bowl, combine the lentils and potatoes with the vegetable mixture, including any cooking juices; toss gently. Add 3 tablespoons lemon juice, the parsley, and pepper. Mix well. Taste and adjust seasonings if necessary. Serve at room temperature.

YIELD: 8 SERVINGS

In Nikki's Kitchen

Winter Stew

Lentils, squash, and cooked greens are a warming combination on a cold fall or winter evening.

1 cup dried lentils
1 large onion, chopped
1 tablespoon grated ginger
3 cups water
1 pound orange squash (acorn, butternut) or pumpkin, peeled and cut into bite-size pieces (3 cups)

1/2 teaspoon cumin
1/2 pound kale, Swiss chard, mustard greens, spinach, arugula, or other dark greens, chopped (about 6 cups lightly packed)
3/4 teaspoon salt
1 lemon, cut into wedges

In a large saucepan, combine the lentils, onion, ginger, and water. Bring to a boil, cover, reduce the heat, and simmer for 20 minutes.

Add the squash or pumpkin and cumin. Replace the cover and simmer about 20 minutes longer, until both lentils and squash are tender.

Add the greens and salt. Cover and cook until the greens wilt, about 5 minutes.

Remove the cover and let cool slightly before serving. Serve with fresh lemon wedges.

YIELD: 4 TO 6 SERVINGS

★ SERVING TEMPERATURES ★

Pay attention to advice regarding the serving temperature of foods, when provided. As with many stews, serving this bean-vegetable mixture warm, rather than piping hot, maximizes its flavor.

The Healthiest Diet in the World

Garden Chili

~

The combination of lentils and cracked wheat makes this a hearty chili. The seasonings are geared to a mild to moderate level of spiciness. Of course, as with most dishes that include hot peppers and chili powder, the heat will vary with the intensity of these ingredients. Those who like hot food can choose the hottest peppers, such as jalapeño or scotch bonnet, and a strong chili powder. Heat seekers can also adjust the level by seasoning their portion with hot sauce to taste. To soften the impact (and add to the nutrition) we always serve a generous spoonful of yogurt on top of each serving and set out an extra bowl of yogurt to add more while eating. Serve with warm tortillas or a crusty bread and salad.

1/2 cup chopped onion
1/2 cup chopped celery
1/2 cup diced red or green pepper
1 cup diced zucchini
1/2 cup cracked wheat (bulgur)
2 tablespoons hot pepper or
  1/2 teaspoon crushed red
  pepper flakes

1 tablespoon chili powder
1 teaspoon dried oregano
2 cups water
1 1/2 cups canned crushed tomatoes
1 cup dried lentils
1/2 teaspoon salt

In a 5-quart pot, combine the onion, celery, sweet pepper, and zucchini. Cover and cook over moderate heat for 5 minutes, until the vegetables start to soften. Add the cracked wheat, hot pepper, chili powder, and oregano. Cook, stirring continuously, for 1 minute.

Add the water, crushed tomatoes, lentils, and salt. Bring to a boil. Cover and cook over low heat for about 50 minutes, until the lentils are tender.

YIELD: **4** SERVINGS

*In
Nikki's
Kitchen*

Black Bean Chili

~

Serve in bowls with a generous topping of yogurt cream. With this chili, we favor 3-Grain Polenta Bread, slices of avocado, and shredded lettuce or Spur-of-the-Moment Carrot Salad.

1/4 cup apple juice, divided	1 teaspoon cumin
1 medium onion, chopped	1 1/2 cups canned crushed tomatoes
1/2 cup chopped red or green pepper	1 cup green beans, cut into 1-inch pieces
2 cloves garlic, minced	1 cup corn kernels (fresh or frozen)
1 1/2 tablespoons chili powder	3 cups cooked black beans, lightly drained but not rinsed
1 hot pepper or 1/4 teaspoon crushed red pepper flakes	

Combine 2 tablespoons apple juice, the onion, sweet pepper, and garlic in a pot. Cook for about 3 minutes, stirring occasionally, until the onion softens. Add the seasonings and cook for 30 seconds. Add the crushed tomatoes, remaining 2 tablespoons apple juice, and the green beans. Cover and simmer over low heat for 10 minutes, until the beans are almost tender. Add the corn and black beans. Cook, uncovered, for 10 minutes, stirring occasionally.

YIELD: 4 SERVINGS

Tempeh-Bean Chili

~

A hot but not fiery chili. Those who like their chili spicy can add fresh chopped jalapeño peppers to taste, along with any of the other suggested garnishes listed. Serve with corn or whole wheat tortillas and shredded lettuce doused with fresh lemon juice.

2 medium onions, chopped	3 cups chopped fresh or drained canned tomatoes
2 cloves garlic, chopped	4 cups cooked kidney or pinto beans, lightly drained
1 medium green pepper, chopped	2 tablespoons dark miso
8 ounces soy or mixed-grain tempeh, coarsely chopped or crumbled (2 cups)	garnishes: fresh chopped cilantro; chopped jalapeño peppers; diced green pepper; diced cucumber; yogurt
2 tablespoons chili powder	
1/4 teaspoon cayenne	
1 teaspoon cumin	
1 teaspoon oregano	

114

The Healthiest Diet in the World

In a 3-quart pot, combine the onions, garlic, and green pepper. Cover and cook over moderate heat for 5 minutes, until the vegetables start to soften. Add the tempeh, chili powder, cayenne, cumin, and oregano. Cook, stirring continuously, for about 2 minutes.

Add the tomatoes and kidney beans. Cover and simmer gently for 20 minutes. In a small bowl, combine a little of the hot chili with the miso; stir to melt the miso. Mix into the hot chili, cover, and let stand off the heat for about 5 minutes to develop the flavors.

Ladle into bowls and let each person garnish to taste with cilantro, jalapeño peppers, green pepper, cucumbers, and yogurt.

YIELD: **4** TO **6** SERVINGS

Quick Cuban-style Black Beans

Spoon this very quick bean sauce over baked sweet potatoes, rice, millet, or corn bread. Top each serving with a generous dollop of yogurt cheese and provide hot sauce at the table for additional seasoning to taste. For a really fast meal, the beans can be served on a base of whole-grain bread.

1/2 cup chopped green pepper
1 small onion, chopped
2 large cloves garlic, chopped
2 tablespoons orange juice
3 cups canned or cooked black beans, undrained (2 15-ounce cans)

2 roasted pimientos, cut into strips
3 tablespoons wine vinegar
1 teaspoon oregano
salt

Combine the green pepper, onion, garlic, and orange juice in a skillet or saucepan. Stir-steam over medium heat for 5 minutes. Add the beans, pimientos, vinegar, and oregano. Bring to a boil and simmer for 5 minutes, until quite hot. Add salt to taste.

YIELD: **4** SERVINGS

*In
Nikki's
Kitchen*

Caribbean Black Beans

Try these black beans garnished with oranges and Spicy Onions on Millet-Polenta patties. Accompany with a refreshing salad that includes yogurt (for example, Yogurt-Cucumber Salad) or a yogurt dressing. Note: The recipe for Spicy Onions follows. Be sure to prepare them well in advance or at the start of meal preparation; the onions need to stand for at least 15 minutes for the flavor to develop.

1/2 cup chopped onion
2 large cloves garlic, minced
2 tablespoons cooking sherry or dry
  red wine
1/2 cup orange juice
1/2 teaspoon cumin

2 cups cooked black beans
1 rounded tablespoon tomato paste
1/2 cup diced tomato
1 orange, peeled and cut into bite-
  size pieces
Spicy Onions (recipe follows)

Combine the chopped onion, garlic, and sherry in a 1 1/2- to 3-quart saucepan. Cook over gentle heat, stirring occasionally, for about 5 minutes, until the onion softens and starts to color. Add the orange juice and cumin and bring to a boil.

Drain the beans to remove excess cooking liquid but do not rinse. Add the beans and any liquid that clings to them to the pot, along with the tomato paste and diced tomato. Mix well and simmer, uncovered, for 10 minutes.

To serve, place the beans in a serving bowl. Arrange the orange pieces and Spicy Onions on top.

YIELD: **4** SERVINGS

Spicy Onions

1 cup thinly sliced onion (Spanish or
  sweet onion like Vidalia preferred)
boiling water

2 tablespoons fresh lime juice
1/2 teaspoon hot pepper sauce
paprika

Place the onion in a bowl and cover with boiling water. Let stand 5 minutes. Drain, rinse with cold water, and pat dry.

Return the onion to the bowl. Add the lime juice and hot pepper sauce and mix well. Let sit at room temperature at least 15 minutes to develop the flavor. If prepared several hours ahead, store in the refrigerator. Return to room temperature before using. Sprinkle liberally with paprika just before serving.

Phyto Fusion

This rich fusion of several notable phytochemicals is adaptable to a choice of beans. We suggest topping each serving with a large dollop of yogurt cheese. Serve with a green salad garnished with tomatoes and Golden Biscuits for a phytochemical feast.

1 cup white wine
1 small to medium cauliflower (1 to 1¹/₂ pounds), broken into florets
2 medium sweet potatoes or yams (about 1¹/₂ pounds), peeled and cut into 1-inch cubes
1 medium onion, chopped
¹/₄ cup chopped parsley

¹/₂ cup bean cooking liquid (or water if needed)
3 cups cooked adzuki beans, red kidney beans, black beans, or black-eyed peas, drained
¹/₄ teaspoon hot pepper sauce or to taste
¹/₂ teaspoon salt or to taste

Pour the wine into a pot large enough to hold the vegetables. Place over medium heat. When warm, add the cauliflorets, sweet potato cubes, chopped onion, and parsley. Cover and cook over low heat for about 20 minutes, until the vegetables are tender. Stir occasionally to promote even cooking.

When the vegetables are cooked, add the bean cooking liquid, beans, hot pepper sauce, and salt. (Adjust salt according to whether or not the beans were presalted.) Simmer, stirring frequently, for about 5 minutes, until the gravy thickens slightly around the vegetables and the beans are heated through.

YIELD: 4 TO 6 SERVINGS

Beans Bourguignonne

A stew that unites root vegetables and hearty red beans in a smooth, mellow mushroom-wine sauce. You may want to serve it in shallow bowls to conserve the gravy, which can be sopped up with whole-grain bread.

1 large onion, cut into crescents
3/4 pound mushrooms (preferably a mix of portobello or cremini and common white mushrooms), sliced (about 4 cups)
1 cup carrot coins
1 pound waxy boiling potatoes (red, new, Yukon Gold, Yellow Finn), cut into 1 1/2-inch chunks
2 cloves garlic, sliced
1 bay leaf

1/2 cup drained canned tomatoes
3/4 cup liquid from canned tomatoes (see note in directions)
1/3 cup dry red wine
3 cups cooked red kidney beans, lightly drained
1/4 teaspoon salt (omit if beans are salted)
freshly ground pepper
1 to 2 tablespoons miso, optional

In a 3- to 5-quart pot, combine the onion and mushrooms. Cook over moderate heat, stirring frequently, for 5 to 8 minutes, until the mushrooms release their juices. Add the carrots, potatoes, garlic, bay leaf, tomatoes, and tomato liquid. (If the tomato liquid is in the form of a thick puree, rather than of broth consistency, dilute with bean cooking liquid or water.) Bring to a boil, cover, and simmer gently for about 15 minutes, until the potatoes begin to yield but aren't yet tender.

Add the wine, beans, and salt if the beans are unsalted. Simmer gently, uncovered, for an additional 10 minutes, or until the potatoes are tender. Remove the bay leaf. Season generously with freshly ground pepper and adjust salt to taste.

For a richer gravy, in a small bowl combine up to 2 tablespoons miso with a little of the hot wine sauce. Stir until the miso melts into the sauce. Add to pot, cover, and let sit for a few minutes before serving.

YIELD: 4 GENEROUS SERVINGS

★ POTATO POINTER ★

When shopping for this recipe, be sure to choose a waxy variety of potato, such as Yukon gold, new, red, Yellow Finn, or "boiling" potatoes, so they don't fall apart.

The Healthiest Diet in the World

Cowboy Beans

With conventional stove-top cooking you need to begin this recipe several hours ahead. However, if you use a pressure cooker, cooking is completed in 45 minutes, demonstrating how practical this tool is when it comes to beans.

1¹/2 cups dried pinto or pink kidney beans
3 cups water
1 medium onion, chopped
2 cloves garlic, chopped
1 medium red pepper, chopped
1 jalapeño pepper, chopped
2 carrots, diced

1 rib celery, chopped
¹/2 teaspoon oregano
1 teaspoon cumin
¹/2 cup tomato juice
1 cup corn kernels (fresh or frozen)
¹/2 teaspoon salt
¹/4 cup minced fresh cilantro or Italian flat-leaf parsley

Combine the beans and water and soak according to basic bean cooking directions. Then bring to a boil for 5 minutes, cover, and simmer for 1 hour.

Add all the vegetables except the corn along with the oregano, cumin, and tomato juice. Cover and cook about 45 minutes longer, or until the beans and vegetables are tender.

Add the corn, salt, and cilantro or parsley, and cook for 5 minutes.

To make in the pressure cooker, combine the rinsed unsoaked dried beans, water, and remaining ingredients except the corn, salt, and cilantro or parsley. Bring to a boil, close the cooker, bring up to pressure, and pressure-cook for 35 minutes. Let the pressure cooker sit off the heat for 5 minutes before gradually releasing the pressure and opening. Add the corn, salt, and cilantro or parsley and simmer for 5 minutes.

YIELD: 4 SERVINGS

119

Rare Root Stew

⌒

This dinner stew features several uncommonly eaten vegetables, such as parsnips, turnips, fennel, leeks, and, if you can find it, celery root (celeriac). Each serving provides about 1 pound of vegetables, generously surpassing the daily recommended minimum.

2 good-size parsnips (at least
  1/2 pound), peeled and cut into
  1-inch pieces
2 good-size carrots (at least
  1/2 pound), peeled and cut into
  1-inch pieces
2 medium turnips (at least
  1/2 pound), peeled, quartered, and
  cut into 1-inch chunks
1 large leek, cut lengthwise, rinsed
  to remove any dirt, and cut into
  1-inch segments
1 fennel bulb, stalks and fronds
  removed, cut into wedges

1 small celery root, peeled and cut
  into wedges
1 stick cinnamon, broken in two
2 large cloves garlic, sliced
1 tablespoon minced fresh ginger
1 medium onion, sliced into rings
1/3 cup apple juice
3 cups cooked red kidney beans,
  lightly drained
1/2 teaspoon salt
1/4 cup chopped parsley

Cut the vegetables so they are approximately equal in size and will cook at the same pace. Place the parsnips, carrots, turnips, leek, fennel, and celery root in a pot with a tight-fitting lid. Bury the cinnamon in the vegetables. Scatter the garlic and ginger on top. Cover with the onion rings. Pour the apple juice over all.

Bring to a boil, cover, and simmer gently for 15 to 20 minutes, until the vegetables start to give a little but aren't yet tender. Stir a few times to promote even cooking. Add the beans and salt. Mix well, replace the cover, and continue to cook until the vegetables are tender, about 10 minutes longer. Check to make sure the stew isn't cooking dry; if necessary, add a little bean cooking liquid or more apple juice.

When done, remove cinnamon pieces, sprinkle the stew with the parsley, and replace the cover until the parsley wilts.

YIELD: 4 SERVINGS

*The
Healthiest
Diet in
the World*

Irish Stew

This recipe employs the technique of braising, or cooking in just enough liquid to keep food moist, adding more as it cooks down if needed. It's important to keep the heat moderate, because cooking too fast (at too high heat) will cause the vegetables to become dry. Serve with generous portions of yogurt cheese spooned into each serving at the table to make a rich, creamy gravy. This is a homey dish that goes nicely with Savory Oat Biscuits or whole-grain bread and a cucumber or cabbage salad.

1 medium onion, cut into small chunks
1 pound Yellow Finn, Yukon Gold, Red Bliss, or new potatoes, cut into bite-size pieces
2 large carrots, sliced into coins

$^1/_2$ teaspoon turmeric
$^1/_2$ to $^2/_3$ cup chickpea cooking liquid
2 cups cooked chickpeas
salt

Place the onion in a heavy 3-quart pot. Set over moderate heat and wilt, stirring frequently, for about 3 minutes.

Add the potatoes to the onion and cook briefly.

Add the carrots, turmeric, and $^1/_2$ cup chickpea cooking liquid or enough to generously cover the bottom of the pot. Cover and cook over moderate heat for 10 minutes. Stir occasionally to keep the cooking even. Add additional liquid if needed to keep moist. The liquid should be of a rich, gravy consistency. Add the chickpeas and salt to taste. Cover and continue to cook for about 5 minutes, or until the potatoes and carrots are fork-tender.

YIELD: **4** SERVINGS

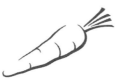

Two Beans, Greek Style

～

Unlike most vegetable dishes, the green beans in this recipe are cooked until very tender and almost pastalike. When cooking vegetables for a substantial length of time in just a small amount of liquid, as you do here, it's very important to choose a heavy pot with a tight-fitting lid; this conserves the juices and keeps food moist during cooking. The soft beans and gravy that result are excellent on cracked wheat or garlic mashed potatoes.

1 pound green beans
1/2 cup dry white wine
1 small onion or 4 scallions,
  chopped
large bunch dill, chopped (at least
  1/2 cup)

1 cup chickpea cooking liquid (or
  water if needed)
2 1/2 cups cooked chickpeas
1/2 teaspoon salt or to taste
1/2 lemon
freshly ground pepper

Trim the ends from the green beans but leave them whole.

Pour the wine into a pot large enough to hold the beans. Place over medium heat. When warm, add the green beans, onion, and dill. Cover and cook over low heat for about 45 minutes, until the green beans are soft and almost falling apart. Stir occasionally to promote even cooking; if the pan seems dry, add more wine or water.

Combine the chickpea cooking liquid and 3/4 cup chickpeas in a blender or food processor. Puree until smooth.

When the green beans are cooked, add the remaining chickpeas, chickpea puree, and salt, adjusting according to whether or not the chickpeas were pre-salted. Bring to a boil over medium heat and simmer, stirring frequently, for about 5 minutes, until the gravy thickens and the chickpeas are heated through.

Remove from the heat. Squeeze in juice from the lemon half and season liberally with freshly ground pepper.

YIELD: 4 SERVINGS

Two Beans with Creamy Walnut Pesto

～

Our recipe White Beans and Carrots with Creamy Walnut Pesto uses the same concept of combining beans, a vegetable, and pesto. In this version, simply switching the beans and the vegetable dramatically changes the character of the meal.

1 pound green beans
1/4 cup dry white wine or water
3 cups cooked chickpeas

3/4 cup Creamy Walnut Pesto
  (page 196)
1 large tomato, cut into wedges

Trim the ends from the green beans and break into 2-inch lengths.

Pour the wine into a large skillet. Place over medium heat. When warm, add the green beans, cover, and cook for 10 minutes, until the green beans are tender but still crisp. Add the chickpeas and heat through.

Remove the beans from the heat. Just before serving, and while the beans are still hot, stir in Creamy Walnut Pesto. Garnish with the tomato wedges.

YIELD: 4 SERVINGS

Chickpea Roast

Mashed chickpeas, highly seasoned with vegetables, make a tasty casserole. Serve plain or with gravy (Sweet Onion, Creamy Mushroom, or Tahini-Mushroom), a favorite tomato sauce, Better Than Ketchup, or Pineapple Salsa. Broccoli Puree is a suitable vegetable accompaniment, as is a baked potato. Leftovers can be used for sandwiches, either cold or reheated.

4 cups cooked chickpeas
3 cloves garlic, chopped
2 onions, chopped
2 tablespoons soy sauce
2 stalks celery, chopped
1 carrot, grated

1/2 teaspoon cumin
1/4 teaspoon turmeric
1/4 teaspoon salt (omit if chickpeas
  are salted)
2 tablespoons tahini
paprika

Preheat the oven to 375°F.

In a large bowl, mash the chickpeas with a potato masher.

Combine the garlic, onions, and soy sauce in a skillet and cook for 5 minutes. Add the celery, carrot, and seasonings and cook 5 minutes more, until the vegetables are crisp-tender.

Add the cooked vegetables and tahini to the chickpeas and mix well. Oil a 1-quart baking dish and fill with the mixture. Sprinkle liberally with paprika. Bake for about 40 minutes, until firm and nicely browned.

YIELD: 4 TO 6 SERVINGS

*In
Nikki's
Kitchen*

North African Chickpeas

This excellent and unusual dish has a nice bite, but those who like foods really spicy may want to double the red pepper flakes. Serve over a cooked grain (whole wheat couscous, bulgur, barley, quinoa, millet), along with a cooling yogurt-based side dish such as Spinach-Yogurt Salad and whole wheat chapatis.

1 medium onion, thinly sliced
1 tablespoon minced garlic
1 tablespoon minced fresh ginger
2 tablespoons red wine or cooking sherry
1 teaspoon cumin
1 teaspoon cinnamon
1 teaspoon paprika
1/2 teaspoon crushed red pepper flakes or to taste
1 cup water or chickpea cooking liquid

1/2 teaspoon salt (reduce if chickpea cooking liquid is salted)
2 medium sweet potatoes (1 1/2 pounds), peeled and cut into bite-size pieces
1/4 cup diced dried apricots
2 cups cooked chickpeas
1/4 cup raisins
2 tablespoons lemon juice
1/4 cup sliced almonds

In a medium saucepan, combine the onion, garlic, ginger, and wine or sherry. Cover and sweat over low heat for 5 minutes. Add the cumin, cinnamon, paprika, and red pepper flakes and cook, uncovered, 1 minute longer. Add the water or chickpea cooking liquid, salt, sweet potatoes, and apricots. Bring to a boil, cover, and simmer until the sweet potatoes are just tender, about 15 minutes.

Add the chickpeas, raisins, and lemon juice. Cook, stirring occasionally, for about 5 minutes, until the chickpeas are hot. Add the sliced almonds.

YIELD: **4 SERVINGS**

Mixed Vegetable Curry with Chickpeas

A mild but very flavorful curry. The mixture of vegetables here is particularly appealing, but you can change the selection if necessary according to availability. For example, zucchini can be omitted and replaced with extra cauliflower or winter squash, sweet potatoes can replace white potatoes, and so on. Accompany with Curried Tomato and Cucumber Salad and brown rice or bread to sop up the juices.

1 large onion, coarsely chopped
2 cloves garlic, minced
1 tablespoon grated fresh ginger
1 teaspoon cumin
1 teaspoon turmeric
1/2 teaspoon cinnamon
1/4 teaspoon crushed red pepper flakes
4 cups coarsely chopped, lightly packed leafy greens (spinach, kale, Swiss chard, romaine)
1/2 cup canned crushed tomatoes
1 1/2 cups chickpea cooking liquid or water

2 cups cooked chickpeas
1 cup cauliflorets
1 cup diced zucchini
1 1/2 cups diced potatoes
1 cup green beans cut into 1-inch segments or green peas (fresh or frozen)
1/2 teaspoon salt (reduce if chickpea cooking liquid is salted)
2 tablespoons almond butter or cashew butter
2 tablespoons fresh cilantro

In a 15-inch skillet, combine the onion, garlic, ginger, cumin, turmeric, cinnamon, red pepper flakes, and greens. Cook over moderate heat, stirring frequently, for 5 minutes. Add the tomatoes, chickpea liquid or water, vegetables, and salt. If using frozen green peas, wait until the end of cooking to add them. Bring to a boil, cover, and simmer over gentle heat for 20 to 30 minutes, until the potatoes are tender.

In a small bowl, stir a little of the hot curry into the almond or cashew butter to melt. Add back to the skillet and simmer over moderate heat, stirring continuously, for 3 to 5 minutes, until the sauce is creamy. Adjust the salt, if necessary, to taste. Sprinkle with the cilantro.

YIELD: 4 TO 6 SERVINGS

In Nikki's Kitchen

Pasta with Fresh Tomatoes, Basil, and Roasted Garlic

No-cook tomato sauces, such as the one this recipe is based on, should be made only with the most flavorful ripe tomatoes and olive oil of the best quality. The dish can be as simple as the one presented here, or modified by adding diced avocado, some chopped red onion, a few sliced black olives, minced roasted hot pepper, or crushed red pepper flakes to taste. The sauce is designed to be paired with small pasta shapes such as spirals, penne, ziti, bow ties, radiatore, or medium shells. Since pasta itself isn't a good source of protein, it should be joined by a first course or accompaniment that features beans and/or yogurt cheese. Suitable choices include Black Bean Hummus, Superior Spinach Dip, Pesto-stuffed Mushrooms, Baked Artichoke Cheese, or a simple dish of cooked chick-peas seasoned with lots of freshly ground pepper.

10 cloves garlic
3/4 pound tomatoes
1/4 cup coarsely chopped fresh basil
  leaves

1 tablespoon chopped capers
1 tablespoon extra virgin olive oil
1 tablespoon balsamic vinegar
1/2 pound whole wheat pasta

To roast the garlic, place the unpeeled cloves in a baking pan in a single layer in an oven or toaster oven at 400°F. Bake 20 to 25 minutes, or until soft and very lightly colored. Remove each clove as it's done. Don't let them become too brown or they'll be bitter. When cool enough to handle, peel and smash gently with the flat side of a knife.

Dice the tomatoes and place in a large bowl, retaining the tomato juices. You should have about 2 cups of tomatoes. Add the roasted garlic, basil, capers, olive oil, and balsamic vinegar. Let stand for 20 minutes or longer for the flavors to blend.

Cook the pasta in a large pot of boiling water until al dente (firm to the bite), or according to personal preference. Drain the pasta and add immediately to the tomato mixture. Toss to blend. Serve warm or at room temperature.

YIELD: 4 SERVINGS

Ravioli and Beans

Plump pillows of ravioli nestled in a bed of beans. The various elements can be made expressly for this dish, or it can be quickly assembled if you have planned ahead by preparing extra ravioli and beans for a previous meal.

10 sun-dried tomatoes
hot water
16 vegetable, cheese, or soy-filled ravioli
1½ cups bean cooking liquid or vegetable broth

2 large cloves garlic, sliced
1 cup lightly packed, coarsely chopped parsley
1 teaspoon salt (omit if beans and liquid are salted)
4 cups cooked white or black beans

Place the sun-dried tomatoes in a shallow bowl. Pour in hot water to just submerge. Let soften while assembling the remaining ingredients.

Bring a large pot of water to a boil for cooking the ravioli (or use precooked ravioli). Cook until tender, about 10 minutes or according to package directions. Drain well and reserve.

In a large pot, bring ½ cup bean cooking liquid to a gentle boil. Add the garlic and simmer for about a minute. Slice the softened sun-dried tomatoes and add to the pot along with their soaking liquid, the parsley, the remaining bean cooking liquid, and the salt. Simmer for 5 minutes.

Add the beans and ravioli and heat through. Spoon onto serving plates, giving each person a generous portion of beans and 4 ravioli.

YIELD: 4 SERVINGS

*In
Nikki's
Kitchen*

Italian Pasta and Vegetable Stew

~

This one-pot meal is quick and easy to make with precooked or canned chick-peas. Serve with Succulent Stuffed Mushrooms and a green salad.

1 cup chickpea cooking liquid or
  water
1 pound small new or red potatoes
1/2 pound green beans
2 large cloves garlic, sliced
1 tablespoon chopped fresh basil or
  1 teaspoon dried basil
1 teaspoon oregano
1 small hot pepper, minced, optional
2 tablespoons tomato paste

2 cups uncooked whole-grain pasta
  (small variety such as spirals,
  penne, rigatoni, wagon wheels)
4 to 6 canned artichoke hearts or
  bottoms, drained and quartered
1/2 teaspoon salt
2 1/2 cups water
3 cups cooked chickpeas
1/4 cup chopped parsley
freshly ground pepper

Pour the chickpea cooking liquid into a 3- to 5-quart pot. Bring to a boil.

Cut the potatoes into manageable-size pieces (about 1 inch). Trim the ends of the beans and, if large, break in half. Add the vegetables, garlic, herbs, and hot pepper, if using, to the boiling liquid. Cover and simmer over medium heat for 15 minutes.

Stir the tomato paste into the vegetables in the pot. When dissolved, add the pasta, artichokes, salt, and enough water to just cover the ingredients. Mix well to submerge the pasta. Cover and simmer gently for 10 minutes. Check halfway through to see if more water is needed. The mixture should be neither soupy nor dry.

Add the chickpeas and parsley, cover, and continue to cook, stirring occasionally, for 5 to 10 minutes longer, until the pasta and vegetables are all tender and the gravy around them is thick and rich. (Remember to keep an eye on the liquid and add more water if necessary.) Season with freshly ground pepper and adjust salt to taste. Serve as is or with grated cheese.

YIELD: 4 SERVINGS

Vegetable Pasta with Cheese

~

An easy way to add more vegetables to the menu is to toss them in with pasta during the last few minutes of cooking, as done here.

1 pound vegetable, cheese, or tofu
  tortellini
1 pound asparagus, cauliflower, or
  broccoli florets
1/4 cup chopped parsley

1 tablespoon olive, flaxseed, or
  hemp oil
1/4 cup grated Parmesan cheese
salt
freshly ground pepper

Bring a large pot of water to a boil for the pasta. Meanwhile, prepare the vegetables, cutting the asparagus into 1-inch lengths or breaking the cauliflower or broccoli into small florets.

Cook the pasta until tender to taste, about 10 minutes or according to package directions. Add the vegetables to the pasta during the last 2 minutes of cooking.

Drain the pasta and vegetables. Do not rinse. Transfer the hot pasta to a serving bowl and toss with the parsley, oil, and cheese, mixing well. Season with salt if needed and lots of freshly ground pepper. Serve additional cheese at the table for those who want it.

YIELD: 4 SERVINGS

NOTE: You can replace the fresh vegetable with 2 cups frozen peas. Don't add until the very end of cooking, just long enough to heat through.

Creamy Vegetable Pasta with Cheese

A few small ingredient changes turn Vegetable Pasta with Cheese into a creamy version that's actually lower in fat (less than 9 grams per serving), although it tastes incredibly rich. Once again, you can replace the fresh vegetable with 2 cups of frozen peas, but don't add them until the very end of cooking, just long enough to heat through.

1 pound vegetable or cheese
  tortellini
1 pound asparagus, cauliflower, or
  broccoli florets
1/4 cup chopped parsley

6 tablespoons Yogurt Cheese
  (page 244)
1/2 cup crumbled feta, blue cheese,
  or goat cheese
freshly ground pepper

Bring a large pot of water to a boil for the pasta. Meanwhile, prepare the vegetables, cutting the asparagus into 1-inch lengths or breaking the cauliflower or broccoli into small florets.

Cook the pasta until tender to taste, about 10 minutes or according to package directions. Add the vegetables to the pasta during the last 2 minutes of cooking.

Drain the pasta and vegetables. Do not rinse. Transfer the hot pasta to a serving bowl and toss with the parsley, Yogurt Cheese, and crumbled cheese. Mix to coat the pasta with the melting cheeses. Season generously with freshly ground pepper.

YIELD: 4 SERVINGS

Portobello Pasta

~

We jokingly call this OsteoPasta, as it's a good source of calcium, vitamin K, and estrogenic phytochemicals, especially when made with tofu. Serve this hearty pasta-vegetable combo in shallow bowls so the flavorful broth isn't lost. It goes well with Creamy Stuffed Italian Artichoke Bottoms and Fennel & Orange Salad— a nice menu for small dinner parties.

2 tablespoons pine nuts or
  pumpkin seeds
3 cups sliced portobello mushrooms
  (about 8 ounces)
8 cloves garlic, sliced
2 tablespoons soy sauce
1/3 cup water
1 small red onion, cut into crescents
3/4 pound dark leafy greens, cut up
  (arugula, escarole, broccoli rabe,
  Swiss chard, spinach, romaine;
  about 8 cups)

2 cups cooked chickpeas or white
  cannellini beans, drained, or
  1 pound firm tofu cut into strips
1/2 cup canned crushed tomatoes
1 cup bean cooking liquid, water, or
  vegetable broth
2 tablespoons balsamic vinegar
3/4 pound whole wheat, kamut,
  spelt, or brown rice angel hair
  pasta, linguine, or other pasta of
  choice
pasta cooking water

Put up a large pot of water to cook the pasta when you begin preparation.

Toast the pine nuts or pumpkin seeds in a dry skillet until just colored; remove from the pan and reserve. If you want to use the same skillet for the rest of the dish, let it cool down a bit before proceeding.

In a 15-inch skillet, combine the mushrooms, garlic, soy sauce, and water. Cover and cook over low heat for 10 minutes. Add the red onion, greens, beans or tofu, crushed tomatoes, bean cooking liquid, and 1 tablespoon balsamic vinegar. Mix well, cover, and cook over moderate heat, stirring occasionally, for about 10 minutes, or until the greens are tender.

Meanwhile, cook the pasta. When just tender, drain and reserve about 1/4 cup cooking water. Add the hot pasta, reserved toasted pine nuts or pumpkin seeds, and the remaining tablespoon of balsamic vinegar to the vegetables. Mix well and cook for just a few minutes, until very hot. If needed, stir in pasta water so there is some broth in the pan. Transfer to serving bowls, making sure the vegetables and broth are evenly divided among them.

YIELD: **4** GENEROUS SERVINGS

Baked Macaroni and Corn

~

This nondairy alternative to classic baked macaroni and cheese can be made with whole wheat or wheat-free pastas (quinoa, rice, corn, kamut, spelt). Take advantage of the oven and serve with baked winter squash. Complete the menu with a green salad.

4 cups uncooked whole-grain spirals, small shells, or elbow macaroni
2 cups diced soft or regular tofu (12 to 16 ounces)
2 cups soy milk
3 tablespoons tahini
1 1/2 teaspoons salt
3 cups corn kernels (fresh or frozen)
paprika

Preheat the oven to 350°F. and bring a large pot of water to a boil for the pasta.

Cook the pasta in boiling water for 6 to 8 minutes, or until slightly underdone. Monitor the cooking time closely, as some nonwheat varieties become mushy and disintegrate if cooked too long. Drain and rinse with cold water to stop the cooking. Drain thoroughly.

Combine the tofu, soy milk, tahini, and salt in a blender or food processor. Puree until smooth. Add the corn and process briefly at high speed.

Place the cooked pasta in an oiled shallow 2-quart or 9 x 13-inch baking dish. Pour the pureed tofu over the pasta. Mix so the pasta is evenly bathed in sauce. Sprinkle liberally with paprika. Bake for 30 minutes, until the sauce is hot and bubbly.

YIELD: **6** SERVINGS

The Healthiest Diet in the World

Pasta with Chickpea-Walnut Sauce

Although this recipe seems to require a lot of steps, it's actually quite easy to make. The sauce is essentially a flavorful chickpea and walnut puree that takes just a few minutes with the aid of a blender or food processor, and the vegetables are tossed in to cook with the pasta during the last few minutes. Prepare a big salad and dinner is done.

1/2 cup walnuts
2 tablespoons cooking sherry or
  dry wine
1/2 cup chopped onion
2 tablespoons chopped garlic
2 cups cooked chickpeas
1 1/2 cups chickpea cooking liquid
  (add dry white wine, vegetable
  broth, or water if needed)

salt
1 pound broccoli, green beans, or
  snow peas
1/2 pound whole-grain pasta
  (linguine, spaghetti, spirals, wagon
  wheels)
crushed red pepper flakes

Bring a large pot of water to a boil for the pasta. Meanwhile, prepare the sauce.

Toast the walnuts lightly in a dry skillet. Transfer to a blender or food processor and grind to a fine meal.

Heat the sherry or wine in a small saucepan. Add the onion and garlic and cook over low heat for about 3 minutes, stirring often, until softened.

Add the cooked onions and garlic to the walnuts in the blender or food processor, along with the chickpeas and cooking liquid. Puree until smooth.

Return the sauce ingredients to the saucepan and cook over moderate heat for 5 to 7 minutes, stirring frequently, until warm and slightly thickened. Taste for salt and add if necessary.

Prepare the vegetable of choice as follows: divide the broccoli into small florets and peel and dice the stems; trim the ends from the green beans and break into 2-inch lengths; trim the ends of the snow peas and leave whole.

Cook the pasta in boiling water for 10 to 12 minutes, until al dente or according to preferred taste. Add the vegetable to the pasta during the last 2 minutes of cooking.

Drain the pasta and vegetable. Transfer to a serving dish and coat generously with the sauce. Serve with any remaining sauce on the side, along with red pepper flakes for individual seasoning.

YIELD: 4 SERVINGS

In Nikki's Kitchen

Linguine with White Bean Sauce

The sauce can be made with canned beans and their liquid if home-cooked beans aren't available. As elsewhere, water or vegetable broth can be added to make up for any deficit. To enhance the flavor, roast some garlic and squeeze out several cloves on top of the pasta before serving. White Pita "Pizza" and a salad of fresh tomatoes dressed lightly with balsamic vinegar and olive oil complete the meal.

2 tablespoons cooking sherry
2 large cloves garlic, minced
1 medium onion, chopped
1 cup diced red pepper
3 stalks celery, sliced 1/4 inch thick
2 cups cooked or canned white beans (cannellini, great northern, or navy)
1 1/2 cups bean liquid (add water or vegetable broth if needed)

1/4 teaspoon crushed red pepper flakes
1/4 cup chopped parsley (flat-leaf preferred)
1/4 cup capers
salt (omit if beans are salted)
freshly ground pepper
10 ounces whole wheat linguine (or other whole-grain pasta)

Bring water to a boil for the pasta while preparing the sauce.

To prepare the sauce, combine the sherry, garlic, onion, red pepper, and celery in a pot large enough to accommodate the cooked pasta. Cover and cook over moderate heat for 5 minutes. Add the beans, bean liquid, red pepper flakes, and 2 tablespoons parsley. Bring to a boil, reduce the heat, and simmer, uncovered, for 10 minutes. Coarsely mash the beans with a potato masher to thicken the sauce. Add the capers. Season with salt if needed and freshly ground pepper to create a highly seasoned sauce. Cook for about 5 minutes longer, until the sauce is creamy.

While the sauce simmers, cook the linguine in rapidly boiling water until al dente, about 10 to 12 minutes. Drain.

Stir the pasta into the hot sauce and mix to coat completely with the sauce and vegetables. Sprinkle with the remaining 2 tablespoons parsley and serve at once.

YIELD: 4 SERVINGS

Multicultural Rice, Beans, and Greens

The ethnic identity of this dish can be easily altered, as explained in the Greek, Southern-style, and Indian versions that follow this initial Italian one. Serve with assorted Grilled or Oven-Roasted Vegetables, or a vegetable-tomato combination.

bean cooking liquid
3 good-size cloves garlic, sliced
3/4 pound arugula, escarole, kale, or broccoli rabe, coarsely chopped (6 to 8 cups)
3 cups cooked brown rice

1/4 cup chopped parsley
3 cups cooked white beans
salt and pepper
Yogurt Cream, optional (page 244)
grated Parmesan cheese, optional

In a heavy 15-inch skillet, heat about 2 tablespoons of the bean cooking liquid, or enough to just cover the bottom of the pan. (If you don't have bean cooking liquid, substitute cooking sherry or vegetable broth). When hot, add the garlic and cook briefly. Add the greens and cook, stirring frequently, until wilted and tender, about 5 minutes. (Broccoli rabe will take a few minutes longer to become tender.)

Add the rice and parsley. Cook, stirring, until warm. Add the beans and a few spoonfuls of cooking liquid. Cook, stirring, until hot. Add additional bean cooking liquid (or a little water or vegetable broth) as needed to make the mixture creamy.

Season with salt and pepper to taste. At serving time, top each portion with a generous dollop of Yogurt Cream and pass grated Parmesan for individual use if desired.

YIELD: 4 TO 6 SERVINGS

VARIATIONS: For *Greek Rice, Beans, and Greens*, replace the parsley with chopped dill and in addition to Yogurt Cream, crumble 2 tablespoons feta cheese on each serving.

For *Southern-style Rice, Beans, and Greens*, use Swiss chard, turnip greens, beet greens, mustard greens, or collards as the green of choice and cooked black-eyed peas instead of white beans. (Collard greens may take 5 to 10 minutes longer to cook.) Serve with a favorite hot sauce for individual seasoning.

For *Indian Rice, Beans, and Greens*, use spinach or mustard greens as the green, replace the parsley with chopped fresh cilantro, and use cooked chickpeas and/or lentils instead of white beans. Top with Curry-Yogurt Cream (page 199).

Baked Tomatoes with Wild Rice Stuffing

～

Stuffed tomatoes look impressive and are really quite easy to make. This recipe can be used as a model for other grain fillings.

2 cups Wild Rice with Mushrooms (page 171)
4 medium-large tomatoes (about 10 ounces each)

1/2 cup Yogurt Cheese (page 244)
1/4 cup chopped parsley

Prepare Wild Rice with Mushrooms according to the recipe directions.

Preheat the oven to 350°F.

Slice the tops from the tomatoes; reserve the tops. Scoop out the insides. This is most conveniently done using a curved grapefruit knife and a serrated grapefruit spoon. Reserve the pulp for another use (see Note). Drain the tomato liquid into the bottom of a shallow baking pan big enough to hold the tomatoes. Invert the tomato shells on a work surface or plate to drain.

Mix the Yogurt Cheese and parsley into the cooked grain. Stuff into the hollowed-out tomatoes. Cover with the tomato tops. Place the tomatoes side by side in the baking pan. Bake for 30 minutes.

YIELD: 4 SERVINGS

NOTE: The reserved tomato pulp should be used within a day. It can be added to salads and soups, used in cooking or for homemade salsa, or simply pureed, seasoned to taste, and simmered for a few minutes to provide a delicate sauce for the stuffed tomatoes or tomorrow's rice, millet, or cracked wheat.

VARIATION: For *Baked Tomatoes with Barley and Mushrooms*, replace Wild Rice with Mushrooms with Barley and Mushrooms (page 173) or another leftover cooked whole grain, using a ratio of 2 cups cooked grain to 1/2 cup Yogurt Cheese for 4 tomatoes. The filling can also be baked in green or red peppers that have been sliced in half lengthwise, precooked for 5 minutes in boiling water, then drained before stuffing. Place the peppers filling up (2 halves per person) in a baking dish and surround with water to a depth of 1/2 inch to keep the pan from scorching.

Accompaniments

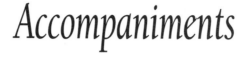

The following recipes are presented as accompaniments, but there's no reason why these vegetable, bean, and grain accompaniments can't be served together as a meal. An alternative way to serve many of the vegetable dishes in this section is as a first course preceding the meal. For more general information on basic preparation of vegetables, beans, and grains, including such techniques as steaming, stir-steaming, stewing, and pressure-cooking, see Cooking Techniques in "Gold Star Basics."

Vegetables

Spring Artichokes

Spring is the season for fresh artichokes. If you need to hold the artichokes after cooking, cover the pot and let them sit off the heat until serving. Any leftovers can be chilled and sliced into salads.

4 medium artichokes with stems	1/2 teaspoon salt
1/2 cup water	1 small onion, cut into thin
3 tablespoons lemon juice	crescents
3 strips lemon peel	6 cloves garlic, sliced

Prepare the artichokes by peeling the stem lightly, cutting off the top third (removing the tips of the leaves), and removing any small tough leaves at the bottom. Cut in half lengthwise and use a grapefruit spoon or small paring knife to scrape away the small hairy leaves (or choke) attached to the heart.

Combine the water, lemon juice, lemon peel, and salt in a broad pot that can hold the artichokes in a single layer. Dip the cut side of each artichoke in this lemon water, then place cut side up, side by side, in the pan.

Scatter the onion and garlic over the artichokes. Bring the liquid to a boil, cover, and simmer over medium heat for about 30 minutes, until the artichokes are easily pierced with a fork. Check periodically during cooking to see that the water isn't boiling too rapidly and evaporating.

Serve 2 warm halves per person, topped with some of the onions and garlic and a little broth.

YIELD: **4** SERVINGS

Roast Asparagus and Peppers

~

A simple way to enjoy fresh spring asparagus.

1 pound asparagus
2 red or yellow peppers

1 tablespoon balsamic vinegar

Preheat the broiler.

Snap off the tough ends of the asparagus. Cut the peppers into $1/2$-inch-wide strips, discarding the seeds and trimming any thick ribs.

Place the vegetables in a single layer on a baking sheet. Broil 5 to 6 inches from the heat for 8 to 12 minutes, turning several times, until the vegetables are tender and lightly charred.

Transfer to a serving dish and sprinkle with the balsamic vinegar. Serve warm or at room temperature.

YIELD: **4** SERVINGS

Orange-Lemon Beets

~

In this unusual dish, sweet earthy beets are studded with tiny pieces of tart raw lemon. You'll be amazed by the tenderness of the lemon peel. What also makes this recipe different is that beets are usually cooked whole without peeling to preserve their color, then peeled and cut as desired afterward. Here we peel and cut the beets first, which adds just a little more work beforehand but dramatically reduces cooking time. Since the cooking medium is part of the recipe, nothing is lost.

1½ pounds red or golden beets
⅓ cup orange juice

1 teaspoon grated fresh ginger
1 small lemon

Scrub the beets, peel, and cut into ½-inch-long matchsticks. (To do this easily, begin by cutting into ⅛-inch-thick slices. Stack several slices and cut into ⅛-inch-wide strips. Cut the strips across into ½-inch lengths.) You should have about 4 cups. Place the beets in a small pot with the orange juice and ginger. Cover and cook over moderate heat for about 15 minutes, until tender.

Cut the unpeeled lemon into very thin slices. Stack the slices and cut into small pieces. You should have about ½ cup.

When the beets are cooked, remove from the heat, transfer to a serving bowl, and, while still hot, mix in the lemon pieces. Serve warm or at room temperature.

YIELD: 4 TO 6 SERVINGS

VARIATION: For *Orange-Lemon Carrots*, replace the beets with carrots.

Broccoli Puree

This creamy, roughly mashed broccoli has a definite bite.

2 pounds broccoli, stems peeled and
  chopped, tops divided into tiny
  florets (about 8 cups)
½ cup water

½ teaspoon salt
4 cloves garlic, minced
2 teaspoons curry powder
½ cup Yogurt Cheese (page 244)

Combine the broccoli, water, and salt in a skillet or saucepan and bring to a boil. Cover and simmer until the broccoli is quite tender, about 15 minutes.

Add the garlic and curry powder and continue to cook, uncovered, mashing with a fork or potato masher until the broccoli is reduced to a rough puree. Add more water if needed to keep moist. Remove from the heat and mash in the Yogurt Cheese. If need be, return to the heat and cook gently, while stirring, until the puree is hot.

YIELD: 4 TO 6 SERVINGS

*In
Nikki's
Kitchen*

Mustard Brussels Sprouts

⌒

Perhaps because the brussels sprouts in this dish are disguised by shredding, even people who claim not to like this vegetable enjoy it in this form.

1 pint (10 ounces) brussels sprouts
2 tablespoons cooking sherry

1 tablespoon prepared mustard

Cut the brussels sprouts into thin shreds.

In a large skillet, heat the sherry until aromatic. Add the mustard and brussels sprouts and stir-cook for 5 to 8 minutes, until tender. Serve at once.

YIELD: **4** SERVINGS

VARIATION: For *Mustard Snow Peas*, use snow peas instead of brussels sprouts.

Stir-Steamed Sesame Cabbage

⌒

Cabbage is always a good companion for tofu or beans. In this recipe, using the rice wine keeps the flavor mellow, while choosing the rice vinegar makes it more tangy. If for some reason you prefer not to add the toasted sesame oil, it can be served on the side as a condiment for individual seasoning at the table. It doesn't take much of the oil to intensify the flavor.

1 1/2 pounds cabbage
2 tablespoons sesame seeds
1 teaspoon Coleman's or Chinese
   mustard powder diluted in
   2 teaspoons water

2 tablespoons Chinese rice cooking
   wine or rice wine vinegar
1 teaspoon toasted sesame oil,
   optional but recommended
salt

Slice the cabbage into strips 1/2 inch wide, and then into 1-inch segments, including the core or "heart." You should have about 8 cups.

Toast the sesame seeds in a dry wok or heavy skillet until lightly colored and aromatic. Watch closely to avoid overbrowning.

Add the cabbage pieces to the hot pan and cook, stirring almost continuously, for about 3 minutes, until the cabbage starts to wilt.

Add the diluted mustard powder and rice wine or vinegar to the cabbage, mix well, cover, and cook over moderate heat for about 5 minutes, until tender but still crunchy.

Remove from the heat and stir in the sesame oil, if using, and a pinch of salt if needed to suit personal taste. Serve hot or at room temperature.

YIELD: **4** TO **6** SERVINGS

Creamy Cabbage with Sesame Seeds

You can make a meal of this dish by pairing it with baked winter squash and cooked kasha.

1 tablespoon sesame seeds	1^1/$_2$ teaspoons soy sauce
olive oil	2 tablespoons whole wheat flour
^{1}/$_4$ cup chopped onion	1 cup soy milk
1 pound cabbage, thinly sliced (about 5 cups)	1 teaspoon prepared mustard

Begin by toasting the sesame seeds in a wok or 15-inch skillet until aromatic. Remove from the pan and reserve.

Add enough oil to just cover the bottom of the pan. Sauté the onion for 3 to 5 minutes, until it starts to color. Add the cabbage, mix well, cover, and steep over moderate heat for 8 to 10 minutes, until tender. Stir occasionally for even cooking.

Stir in the soy sauce. Sprinkle the flour evenly over the cabbage and mix well. Gradually stir in the soy milk and mustard. Cook for a few minutes over moderate heat, stirring continuously, until the sauce thickens and comes to a gentle boil.

Remove from the heat, sprinkle with the toasted sesame seeds, and serve immediately.

YIELD: **4** SERVINGS

In Nikki's Kitchen

Stewed Red Cabbage

~

This unusual combination of ingredients produces a sensational fusion of flavors and an excellent array of phytochemicals. For a nondairy version and a slightly different effect, omit the Yogurt Cheese.

1 pound red cabbage	1/2 cup orange juice
1 medium onion, thinly sliced	2 tablespoons tomato paste
4 cloves garlic, chopped	3 tablespoons Yogurt Cheese
1/2 teaspoon salt	(page 244)

Cut the cabbage into very thin strips. There should be about 5 cups.

In a deep pot, cook the onion over medium heat for about 5 minutes, stirring occasionally, until wilted. Add the garlic and cook briefly. Stir in the cabbage and salt. Cook for 3 to 5 minutes, until it begins to wilt.

Add the orange juice and tomato paste and mix well. Cover and cook, stirring occasionally, until the cabbage is very tender, about 20 minutes.

Remove from the heat and immediately add the Yogurt Cheese, stirring until completely absorbed into the cabbage.

YIELD: 4 TO 6 SERVINGS

Asian Sesame-Ginger Carrots

~

Crunchy cooked carrots accented by sesame seeds, orange, and ginger.

6 medium carrots	1 tablespoon minced orange peel
1 tablespoon sesame seeds	1 tablespoon minced fresh ginger
2 tablespoons cooking sherry	

Shred the carrots using the coarse blade of a food processor or a hand grater. You should have about 3 cups.

Toast the sesame seeds in a dry skillet for 1 to 2 minutes, until aromatic. Watch closely to avoid burning. Remove the pan from the heat and let cool slightly (if the pan is too hot the sherry will sputter when added). Add the cooking sherry, orange peel, ginger, and carrots to the skillet. Cook over medium heat for about 8 minutes, stirring almost continuously, until the carrots are piping hot and just tender. Serve at once.

YIELD: 4 SERVINGS

Mexican Chili Carrots

Crunchy carrots with a gentle bite.

6 medium carrots	1 clove garlic, minced
1 tablespoon pumpkin seeds	1/2 teaspoon cumin
2 tablespoons orange or apple juice	2 teaspoons chili powder
1 tablespoon minced orange peel	1/4 teaspoon salt

Shred the carrots using the coarse blade of a food processor or a hand grater. You should have about 3 cups.

Toast the pumpkin seeds in a dry skillet for 1 to 2 minutes, until lightly colored and beginning to pop. Watch closely to avoid burning. Remove the pan from the heat and let cool slightly (if the pan is too hot the juice will sputter when added). Add the juice, orange peel, garlic, cumin, chili powder, salt, and carrots to the skillet. Cook over medium heat for about 8 minutes, stirring almost continuously, until the carrots are piping hot and just tender. Serve at once.

YIELD: **4** SERVINGS

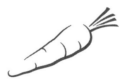

*In
Nikki's
Kitchen*

Braised Cauliflower with Currants and Pine Nuts

～

The cauliflower in this slightly sweet, delicate sauce gets its creaminess from your choice of nut butter or Yogurt Cheese. Serve with a bean entrée and cooked grain, or use this cauliflower as a topping for grains or pasta and complete the menu with a bean salad or accompaniment.

1 medium head cauliflower (about 2 pounds)
2 tablespoons pine nuts
1 medium red onion, chopped
4 cloves garlic, sliced
1 cup orange juice

1/2 cup canned crushed tomatoes
1/4 cup currants
3 tablespoons almond, cashew, or peanut butter or 1/2 cup Yogurt Cheese (page 244)

Divide the cauliflower into small florets. You should have about 5 cups.

Set a 15-inch skillet over medium heat and toast the pine nuts until golden. Shake the pan frequently and watch closely to avoid burning. Remove from the pan and reserve.

Combine the cauliflorets, onion, garlic, orange juice, tomatoes, and currants in the skillet. Mix well to coat the cauliflower with the sauce. Bring just to a boil, cover, and simmer over low heat for about 15 minutes, until the cauliflower is tender. Stir occasionally to promote even cooking. When done, remove the cover and cook a few minutes longer, stirring to thicken the sauce just a little. If you aren't ready to eat at this point, cover and let stand off the heat until just before serving. If the cauliflower is no longer hot, reheat briefly. Just before serving, remove from the heat and stir in the nut butter or Yogurt Cheese, mixing until creamy. Toss in the pine nuts.

YIELD: 4 TO 6 SERVINGS

Pink Cauliflower Oreganata

In this dish, cauliflower acquires its pale pink color from the tomato pieces and its perky flavor from the oregano.

1 small to medium cauliflower
   (1½ to 2 pounds)
1 small onion, chopped
3 tablespoons cider vinegar
2 tablespoons water

1 medium to large tomato, diced
½ teaspoon oregano
1 teaspoon basil
½ teaspoon salt

Divide the cauliflower into small florets. You should have 4 to 5 cups.

In a large heavy skillet, combine the cauliflorets, onion, 2 tablespoons cider vinegar, and the water. Cover and cook over moderate heat, stirring occasionally, for about 15 minutes, or until the cauliflower is tender.

Add the tomato, oregano, basil, salt, and remaining tablespoon cider vinegar. Cook for a few minutes, until hot.

YIELD: **4** SERVINGS

Cauliflower with Tahini Gravy

~

The use of tahini in gravies imparts an excellent creamy texture along with some desirable fats.

2 pounds cauliflower or 1¹/2 pounds
  cauliflorets
¹/2 cup water
1 tablespoon soy sauce
1 small onion, coarsely chopped
2 large cloves garlic, sliced

¹/4 cup chopped fresh dill or parsley
¹/3 cup vegetable broth or water
2 tablespoons tahini
1 tablespoon lemon juice
salt

If using whole cauliflower, break into florets. You should have 5 to 6 cups.

Pour the water and soy sauce into a shallow skillet large enough to hold the florets. Add the onion, garlic, dill or parsley, and cauliflower. Cover and cook over moderate heat for 12 to 15 minutes, or until the cauliflorets are just tender.

Transfer the cauliflorets to a serving dish, leaving the liquid and seasonings in the pan. Using a fork, beat the vegetable broth or water into the tahini until smooth. Add to the liquid in the pan along with the lemon juice. Place over moderate heat and simmer 5 minutes, stirring continuously, until hot and slightly thickened. Season with salt to taste.

Pour the gravy over the cauliflower in a serving dish. Mix well. Serve while still hot.

YIELD: 4 SERVINGS

VARIATION: For *Green Beans with Tahini Gravy*, replace the cauliflower with 1 pound green beans. Trim the ends from the beans, but leave whole. Proceed as above, cooking the beans for about 15 minutes.

*The
Healthiest
Diet in
the World*

Vegetables Baked in Red Wine

~

Wine provides a flavorful medium for cooking vegetables.

1 medium head cauliflower (2 to
  2¹/₂ pounds, untrimmed, or 7 to
  8 cups florets)
2 medium baking potatoes
  (8 ounces each)
1 large sweet potato (about
  ³/₄ pound)

4 shallots (individual bulbs)
4 cloves garlic
1 cup dry red wine
1 teaspoon rosemary
1 teaspoon salt
freshly ground pepper

Preheat the oven to 400°F.

Divide the cauliflower into florets. Scrub the potatoes and cut into quarters lengthwise; cut each quarter across into 3 pieces. Peel the sweet potato and cut in the same manner. Remove the papery skins from the shallots and garlic; cut into thin slices. Place the cauliflorets and potatoes in a baking dish that can hold the vegetables in a single layer. It's okay for them to be snug, but don't pile them up. A 9 × 13-inch or shallow 2-quart casserole should be adequate. Scatter the sliced shallots and garlic over the vegetables.

Combine the wine, rosemary, and salt. Pour over the vegetables. Cover the baking dish and bake for 20 minutes. Remove the cover. Season the vegetables with lots of freshly ground pepper. Stir so that all surfaces are coated with the wine. Return to the oven and bake, uncovered, for about 45 minutes, or until the vegetables are tender. Stir occasionally to coat all surfaces with the wine and promote even cooking. If the wine has cooked out before the vegetables are done, add a little more wine or water to finish the cooking and keep the pan from scorching.

YIELD: 4 TO 6 SERVINGS

147

*In
Nikki's
Kitchen*

Braised Leeks

~

Serve as an accompaniment to a meal or as part of an assorted appetizer plate.

4 good-size leeks
1 quart water
1 teaspoon salt
2 tablespoons pine nuts

2 large cloves garlic, chopped
2 tablespoons balsamic vinegar
1/4 cup reserved leek cooking water

Trim the dark green tops from the leeks and discard. Slice the leeks in half length-wise and wash well under cold running water to remove any dirt lodged between the layers. Cut into 3-inch sections.

Bring the water to a rolling boil. Add the salt and leeks and cook for 5 minutes. Remove the leeks with a slotted spoon or tongs, run under cold water to refresh and stop further cooking, and drain. Reserve 1/4 cup leek cooking water.

In a large skillet, toast the pine nuts until they just begin to color. Add the garlic, leeks, and balsamic vinegar and shake the skillet to coat the leeks with vinegar. Place over high heat and cook for 1 to 2 minutes, stirring or shaking the pan continuously, to slightly sear the leeks.

Reduce the heat, add the reserved leek cooking water, and cook until the liquid is almost evaporated.

Serve hot or at room temperature.

YIELD: **4** SERVINGS

VARIATION: For *Braised Celery Stalks*, replace the leeks with 8 celery stalks. Cut into 3-inch sections and slice any wide pieces in half lengthwise. Proceed as for Braised Leeks.

Corn Picadillo

~

This sprightly vegetable dish appeals to both the eye and the palate. It's most flavorful when made with fresh sweet summer corn cut right off the cob; however, it can be made with frozen corn, too. A good accompaniment to grilled tofu or tempeh entrées, along with a cooked whole grain.

1 tablespoon cooking sherry
1/2 cup chopped onion
1/4 cup chopped green pepper
1 large tomato, diced
2 cups corn kernels (cut from 2 big or 4 small ears, or frozen)

2 tablespoons chopped green or black olives
2 tablespoons currants or chopped raisins
1 tablespoon chopped fresh basil

Heat the cooking sherry in a large shallow skillet. Add the onion and green pepper. Cook over medium heat for about 5 minutes, stirring occasionally, until the onion softens. Add the remaining ingredients. Continue to cook for about 8 minutes, until the corn is cooked and everything is hot.

YIELD: **4** SERVINGS

Smothered Eggplant

Rich, creamy yogurt melds with smoky strands of eggplant to create a cooling vegetable accompaniment that's suited to many different cuisines. This is a recipe for cooks who don't mind getting their hands dirty, as the preparation of the eggplant requires a "hands-on" approach.

1 large or 2 small eggplants (about
  2$^1/_2$ pounds)
2 cloves garlic
1 cup Yogurt Cheese (page 244)

3 tablespoons lemon juice
$^1/_4$ teaspoon salt
1 teaspoon paprika

Broil the eggplants over a gas, wood, or charcoal flame until the skin is charred and the inside is quite soft. Turn several times so that all sides cook. This will take about 10 to 20 minutes, depending on the size of the eggplant and the flame. After cooking, let sit until cool enough to handle. Remove the skin and "string" the eggplant by peeling off sections with your fingers from the stem to the blossom end. Make each "string" the width of a finger or less. Discard any seeds.

In a shallow serving bowl, mash the garlic with a mortar or the back of a spoon. Add a little Yogurt Cheese and mash together. With a fork, beat in the remaining Yogurt Cheese, the lemon juice, salt, and paprika. Add the stringed eggplant and mix well. Serve at room temperature or chilled. Just before serving, sprinkle a little more paprika on top for appearance.

YIELD: **4** TO **6** SERVINGS

*In
Nikki's
Kitchen*

Spicy Italian Greens

~

This recipe is designed for "bitter greens," although romaine lettuce can be used combined with Italian parsley. A dollop of yogurt cheese on top of each serving provides a nice contrast. To turn this into a main dish, add 3 cups cooked chickpeas, white beans, or lentils at the end and heat through. If desired, serve over some small-size pasta, such as bow ties, wagon wheels, spirals, or shells. Another option is to mix the cooked greens (with or without the beans) with tortellini.

1 1/2 pounds leafy greens (beet greens, broccoli rabe, Swiss chard, chicory, escarole, frisée, kale, or romaine mixed with 1/2 cup Italian flat-leaf parsley)
2 large cloves garlic, minced

1/2 cup canned crushed tomatoes or tomato puree
1/2 teaspoon crushed red pepper flakes
2 tablespoons capers

Wash the greens well and chop coarsely. You should have about 12 cups.

Combine the greens with the remaining ingredients in a large heavy skillet or pot large enough to hold them. Cook, uncovered, for about 5 minutes, or until the greens wilt. Stir as needed for even cooking.

Cover and cook until the greens are tender, about 10 minutes depending on the greens.

YIELD: 4 TO 6 SERVINGS

Country Greens

~

Greens and mushrooms are good companions. Feel free to try this with other greens such as spinach, kale, beet greens, collards, or romaine, and other varieties of cultivated or wild mushrooms. And if you can't find shallots, use red onion instead.

1 1/2 pounds red or white Swiss chard
6 ounces cremini mushrooms

1/3 cup sliced shallots
2 tablespoons lemon juice
salt and pepper

Wash the greens well, remove the tough stems, and cut crosswise into 1/2-inch-wide strips. You should have about 12 cups.

Clean the mushrooms and slice the caps and stems. You should have about 2 cups.

In a pot large enough to hold the greens, cook the mushrooms over moderate heat for 5 to 8 minutes, stirring occasionally to prevent sticking, until they wilt and release their juices. Add the shallots and cook 1 to 2 minutes.

Add the greens to the pot and mix until they begin to wilt and cook down. (Tongs are a good tool for this job, or chopsticks if you're adept at using them.)

Cover the pot and cook over low heat for 5 to 10 minutes, until the greens are tender. Remove from the heat, add the lemon juice, and season with salt and pepper to taste.

YIELD: 4 SERVINGS

Sesame Green Beans

~

Sesame seeds enhance almost any vegetable. If you agree, try this recipe with steamed cauliflower and broccoli florets.

1 pound green beans
1 tablespoon sesame seeds
1 tablespoon lemon juice

1 teaspoon toasted sesame oil
salt and pepper

Steam the beans for 5 to 8 minutes, until tender but still crunchy.

Toast the sesame seeds in a dry skillet for a few minutes until aromatic.

Transfer the warm beans to a serving bowl and toss with the lemon juice, sesame oil, toasted seeds, and salt and pepper to taste.

YIELD: 4 SERVINGS

Blackened Green Beans

~

These crisply cooked beans have a subtle smoky taste and a hint of spiciness. If you like really hot food, use a potent chili powder or add a pinch of cayenne. If you're sensitive to sodium, this dish may not be a good choice; even with a reduced-sodium soy sauce it packs 300 mg sodium per serving. And a final note for whoever is on cleanup—let the blackened pan soak for a while and it will clean with ease.

1 pound green beans
2 tablespoons soy sauce
4 cloves garlic, chopped

1 teaspoon chili powder
2 to 3 tablespoons water

Trim the ends from the green beans but leave whole.

Combine the beans and soy sauce in a wok or large skillet. Cook over high heat, stirring continuously, for 5 to 10 minutes, until the beans are singed and the soy sauce evaporates. Add the garlic during the last minute or so.

Remove the pan from the heat. Immediately add the chili powder and water, 1 tablespoonful at a time, stirring to dissolve the blackened soy in the pan. Do this carefully, as there will be some sputtering.

YIELD: 4 SERVINGS

VARIATIONS: For *Blackened Carrots*, cut 1 pound carrots into 2-inch-long matchsticks (about 3 cups) and follow the directions above. Likewise, *Blackened Asparagus* can be made by breaking 1 pound stalks into 2-inch lengths (about 4 cups), while the same amount of broccoli stems, peeled and cut into 2-inch-long matchsticks, makes great *Blackened Broccoli*.

Mushrooms with Carrots

~

The mild flavor of cultivated mushrooms is vitalized by the sweetness of the carrots, mediated by the sweet-tart taste of the vinegar.

3 medium carrots, cut into 1/4-inch
  cubes
1/4 cup water
1 small onion, minced
3/4 pound mushrooms, sliced
  (4 cups)

1 teaspoon dried oregano
1/4 teaspoon salt
2 tablespoons balsamic vinegar

Combine the carrots and water in a large skillet, bring to a boil, cover, and cook until barely tender, about 5 minutes. Add the onion and cook, uncovered, for about 5 minutes, until the onion is wilted and the liquid evaporates. Add the mushrooms and cook, stirring several times, until the mushrooms are tender and have released their juices, 8 to 10 minutes. Add the oregano, salt, and vinegar. Boil gently for about 3 minutes.

YIELD: **4** SERVINGS

★ **SLICING MUSHROOMS** ★

When you have a lot of mushrooms to slice, one of the easiest ways to go about it is to use an egg slicer.

Glazed Plantains

Plantains go well with South American dishes. This particular sweet-and-spicy version can be paired with Black Bean Soup, Quick Cuban-style Black Beans, or Picadillo, among others.

2 large ripe plantains (about
  1¹/₂ pounds)
2 tablespoons fruit juice–sweetened
  orange marmalade

³/₈ teaspoon cayenne
¹/₂ cup orange juice

Peel the plantains and slice into ¹/₄-inch-thick rounds.

Melt the marmalade in a large skillet over medium heat. Stir in the cayenne and orange juice. Add the plantains and cook over low heat for 5 to 8 minutes, turning to coat both sides. When done, the plantains will be tender and covered with a thick glaze.

YIELD: **4 TO 6** SERVINGS

Mashed Potatoes with Garlic

~

Low in fat, but not in flavor.

1 small leek, optional
1¹/2 pounds potatoes, cut into
  1-inch chunks
8 cloves garlic, thinly sliced
¹/2 cup water

¹/2 cup soy milk
¹/2 teaspoon salt or to taste
pepper
paprika

If using the leek, cut in half lengthwise, wash well to remove dirt, and chop.
  Combine the vegetables in a pot with the water. Bring to a boil. Cover and cook over low heat for 20 minutes, or until the potatoes are very tender. Remove the peel or leave it on, according to personal preference and the thickness of the skins.
  Using a potato masher, mash the vegetables along with any liquid remaining in the pot. Then with a fork, whisk, or electric mixer, gradually beat in the soy milk until light and fluffy. Season to taste with salt and pepper. Sprinkle surface generously with paprika.

YIELD: **4** SERVINGS

Chunky Red Chili Mashed Potatoes

~

Pale red in color, with a subtle hint of tomato and spiciness.

1¹/2 pounds potatoes
¹/2 cup water
¹/2 cup Yogurt Cheese (page 244)
2 scallions, thinly sliced, or 3
  tablespoons minced chives

1 teaspoon chili powder
1¹/2 tablespoons tomato paste
salt

Cut the potatoes into 1-inch chunks. Combine in a pot with the water. Bring to a boil, cover, and cook over low heat for 20 minutes, or until tender.
  Drain the potatoes. Remove the peel or leave it on, according to personal preference and the thickness of the skins. Add the Yogurt Cheese, scallions, chili powder, and tomato paste. Coarsely mash with a potato masher until uniformly blended. Season with salt to taste.

YIELD: **4** SERVINGS

Mashed Potatoes with Celeriac

Celeriac, sometimes called celery knob or celery root, has a taste similar to celery, but with a sweet undertone. Combined with potatoes, it makes a flavorful "mashed potato" with a lighter texture. Celeriac is low in carbohydrates, so this dish has 8 grams fewer carbohydrates than an all-potato version. It also contains an insignificant amount of fat (less than 1/2 gram). If celeriac is unavailable, substitute peeled eggplant for a similar low-carbohydrate result and a novel flavor.

1 pound potatoes (3 cups cubed)	2 tablespoons light miso or
1/2 pound celeriac (2 cups cubed)	1/2 teaspoon salt
1/4 cup white wine	freshly ground pepper
1/4 cup water	

Peel the potatoes or not, according to personal preference and the thickness of the skins. Cut into 1-inch chunks. Trim the knobby portions of the celeriac and remove the peel using a potato peeler and small paring knife where necessary. Cut the celeriac into 1-inch chunks.

Combine the vegetables in a pot with white wine and water. Bring to a boil. Cover and cook over low heat for 20 minutes, or until the vegetables are very tender.

Drain the vegetables, reserving any liquid. Transfer to a food processor, add the miso or salt, and whip until smooth, light, and fluffy, adding the reserved liquid as needed. Season generously with freshly ground pepper.

YIELD: 4 SERVINGS

Potatoes Pepperonata

~

Potatoes stewed with peppers and onions are comforting and comely. A Mediterranean classic that goes with Italian, Spanish, Greek, or even traditional American cooking.

1 large red onion, chopped
2 cloves garlic, chopped
1/2 cup diced tomato
2 red peppers (5 to 6 ounces each),
  cut into thin strips

2 medium potatoes (1 pound total),
  cut into 3/4-inch cubes
1/2 teaspoon salt
freshly ground pepper

Combine the onion, garlic, and tomato in a 4-quart pot with a tight-fitting lid. Cover and place over low heat for 10 minutes.

Add the red peppers, potatoes, and salt. Replace the cover and continue to cook, stirring occasionally, for 20 minutes, or until the potatoes are done. The vegetables should expel enough of their own juices to cook the potatoes. However, if the mixture seems dry, a little water should be added. Season with a generous amount of freshly ground pepper before serving.

YIELD: **4 SERVINGS**

Louisiana Sweet Potatoes

~

Cajun carotenoids.

4 medium sweet potatoes, peeled
  and diced (7 to 8 cups)
2 teaspoons paprika
2 teaspoons chili powder

1 teaspoon dried mustard powder
1 tablespoon soy sauce
2 tablespoons water

Place the sweet potato cubes in a pot with water to cover. Bring to a boil and simmer 10 to 12 minutes, until just cooked but still firm. Drain.

In the pot the potatoes were cooked in, combine the paprika, chili powder, mustard powder, and soy sauce. Place over moderate heat and cook, stirring, for 1 minute.

Add the water to the pan with the seasonings to dilute. Add the potatoes and mix until well coated with the spices. Cook for 3 to 5 minutes, stirring frequently, until hot.

YIELD: **4 SERVINGS**

Zucchini à l'Orange

〜

The sprightly flavors of orange and mint do an excellent job of making summer squash come alive.

2 tablespoons pumpkin seeds
1½ pounds zucchini or yellow crookneck squash (2 to 4 squash, depending on size)
¼ cup orange juice
1 teaspoon minced orange rind
2 tablespoons chopped fresh mint or 2 teaspoons dried mint

¼ teaspoon salt
2 oranges, peeled, separated into segments, and each section cut in half
½ teaspoon paprika

Toast the pumpkin seeds in a dry skillet until they pop. Set aside.

Cut the squash into thin sticks, about ¼ inch wide and 2 inches long. Combine in the skillet with the orange juice, orange rind, mint, and salt. Stir-steam over medium-high heat for 3 to 5 minutes, until just tender. Stir in the orange pieces and cook briefly to just warm through. Remove from the heat, top with the toasted pumpkin seeds, and sprinkle evenly with the paprika.

YIELD: 4 SERVINGS

★ STIR STEAMING ★

Stir-steaming: The process of cooking a vegetable quickly in a small amount of liquid over medium-high to high heat while stirring. Similar to stir-frying but using a flavorful liquid instead of oil.

In Nikki's Kitchen

Wine-simmered Vegetables

~

Wine-simmering is an easy way to prepare vegetables that will be used as a side dish, served over grains, or dressed with a sauce. It's a nice alternative to steaming. Wine-simmering works best for vegetables that are cut in bite-size pieces. Try green beans; carrot coins; 2-inch-long, 1/4-inch-thick matchsticks made from carrot, zucchini, peeled broccoli stems, celery; bite-size cauliflorets or broccoli florets; snow peas; or fennel wedges. Several vegetables can be combined in the pan.

dry red or white wine   **vegetable(s) of choice**

Choose a heavy skillet large enough to hold the vegetables. Pour enough wine into the skillet to cover the bottom to a depth of 1/4 inch. Place over moderate heat. When the skillet is hot and vapors start to rise from the wine (but prior to boiling), add the vegetables to the skillet. Cover and cook over low to moderate heat for 10 minutes. Taste for doneness, cooking a few minutes longer if necessary, according to preference.

Basic Baked Vegetables

~

Sometimes the simplest approaches are overlooked. Many tuberous vegetables are suitable for baking. Below we provide directions for some standards, as well as some novel ideas. Although the preferred oven temperature for each vegetable is specified, they're generally adaptable to a range of baking temperatures, from 350 to 425°F. This makes them compatible with other things that might also be in the oven. A good habit to develop is that of preparing extras to use in salads, cooked vegetable dishes, for snacks, or even for breakfast.

Allow one good-size vegetable per serving (or half in the case of winter squash). Follow the directions outlined below for preparing and timing individual vegetables. Bake until tender and easily pierced with a fork.

When it comes to the garnish, it can be as easy as a generous slathering of yogurt cheese, or you can be more adventurous. For example, both winter squash and sweet potatoes are terrific topped with flavorful cooked beans, while baked beets make a surprising treat with Lemon-Tahini Dressing.

The Standard Baked Potato

Preheat the oven to 400°F. Scrub the potato clean and cut out any sprouts or eyes. Dry well with paper towels. Pierce in several places with a fork to prevent bursting in the oven. Place on a baking sheet or directly on the rack of the oven. Bake until the potato yields readily to gentle pressure with a mitted hand, or until a skewer will easily pierce through the center. A medium 8-ounce potato will take about 45 minutes. Naturally, larger potatoes will take longer to bake than smaller ones. If you spike the potato with a metal kebab skewer, baking time will be reduced by about one-third.

Baked Sweet Potatoes and Yams

Preheat the oven to 375°F. Scrub the potatoes and dry them with paper towels. Prick in several places with a fork to prevent bursting in the oven. Place on a baking sheet or directly on the rack of the oven. Bake until the potatoes yield readily to gentle pressure with a mitted hand, or until a skewer will easily pierce through the centers. Sweet potatoes bake a little faster than white potatoes. A medium 8-ounce sweet potato will take about 40 minutes.

Baked Beets

Beets are as easy to bake as potatoes, but they aren't commonly served this way. Preheat the oven to 400°F. Cut off any beet greens and put aside for another dish. Scrub the beets well and dry. Cut off the stem right to the top of the beets; cut off the roots. Do not peel. Place the beets in a baking dish and cover tightly with a lid or foil. Alternatively, beets can be enclosed entirely in foil.

Bake until tender and easily pierced with a sharp knife. This will take 1 hour or more, depending on size. After cooking, when the beets are cool enough to handle, slide the skins off. Serve whole or cut into pieces. Eat plain or dress as desired. Baked beets are delicious topped with Curry-Yogurt Cream, Lemon-Tahini Dressing, or Orange-Parsley Dressing.

Baked Winter Squash

Orange-fleshed winter squash include hubbard, acorn, butternut, buttercup, and several other specialty varieties, as well as pumpkin.

Preheat the oven to 350 to 375°F. Cut the squash in half from stem to blossom end. Scoop out the seeds. If particularly large, cut the halves into more manageable pieces.

Place the cut side down in a shallow baking dish and surround with about 1/2 inch water to prevent scorching. Bake for 30 to 40 minutes, or until barely tender.

Invert the squash and return to the oven for 10 to 15 minutes, until the flesh is tender. During this final stage of baking, a light sprinkling of cinnamon or nutmeg can be used for seasoning.

In Nikki's Kitchen

Baked Onions

The inspiration for these onions came from the cookbook *La Cucina Fresca* and it's a dish we frequently serve when entertaining. Although both white and red onions are suitable for baking, the red have more visual appeal.

Preheat the oven to 375°F. Place unpeeled, whole onions in a shallow baking pan just large enough to hold them comfortably. Bake for about 1 hour, or until soft to the touch. Remove from the oven, and when cool enough to handle, cut into quarters almost down to the root so that the onions open like flowers with the bottoms still intact.

Place the baking pan that held the onions on top of the stove and add a few tablespoons of balsamic vinegar. Heat while scraping any caramelized onion juices off the bottom of the pan, incorporating them into the vinegar. Cook until syrupy, then spoon over the onions.

Baked Yucca

Yucca is a popular tuber in Latin America and in Hispanic communities in North America. Some people know it by the alternate names cassava and manioc, and others have tasted it as tapioca. Yucca is a terrific source of potassium and magnesium, a good source of folate and vitamin C, and surprisingly rich in calcium. Cooked, it has an unusual dry, slightly sweet flesh. While most commonly peeled, cut into chunks, and boiled, we prefer it baked. When choosing a yucca, pick one with the barklike brown skin as intact as possible (there are often some bare patches). Any flesh that shows through should be pale pink or tan on the surface and white as coconut beneath. Avoid specimens with grayish fibers, discolored patches, or soft spots.

Preheat the oven to 375 to 400°F. If the yucca is coated with wax, scrape under hot water with a paring knife to remove. Place on a baking sheet and bake until tender. The time will vary with the size of the yucca and is approximately the same as for baked potatoes. A small, 7- to 8-ounce yucca will take 30 to 40 minutes.

Oven-Roasted Vegetables

Roasting is an excellent way to intensify the flavor of vegetables, and although most cooks don't realize it, no added fat is required. The fragrance of the vegetables permeates the kitchen as they cook, and they emerge from the oven tender and golden. If roasting several vegetables together, keep their individual cooking times in mind; the objective is to have them all done at about the same time. The way to go about this is to add them at appropriate intervals according to the estimated times given below, or to cut longer-cooking vegetables into pieces to reduce their cooking time and match that of quicker-cooking ones.

Don't crowd the pan when roasting, as this encourages vegetables to steam and inhibits browning. As the directions below demonstrate, it isn't necessary to coat vegetables with oil for roasting. However, for increased browning and deeper flavor, you can toss them in a little olive oil infused with herbs or spices before placing them in the pan. A modest but adequate ratio is to use 1 tablespoon of oil per cup of vegetables. For flavor, add 1 to 2 teaspoons oregano, rosemary, thyme, chili powder, curry powder, or other favorite seasoning, or a good pinch of cayenne per tablespoon of oil.

A generous serving of roasted vegetables makes a good accompaniment to beans, and is practically a meal in itself on top of pasta, polenta, or cooked grains. If this is your intent, be sure to include protein, either separately or by topping the vegetables with a generous amount of yogurt cheese or a protein-providing sauce like Spicy Orange-Nut Sauce, Chickpea Pesto, or Agliata. You can turn leftovers into salad by tossing them with lemon juice or balsamic or red wine vinegar and herbs.

Following the basic steps outlined below is a list of different vegetables with advice on preparing and timing.

Preheat the oven to 500°F. Generously oil baking sheet(s) or shallow roasting pan(s) with olive oil, making sure you have enough space to place the vegetables without crowding. Spread the vegetables in the pan(s) in a single layer. You may want to organize the vegetables according to baking time in order to add or remove them at appropriate intervals.

Scatter any seasonings you want to use on top of the vegetables, including slivered garlic, rosemary, and oregano. Place in the oven. Check on the vegetables occasionally and use a metal spatula to move them to promote even roasting and prevent sticking. Cook as indicated in the timetable below, or until the vegetables reach the desired degree of tenderness.

When done, arrange on a platter and season to taste with freshly ground pepper. Depending on their intended use, you can also flavor them with soy sauce or balsamic vinegar.

*In
Nikki's
Kitchen*

PREPARATION AND TIMETABLE FOR OVEN-ROASTING VEGETABLES

Vegetable	Preparation	Roasting Time (minutes)
asparagus	break off tough ends; leave whole	20
beets	peel or not; cut into 1/2- to 1-inch pieces	40
brussels sprouts	cut in half lengthwise (through stem)	20 to 25
carrots	peel and cut lengthwise into quarters	30 to 40
eggplant	sliced 1/2 inch thick cut into 1-inch cubes	15 30 or until interior is quite soft and surface well browned
fennel	cut into 1/2-inch-thick wedges	15 to 20
mushrooms	leave whole	20
onions	cut into 1-inch-thick crescents	15
potatoes 　small new or red 　large white	quartered cut into 1 1/2-inch pieces sliced 1/4 inch thick	30 30 to 40 30 or until surface is golden and crisp
sweet potatoes	peeled, sliced, or cut into 1-inch chunks cut into sticks resembling french fries	30 15 to 20
zucchini	cut lengthwise into quarters	30 to 40, turning several times in order to brown cut surfaces

Guidelines for Grilling Vegetables (and Fruit)

~

Many vegetables lend themselves to grilling. Depending on how ambitious you are, they can be marinated beforehand, or basted during grilling, or grilled plain and, if desired, dressed afterward.

For marinating, we recommend Spicy Marinade or the marinade in Asian Grill. Allow the vegetables to bathe in the marinade for at least 30 minutes (see the options below). Marinations of more than 2 hours should be done in the refrigerator.

If you prefer basting to marinating, try Sweet Mustard Basting Sauce.

The easiest approach to grilling is to simply put the prepared vegetables on the grill and, if desired, season them afterward. Of course, you may find they taste so good plain that nothing else is necessary. Our favorite tactic is to sprinkle the vegetables while still hot from the grill with a little balsamic vinegar. This works particularly well with slices of grilled zucchini, eggplant, mushrooms, carrots, broccoli trees, and cauliflower. Sometimes we use soy sauce instead.

Cooking time will vary with the heat of the fire, the distance at which foods are placed, and their position on the grill. A common mistake people make is to grill foods too hot or too close to the flame. As a result, the food chars on the outside before it has a chance to cook. The table below indicates relative cooking times. It's important to stay at the grill so you can watch and turn foods or move them to other parts of the grill as needed. Cook until seared on all sides with grill marks.

If you want, you can impart flavor and aroma by adding a handful of fresh or dried herbs, tea leaves, or dried citrus peels to the fire.

Because vegetables can easily slip between the grill grates, a mesh grill rack is a worthwhile tool to have. Long tongs with heatproof handles are the best implement for moving and turning. Lightly oiling the rack by wiping with a folded paper towel dipped in oil will keep vegetables from sticking.

Gauging the amount of vegetables to cook is tricky. Since grilled vegetables are so tasty, people tend to eat a lot, especially if you serve an assortment. This, of course, is an excellent outcome. We suggest choosing 4 to 6 items and planning the following amounts per serving: 3 to 4 mushrooms; 1/2 onion; 5 to 6 ounces cauliflower or broccoli; 1/2 large sweet potato; 8 ounces or half of a 1-pound eggplant or acorn squash; 1 small zucchini or crookneck squash; 2 plum tomatoes; 1/2 sweet red or green pepper.

While you're at it, you should also try grilling fruit. We suggest peaches, nectarines, and pineapple.

PREPARATION AND TIMING GUIDELINES FOR GRILLING VEGETABLES AND FRUIT

Food	Preparation	Time (minutes per side)	Options
broccoli	peel stalks and slice into thin trees	3 to 5	marinate 1 hour or more, baste, or cook plain and sprinkle with soy sauce or balsamic vinegar
carrots	peel and cut lengthwise into 1/4-inch-thick pieces	5 to 8	marinate 1 hour or more, baste, or cook plain and sprinkle with balsamic vinegar
cauliflower	divide into florets or 1/4-inch-thick slices	7 to 10	marinate 1 hour or more, baste, or cook plain and sprinkle with balsamic vinegar
corn	leave whole in husks	turn frequently and cook until husk is charred; 15 to 20 total	after cooking remove husks and silk and place back on grill to brown kernels slightly
eggplant	cut into 1/4-inch-thick rounds	5	marinate 30 minutes or longer, baste, or cook plain and sprinkle with soy sauce or balsamic vinegar
mushrooms	thread whole on skewers or place directly on mesh grate	3 to 5	marinate 30 minutes or longer, baste, or cook plain and sprinkle with soy sauce or balsamic vinegar
onions	cut into halves, wedges, thick slices, or thread chunks on skewers	5	marinate 30 minutes or longer, or cook plain

Food	Preparation	Time (minutes per side)	Options
summer squash (crookneck, pattypan, zucchini)	cut lengthwise into 1/4-inch-thick slices	3 to 5	marinate 30 minutes or longer, baste, or cook plain and sprinkle with soy sauce or balsamic vinegar
sweet potatoes	peel and slice 1/4 inch thick	7 to 10	marinate 30 minutes or longer, baste, or cook plain; can cover or make a foil tent to promote cooking
sweet red or green peppers	cut into halves, strips, or 1- to 2-inch wedges for skewers	3 to 5	cook plain
tomatoes, plum preferred	cut in half lengthwise	3 to 5	cook plain
winter squash	cut into 1/4-inch-thick rounds; remove seeds; with a vegetable peeler or paring knife, remove as much peel as possible	7 to 10	marinate 30 minutes or longer, baste, or cook plain; can cover or make a foil tent to promote cooking
peaches, nectarines	divide into halves	3 to 5	cook plain; dust with cinnamon after cooking
pineapple	cut into 1/2-inch-thick slices; use a paring knife to remove as much peel as possible	5	cook plain; dust with cinnamon after cooking

In Nikki's Kitchen

Beans

Guidelines for preparing beans are found in "Gold Star Basics." In order to make beans more convenient to use, cook ample amounts ahead at one time. Other quick options include pressure cooking (see Cooking Techniques, on page 249) and canned beans, which are acceptable for dishes that call for pre-cooked beans. When bean cooking liquid is specified in a recipe, canning liquid can be used in its place. If the beans are presalted, be sure to make adjustments in the recipe. If the canning medium is inadequate or unsuitable, it can be extended or replaced with water or vegetable broth.

In addition to these bean accompaniments, the numerous bean-based entrées in "Main Dishes" can be served as side dishes. As side dishes, the yield will generally provide 1 1/2 to 2 times the indicated servings.

Black-eyed Peas Tripoli

Ready in less than 10 minutes, this black-eyed pea dish is well flavored with cilantro and enjoys the crunchy texture of lightly cooked celery. The recipe can also be prepared with lentils (especially the firmer French lentils), small lima beans, or small white navy or pea beans. For a terrific Middle Eastern meal, serve with cracked wheat, Tomato Couscous, or Warm Bulgur Salad. Add a green or orange vegetable and/or salad. Also good with yogurt or yogurt cheese in the form of Cold Cucumber-Yogurt Soup, Yogurt-Cucumber Salad, or any variety of White Pita "Pizza."

1 small onion, chopped	1/2 teaspoon salt (reduce if beans are salted)
2 cloves garlic, sliced	
1/4 cup bean cooking liquid or water	freshly ground pepper
3 cups cooked black-eyed peas	1 to 2 tablespoons olive, flaxseed, or hemp oil, optional
2 stalks celery, chopped	
1/2 cup chopped fresh cilantro	lemon wedges

In a pot large enough to hold the beans, combine the onion, garlic, and bean cooking liquid or water. Cover the pot and stew over moderate heat for 5 to 8 minutes, until the onion is just tender. Add the beans, celery, cilantro, and salt. Cook uncovered, stirring frequently, for 2 to 3 minutes. Remove from the heat, season liberally with freshly ground pepper, and drizzle with the oil if desired. Serve with lemon wedges at the table for individual seasoning.

YIELD: **4 SERVINGS**

Split Peas in Creamy Mustard Sauce

~

These rich, flavorful split peas are best accompanied by a grain (perhaps Nutted Rice with Raisins) and a sprightly yogurt salad such as Carrot Raita. Whole wheat chapatis are excellent for scooping up the components of this meal.

2 cups dried green split peas	1/2 teaspoon turmeric
6 cups water	2 tablespoons finely chopped ginger
2 bay leaves	3 tablespoons prepared mustard

Combine the split peas with the water and bring to a boil. Add the bay leaves, turmeric, and ginger. Cover and simmer over low heat for about 45 minutes, or until the peas are just tender but not breaking apart. Stir occasionally during cooking and test frequently near the end so the peas don't overcook.

When the peas are cooked, remove and discard the bay leaves. Stir in the mustard and cook, stirring continuously, for 1 to 2 minutes, until the mustard melts into the sauce and turns it rich and creamy. Cover the pot, remove from the heat, and let sit for about 10 minutes, allowing the flavors to develop before serving.

YIELD: 4 TO 6 SERVINGS

Channa Dahl

~

This Indian-style bean puree can be served as a side dish at an Indian meal, spooned over baked potatoes or a cooked grain for an entrée, or served at room temperature as a dip with whole wheat chapati wedges and raw or lightly steamed vegetables (see the variation following the recipe). With cooked or canned chickpeas, it's ready to eat in under 5 minutes. Our preference in prepared curry powders is Madras, which has a nice flavor and is relatively mild. The spiciness of the dish may vary with other curry powder blends.

2 cups cooked chickpeas, drained	1 tablespoon curry powder
1 cup chickpea cooking liquid, water, or vegetable broth	1/2 teaspoon cumin
2 cloves garlic	salt

Combine all ingredients except the salt in a blender or food processor. Puree until smooth. Transfer to a small saucepan and cook 2 to 3 minutes to warm through. Salt to taste; if the beans or liquid were presalted, you shouldn't need more salt.

YIELD: 2 CUPS; 4 SERVINGS

VARIATION: To turn this into *Curried Hummus*, reduce the chickpea cooking liquid to 1/2 cup. It can be made well ahead of time and chilled.

Spring Chickpeas

~

This very cheerful dish has a clean, sprightly taste of fresh seasonal vegetables. Cheese eaters will enjoy it topped with crumbled feta or goat cheese. For a spring meal, begin with Cold Cucumber-Yogurt Soup. Couple the chickpeas with a flavorful grain dish and salad with Lemon-Tahini Dressing. (As an alternative to the soup, accompany with Sweet Red Pepper Quick White Pita "Pizza.")

1 large clove garlic, chopped
1 large onion, cut into thin crescents
2 carrots, cut into thin coins
1/4 cup chickpea cooking liquid
1/2 pound sugar snap or snow peas,
   cut into 1-inch segments (2 cups)

2 1/2 cups cooked chickpeas
2 tablespoons chopped parsley
1/4 teaspoon salt or to taste
freshly ground pepper

In a medium saucepan, combine the garlic, onion, carrots, and cooking liquid. Bring to a boil and cook, uncovered, until the carrots are tender, 5 to 8 minutes.

Add the peas and cook for 3 to 5 minutes, stirring frequently, until the peas are cooked but still crisp. Add the chickpeas, parsley, and salt to taste, adjusting according to whether the chickpeas were presalted or not. Cook quickly until heated through.

Remove from the heat and season liberally with freshly ground pepper. Serve at once or cover until serving time.

YIELD: **4** SERVINGS

Lemony Limas

~

Lots of fresh lemon melds nicely with the delicate flavor of lima beans. The beans should be cooked ahead. With a pressure cooker this can be done in less than 20 minutes. You'll need about 1/2 pound dried beans for this dish, but it always make sense to cook extra for another use. In fact, Lemony Limas store well in the refrigerator and make an excellent cold salad or filling for pita bread, so you may want to multiply the recipe for planned leftovers. Serve with a platter of Grilled or Oven-Roasted Vegetables and a simple grain, or with Baked Tomatoes with Wild Rice Stuffing and an ample green salad.

1 medium onion, chopped

2 cloves garlic, sliced

1/4 cup bean cooking liquid or water

1/4 cup lemon juice

1 teaspoon minced lemon peel

1/2 teaspoon salt (reduce if beans are salted)

1 stalk celery, chopped

1/4 cup chopped parsley

3 cups cooked baby lima beans

1 tablespoon olive, flaxseed, or hemp oil, optional

In a pot large enough to hold the beans, combine the onion, garlic, and bean cooking liquid or water. Cover the pot and stew over moderate heat for 5 to 8 minutes, until the onion is just tender. Add the remaining ingredients, except the oil. Simmer, uncovered, for 2 to 3 minutes.

Remove from the heat, and drizzle with the oil if desired. Serve warm or at room temperature. Leftovers can be chilled for a tasty salad.

YIELD: 4 SERVINGS

VARIATION: For *Lemony Lentils*, prepare with precooked lentils. French lentils are the best choice as they maintain their shape well.

Soybeans Southern Style

An especially good way to prepare the canned soybeans available in natural food stores. For an excellent Southern dinner, serve with Mashed Potatoes with Celeriac or corn on the cob, Creamy Miso-Mustard Coleslaw or Country Greens, and Golden Biscuits, corn bread, or even tortillas.

1 large onion (Vidalia, Walla Walla, or other sweet type preferred), chopped

1 tablespoon soy sauce

1 1/2 cups diced canned tomatoes, lightly drained

1 1/2 tablespoons molasses

1 1/2 tablespoons cider vinegar

3 cups cooked soybeans

hot pepper sauce to taste

Combine the onion and soy sauce in a saucepan, cover, and cook over low heat for 5 minutes. Add the tomatoes, molasses, and vinegar. Simmer, uncovered, for 5 minutes. Add the soybeans and the hot sauce to taste. Cover and simmer for about 10 minutes, until the soybeans are quite hot and surrounded with sauce. Because soybeans hold their shape, longer cooking won't harm the dish, nor will reheating.

YIELD: 4 SERVINGS

Grains

Grains should be served often as an accompaniment to vegetable, tofu, tempeh, and bean dishes. The guidelines for preparing a variety of whole grains are found in "Gold Star Basics." The recipes in this section illustrate how grains can be easily adorned. In addition, you'll find a variety of sauces and toppings to put on plain grains in "Sauces and Toppings."

Nutted Rice with Raisins

The directions begin with cooking the rice; however, this aromatic dish can be prepared by warming up 3 cups of precooked brown rice and continuing with the recipe as directed. You could also save time by pressure-cooking the rice (see Cooking Techniques, on page 249, in "Gold Star Basics").

1 cup uncooked brown rice
2 cups water
2 tablespoons pumpkin seeds

1/4 cup raisins
1/4 cup sliced almonds
1/4 teaspoon cinnamon

Combine the rice and water in a pot, bring to a boil, cover, and cook over low heat for about 45 minutes, until the grain is tender and the liquid is completely absorbed.

Place the pumpkin seeds in a dry skillet, set over medium heat, and toast until they begin to brown and pop.

Add the toasted seeds, raisins, almonds, and cinnamon to the warm rice and toss gently with a fork or chopsticks. Replace the cover until ready to serve.

YIELD: 4 SERVINGS

Tomato Couscous

Quick, easy, flavorful, and rich in lycopene (see Chapter 4).

1 1/2 cups water
1 1/2 cups tomato juice

2 cups whole wheat couscous or fine
    bulgur
salt

Combine the water and tomato juice in a pot and bring to a boil. Sprinkle in the grain, stir once, cover, and cook for 5 minutes. Remove from the heat and let sit 10 minutes. Fluff with a fork, season to taste with salt, and serve.

YIELD: 4 SERVINGS AS UNDERLAYER; 6 SIDE-DISH SERVINGS

Wild Rice with Mushrooms

Although used like a grain, wild rice is actually neither rice nor grain, but the seed of a native American grass. Wild rice is generally combined with real rice in recipes, perhaps because it's expensive. However, we think it's worthy of being featured alone, and since it quadruples in volume with cooking, a little goes a long way. Using a pressure cooker speeds up the preparation of this dish.

1 small onion, chopped	1 tablespoon soy sauce
3 ounces wild or cultivated mushrooms, coarsely chopped (1 cup)	2 tablespoons water
	1/2 cup wild rice
	1 1/4 cups boiling water

Combine the onion, mushrooms, soy sauce, and water in a pot. Cover and cook over moderate heat for 5 minutes, until the onion is tender and the mushroom juices run freely.

Add the wild rice and boiling water. Cover and simmer gently for 50 minutes, until the liquid is absorbed and the rice is tender.

To make in a pressure cooker, cook the onion, mushrooms, and soy sauce in a covered pressure cooker as directed above, making sure the pressure valve isn't engaged. Add the rice and 1 cup cold water. Close the cooker, engage the pressure valve, and bring to pressure over high heat. Lower the heat to just maintain pressure and cook for 25 minutes. Remove from the heat, let sit 5 minutes, then reduce the pressure fully by opening the steam-release valve, or running older models under cold water. If the liquid isn't completely absorbed, cover the pot to conserve heat and let the rice absorb what remains, or uncover and cook over low heat to evaporate.

YIELD: 2 CUPS; 4 SERVINGS

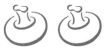

In Nikki's Kitchen

Kasha with Stewed Onions

⌣

Kasha and onions are a classic duo and an especially healthful one, as both the grain and the vegetable are rich in the phytochemicals called flavonoids, discussed in Chapter 4. You can further embellish this dish with a topping of yogurt cheese or Creamy Mushroom Gravy. Other variations include adding a cup of sliced mushrooms to cook along with the onions, or replacing half the kasha with bow-tie noodles for the famous dish kasha varnishkas.

1 cup kasha (toasted buckwheat groats)
2 cups boiling water
1/2 teaspoon salt

2 large onions, chopped
2 teaspoons soy sauce
2 tablespoons water

Combine the kasha with the boiling water and salt in a saucepan, cover, and simmer over low heat for about 30 minutes, until the liquid is completely absorbed and the grain is tender.

In a heavy skillet, combine the onions, soy sauce, and 2 tablespoons water. Place over medium heat. When hot, cover, reduce the heat as low as possible, and steep 10 to 15 minutes, stirring occasionally, until the onions have a rich, velvety texture. If the onions become dry at any time during cooking, add more water, 1 tablespoonful at a time, as needed. If the onions are prepared in advance, they can be covered and left off the heat and reheated briefly just before serving.

Spoon the onions over the cooked kasha at serving time.

YIELD: **4** SERVINGS

Oat Pilaf

⌣

A quick, easy accompaniment with a moist texture reminiscent of stuffing. This is a good way to incorporate more water-soluble grain fiber into the diet (see Golden Guideline #1).

1 egg
2 cups oats
1 cup water, broth, liquid from canned tomatoes, or a mixture of 1/4 cup tomato juice and 3/4 cup water

1 1/2 tablespoons soy sauce (reduce if liquid is salted)
4 scallions, sliced
3/4 cup frozen green peas

Crack the egg in a saucepan and beat lightly until mixed. Stir in the oats and mix until completely coated with egg. Place over medium heat and cook, stirring almost continuously, until the surface of the oats is dry.

Add the liquid, soy sauce, scallions, and green peas. Bring to a boil, reduce the heat, and simmer gently, uncovered, for 5 to 8 minutes, until the liquid is absorbed. Stir with a fork occasionally during cooking. When cooking is completed, cover, remove from the heat, and let sit until serving.

YIELD: 4 CUPS; 4 SERVINGS

Barley and Mushrooms

Hulled barley is the whole-grain form, which isn't the same as the more common pearl barley. It has a richer flavor and an appealing chewiness. Barley takes a while to cook, but the time can be substantially reduced with a pressure cooker.

12 ounces mushrooms, sliced
  (4 cups)
1 cup chopped onion
1 tablespoon soy sauce
2 tablespoons water

1 1/2 cups hulled barley
4 cups boiling water
1/2 teaspoon salt
freshly ground pepper

Combine the mushrooms, onion, soy sauce, and 2 tablespoons water in a large pot. Cook over moderate heat, stirring occasionally, for 5 to 8 minutes, until the mushroom juices run freely. Stir in the barley and cook 1 minute.

Add the boiling water, cover, and cook over low heat 1 1/4 to 1 1/2 hours, or until the barley is tender. Stir occasionally to check progress. When done, the barley will be chewy but no longer hard. Add salt toward the end of cooking.

When cooking is complete, season generously with freshly ground pepper.

To make in a pressure cooker, combine the mushrooms, onion, soy sauce, barley, and 3 cups cold water. Cover, bring up to pressure, and pressure-cook for 50 minutes. Remove from the heat and let sit 5 minutes before gradually releasing the pressure with the quick-pressure-release valve (otherwise, let cool naturally). Season to taste with salt and pepper. Stir well to incorporate any remaining liquid, which the grain will continue to absorb as it sits.

YIELD: 4 1/2 CUPS; 4 TO 6 SERVINGS

★ THE G-FORCE OF BARLEY ★

Barley has a low G-Force compared with most grains (see G-Force Ratings in chapter 1). This makes it an excellent choice for people who are concerned about eating too much carbohydrate. Barley is also high in beta glucan, the soluble dietary fiber that helps reduce blood cholesterol.

Millet Polenta

~

The standard ratio for cooking millet is 3 cups liquid per 1 cup grain. When cooked with additional water in the manner presented here, millet develops the rich, creamy texture of cornmeal polenta. An advantage of using millet is that it offers substantially more protein (about 8.4 grams per cooked cup versus 2.2 grams for cornmeal). Serve topped with a favorite saucy bean dish, for example, White Beans with Swiss Chard, or with Creamy Garden Vegetables, Italian Style. For an impressive appetizer, top with grilled portobello mushrooms flavored with balsamic vinegar.

4 cups water
1 cup millet
1/2 teaspoon salt

2 cloves garlic, minced, optional
freshly ground pepper

Bring the water to a boil in a saucepan. Add the millet, salt, and garlic, if using. Cover and cook over low heat for 20 minutes.

Uncover the pot and continue to cook, stirring frequently, for 10 to 15 minutes, until the polenta becomes thick and has a soft, creamy texture. Season to taste with salt and pepper.

YIELD: 4 SERVINGS AS AN UNDERLAYER; 6 APPETIZER SERVINGS

Millet Polenta Patties

~

These broiled polenta patties are an excellent base for beans. Depending on the size of the meal, plan to serve 2 to 3 patties per person. According to the capacity of your oven, you may need to broil the patties in 2 batches. This final step can be done immediately following preparation, or the patties can be put together as long as a day in advance and refrigerated.

3 cups water
1 cup millet
1/2 teaspoon salt

1/2 cup shredded zucchini
1/2 cup shredded carrot
freshly ground pepper

Bring the water to a boil in a saucepan. Add the millet and salt, cover, and cook over low heat for 20 minutes.

Uncover the pot and continue to cook, stirring frequently, for about 10 more minutes, until the millet becomes quite thick and has a soft, creamy texture. Remove from the heat and stir in the shredded vegetables. Season to taste with salt and pepper.

Wipe a large baking sheet with olive or canola oil. Using 1/3 cup of polenta at a time, shape into patties on the oiled baking sheet. The patties can be broiled at once or prepared ahead, covered, and refrigerated at this point until needed.

To finish cooking, heat the broiler and place the baking sheet of polenta patties 4 to 6 inches below the heat. Cook about 5 minutes on each side, or until very lightly browned. Serve at once.

YIELD: 12 PATTIES; 4 TO 6 SERVINGS

Sunflower-Rice Patties

Serve these patties as an accompaniment or a light entrée. Size them based on intended role (and according to appetites). Allot 1/2 cup mixture for large-size patties or 1/3 cup for slightly smaller ones. Especially tasty garnished with Creamy Tomato Topping and joined by a bean soup or chili.

3 cups cooked brown rice
2 eggs, lightly beaten
1/2 teaspoon salt
1/4 cup flaxseed meal (page 239)
1/2 cup minced onion

1/4 cup minced green pepper
1/4 cup finely chopped parsley
1/4 cup sunflower seeds
canola oil or other cooking oil

In a large mixing bowl, combine all ingredients except the oil. Mix well.

Wipe the bottom of a large heavy skillet or griddle with oil and place over medium-high heat. You will probably need to cook this amount in 2 batches, unless you have a large griddle. When the surface of the pan is hot, arrange the rice mixture in mounds, using from 1/3 to 1/2 cup for each patty. Flatten each mound lightly with a spatula. Cook until golden brown on each side, turning once. Be sure to let the bottom brown before turning, as at this point the patties will hold together nicely. It will take about 8 minutes per side, but timing will vary with the heat and the pan.

YIELD: 8 TO 12 PATTIES; SERVES 4 TO 6

Vegetable-Corn Cakes

~

These delicate corn pancakes provide a nourishing accompaniment that takes the place of bread. Plan on 2 corn cakes per person, but if preferred as an entrée, figure on 4 per serving. Garnish with Pineapple Salsa, Salsa Cruda, or other favorite salsa and use as an accompaniment to cooked black beans and rice or sweet potatoes. Another option is to make the beans and salsa one, by choosing Black Bean Salsa. Note that a nonstick pan is essential for this recipe.

1 cup cornmeal	6 ounces firm tofu, cut into $1/4$-inch
$2^1/2$ teaspoons baking powder	cubes (1 cup)
1 cup soy milk	$1/3$ cup chopped red pepper
1 tablespoon light miso	$1/2$ cup corn kernels (fresh or frozen)
1 teaspoon canola oil	1 scallion, thinly sliced

Combine the cornmeal and baking powder in a mixing bowl. Add the soy milk, miso, and oil. Mix gently but thoroughly, so that the miso is distributed throughout, the cornmeal is completely moistened, and no lumps remain. Fold in the tofu and vegetables.

Heat a nonstick frying pan or griddle. When hot, drop the batter by one-quarter cupfuls onto the hot pan. Cook until brown on both sides; turn just once and do it gently to keep the delicate corn cakes from breaking apart. If preparing more than 1 panful, place the cooked corn cakes on a clean cloth napkin or dish towel and fold it around them to keep warm. If reheating is necessary, return to the pan briefly before serving.

YIELD: 8 CORN CAKES; 2 TO 4 SERVINGS

Salads and Salad Dressings

One of the easiest ways to add more vegetables to the daily menu is by serving a large tossed salad with meals. At its simplest, a salad can be composed of nothing more than greens. To add interest, start with a base of lettuce (loose-leaf or romaine) and jazz it up with some arugula, endive, radicchio, mesclun (mixed baby greens), mizuna, escarole, chicory, watercress, and such. It isn't much more effort to toss in some sprouts, carrot and cucumber slices, strips of sweet red or green pepper, diced celery, raw mushrooms, tomato wedges, grated red cabbage or raw beets, a handful of cooked beans, or some leftover cooked vegetables. A few olives, capers, or toasted pine nuts or pumpkin seeds make salads impressive with little effort.

With so many distinctive ingredients, your salad may not need any dressing at all. However, since the salad dressing recipes in this section are good in every sense of the word—tasty, replete with nutrients and phytochemicals, and made with the right fats or low in fat—feel free to use them to dress salads amply. Those with fat not only supply essential fatty acids, but can help you achieve a suitable fatty acid balance. In general, for side-dish salads plan on about 2 tablespoons dressing per serving; for main-dish salads allow at least 1/4 cup dressing per serving.

Creamy Miso-Mustard Coleslaw

⁓

As with all coleslaw recipes, you can vary this one by adding shredded carrots, slivered green pepper, or minced celery.

**1¹/₂ pounds cabbage, shredded
(about 7 cups)**

**³/₄ cup Creamy Miso-Mustard
Dressing (page 193)**

In a large bowl, combine the cabbage and dressing. Mix well until the dressing is evenly and thoroughly incorporated.

YIELD: ABOUT 5 CUPS; 4 TO 6 SERVINGS

Brussels Slaw

⁓

Although often disliked due to their strong sulfurous odor when cooked, brussels sprouts make excellent eating when served raw in the manner of coleslaw. They are a member of the same vegetable family as cabbage and broccoli and thus provide the same important cancer-protective phytochemicals, as well as being among the best sources of folate, vitamin C, vitamin K, potassium, and vegetable fiber (see Chapter 4).

**1 pint (10 ounces) brussels sprouts
¹/₂ cup yogurt
1 slightly rounded tablespoon
grainy mustard**

**1 tablespoon flaxseed or hemp oil
¹/₄ cup walnut pieces**

Cut the brussels sprouts into thin shreds. You should have a little more than 3 cups.

In a serving bowl, mix the yogurt with the mustard until evenly blended. Using a fork, beat in the oil. Add the cut brussels sprouts and walnut pieces to the dressing and mix well.

YIELD: 4 SERVINGS

*The
Healthiest
Diet in
the World*

Moroccan Carrot Slaw

A shredded carrot salad with a kick.

2 cups shredded carrots (4 to 5
   medium carrots)
3 tablespoons fresh orange juice
1/2 cup loosely packed cilantro
   and/or Italian flat-leaf parsley
1/2 teaspoon paprika

1/4 teaspoon cumin
1/8 teaspoon cayenne
1/8 teaspoon salt
1 tablespoon flaxseed, hemp, or
   olive oil

Place the carrots in a serving bowl. Combine the remaining ingredients in a
blender or food processor and puree. Pour the dressing over the carrots and
mix well.

Serve at once, hold 1 to 2 hours at room temperature, or refrigerator for service within a day or two.

YIELD: **4** SERVINGS

Spur-of-the-Moment Carrot Salad

Shredded carrots mixed with a favorite dressing provide a quick, last-minute
accompaniment to almost any meal.

1 1/2 cups coarsely shredded
   carrots (3 medium carrots)
1/4 cup slivered green
   pepper

1/4 cup Orange-Parsley Dressing
   (page 188), Tomato-Basil Dressing
   (page 188), or Piquant Mustard-
   Tomato Dressing (page 189)
1 tomato, cut into thin wedges

Combine the carrots and green pepper in a mixing bowl. Add the dressing of
choice and mix well. Divide among 4 individual serving plates. Place a few
tomato wedges alongside the dressed carrots.

YIELD: **4** SERVINGS

*In
Nikki's
Kitchen*

Carrot Raita

~

Grated carrots and yogurt unite in a salad that's soothing and spicy at the same time.

2 cups yogurt
1/2 teaspoon salt
2 carrots, coarsely grated

1/2 teaspoon cumin
1/4 teaspoon cayenne

In a serving bowl, stir the yogurt and salt into the carrots until evenly mixed. Sprinkle the cumin and cayenne on top.

YIELD: **4** SERVINGS

Roasted Corn Salad

~

Dry roasting corn kernels enhances the flavor of this salad, which also depends on fresh corn. Admittedly, it's a bit time consuming to roast all the components for this dish; to save steps, the hot peppers can be roasted in the oven along with the garlic, which takes longer than the broiler or open flame technique but requires less attention. Roasted Corn Salad is a good choice with bean, tofu, or tempeh entrées, or as a lively accent on a mixed vegetable plate.

2 long hot peppers
4 cloves garlic
4 ears corn (about 4 cups kernels)
1/2 cup chopped cucumber

2 scallions, thinly sliced
1/4 cup orange juice
1 teaspoon minced orange peel
1/4 teaspoon salt

Roast the hot peppers according to your preferred method (broiler, open flame, or oven—see "Gold Star Basics," page 242). Roast the garlic in the oven at 400°F. for about 20 minutes (see the directions for Roasted Garlic Cloves on page 242). When done, wrap the hot peppers in a clean towel to steam for a few minutes. When cool enough to handle, peel the peppers, remove the seeds, and chop. Mash the garlic.

Meanwhile, cut the corn kernels off the cob. Place a heavy cast-iron skillet over medium heat. When very hot, add the corn kernels and roast over fairly high heat, tossing frequently, until the kernels are lightly colored and starting to pop. This should take 15 to 20 minutes. Do not crowd the corn in the pan. If you don't have a large enough skillet (15 inches at least), roast in 2 batches. When cooked, transfer the corn to a serving bowl.

Add the roasted hot peppers, garlic, cucumber, scallions, orange juice and peel, and salt to the corn. Mix well. Serve at once or let sit at room temperature until serving time. Extra salad can be kept for several days in the refrigerator, but bring to room temperature to serve.

YIELD: 3 CUPS; 4 TO 6 SERVINGS

Cucumber-Tomato Salsa

For a lively hors d'oeuvre, spoon this spicy salsa on top of Baked Tortilla Crisps and top with yogurt cheese seasoned lightly with tomato juice (3 tablespoons juice per 1/2 cup yogurt cheese). The salsa can be made with less hot pepper according to taste preferences, and if prepared to accompany a spicy entrée, you may want to skip the hot pepper altogether. Although cilantro gives the salsa a more authentic flavor, parsley can be substituted for those who don't care for cilantro's distinctive taste.

1 cup chopped plum tomatoes
2 cups chopped cucumber (peel if
  skin is waxed)
1/4 cup minced scallions
1 tablespoon fresh lemon juice

1 jalapeño pepper, seeded and finely
  chopped
1/2 teaspoon salt
1/4 cup minced cilantro or Italian
  flat-leaf parsley

Combine all ingredients in a serving bowl. If made well in advance, cover and refrigerate until serving.

YIELD: 3 CUPS; 6 SERVINGS

★ PEPPER POINTER ★

When handling hot peppers, it's a good idea to wear rubber gloves. Thin surgical gloves are easy to work in. Avoid touching your skin or eyes. Rinse the knife and work surface before removing your gloves.

In Nikki's Kitchen

Yogurt-Cucumber Salad

~

This cooling salad, a standard in our repertoire, works in almost any menu. It can be varied by substituting 2 to 4 tablespoons fresh mint, parsley, or dill for the dried herb, by adding 1/2 teaspoon cumin instead, or with 2 thinly sliced scallions and/or a minced clove of garlic. Although simple to put together at the last minute, if the salad is prepared half an hour or more ahead the flavors have a chance to blend and develop. If prepared more than 1 hour before serving, refrigerate.

1/2 to 1 tablespoon crushed
  dried mint
1 cup yogurt

1 1/2 cups peeled, thinly sliced
  cucumber
small lemon wedge

In a serving bowl, beat the mint into the yogurt with a fork, gauging the amount by personal taste. Stir in the cucumber and squeeze in a little lemon juice.

YIELD: 4 SERVINGS

Fennel & Orange Salad

~

Pair this very refreshing salad with grain, pasta, or bean entrées.

1 large fennel bulb
2 navel oranges
1/2 small red onion, thinly sliced

black olives
balsamic vinegar
freshly ground pepper

Remove the stalks and feathery leaves (fronds) from the fennel. Discard the stalks. Set aside about 1 tablespoon chopped fronds; reserve the remainder for another use. Cut the fennel bulb in half lengthwise. Slice the fennel into thin wedges. Arrange on a serving plate.

Peel the oranges and separate into segments. Do this over the fennel plate so that any juice will be conserved. Intersperse orange segments with the fennel.

Scatter the onion slices over all. Garnish with the olives. Dress with a splash of balsamic vinegar and a generous amount of freshly ground pepper. Scatter the reserved fennel fronds on top. Serve at room temperature.

YIELD: 4 TO 6 SERVINGS

Warm Mushroom Salad

For a salad that's both economical and flavorful, a combination of half cultivated white and half exotic mushrooms works well. Of course, you can prepare this dish using only the exotics: cremini, shiitake, portobello, oyster, and chanterelle mushrooms. Or make it exclusively with the common white mushrooms.

2 cups sliced mushrooms (6 ounces)
2 tablespoons chopped shallots or scallions
1 large clove garlic, minced
2 tablespoons balsamic vinegar
1 cup diced tomato
1/4 teaspoon salt
4 to 6 cups mixed greens

Combine the mushrooms, shallots or scallions, garlic, and vinegar in a skillet. Sauté for 5 minutes, or until the mushroom juices run freely. Remove from the heat. Add the tomato and salt.

Divide the greens on 4 individual serving plates. Top with the warm mushroom-tomato mixture, spooning the juices in the pan over all. Serve immediately.

YIELD: 4 SERVINGS

In Nikki's Kitchen

Curried Tomato and Cucumber Salad

～

The seasoned vegetables for this salad can be prepared in advance and held at room temperature for about 1 hour or refrigerated for several hours, but wait until just before serving to add the yogurt.

2 teaspoons curry powder
1/2 teaspoon cumin
1 1/2 cups diced tomato
1 1/2 cups peeled diced cucumber
2 cloves garlic, minced

3 tablespoons chopped fresh
  cilantro
1/4 teaspoon salt
1 cup yogurt

Place the curry powder and cumin in a dry skillet. Set over low heat and stir for about 1 minute, until aromatic. Remove from the heat.

In a serving bowl, combine the tomato, cucumber, garlic, and cilantro. Add the toasted seasonings and salt. Mix well.

Just before serving, stir in the yogurt.

YIELD: **4** TO **6** SERVINGS

Orange-Arame Salad

～

Arame is a shredded, dark brown sea grass with a mild aroma and flavor. It's a good introduction to sea vegetables, as it tastes the least strongly of the sea. If not available locally, mail order sources for arame and other seaweeds are listed in "Resources."

1 cup arame
1 cup orange juice
a few slices of red onion

2 small oranges
1/2 cup coarsely chopped walnuts

Combine the arame and orange juice in a small saucepan and let sit for 5 to 10 minutes to soften. Bring to a boil and simmer for 5 minutes. Remove from the heat, add the onion slices, and let cool to room temperature.

Using a sharp paring knife, peel and section the oranges according to the directions on page 183. Do this over a shallow serving bowl to catch any juices.

Transfer the arame mixture to the bowl. Top with the orange segments. Sprinkle the walnuts on top.

YIELD: **4** SERVINGS

Spinach-Yogurt Salad

~

You can hold this salad at room temperature for about 1 hour in cool weather, but if made well in advance or in hot weather, refrigerate until ready to serve.

1/2 pound spinach
2 tablespoons lemon juice
1/4 teaspoon salt

1 cup yogurt
1 teaspoon dried mint

Wash the spinach well and drain afterward to remove as much water as possible. Discard any tough stems. Place in a pot, cover, and cook over moderate heat for 5 to 10 minutes to wilt.

Cool the spinach enough to handle. Squeeze out as much moisture as possible. (The liquid can be saved for soup stock.) Chop. You should have about 1 cup.

In a serving bowl, combine the chopped spinach with the lemon juice, salt, and yogurt. Mix well. Sprinkle the mint on top.

YIELD: 4 SERVINGS

Basil-Bean Salad

~

This basic recipe can be followed with almost any bean and using dressings other than Tomato-Basil. For a more elaborate salad, add 1/2 cup cooked fresh or thawed frozen corn kernels.

2 cups cooked chickpeas, white
beans, pink beans, or black beans,
well drained
1/2 cup chopped celery or sweet red
or green pepper

1/2 cup Tomato-Basil Dressing
(page 188)

Combine all ingredients and let marinate in a covered bowl for 1 hour at room temperature. If prepared more than an hour or so ahead, refrigerate until serving. Keeps for several days.

YIELD: 4 SERVINGS

Black Bean Salsa

Serve this salsa as a side dish or topping for grains and/or vegetables. Canned beans are perfectly acceptable here. Regarding the hot pepper: For a spicy salsa use jalapeño; for a less spicy dish choose serrano or hot chile pepper. If preferred, omit the fresh hot pepper and season to taste with prepared hot pepper sauce.

2 cups cooked black beans, rinsed and drained
1/4 cup minced red or sweet white onion (such as Vidalia or Walla Walla)
1/2 cup minced green pepper
1 cup diced tomato

1 large clove garlic, minced
1 teaspoon cumin
1/4 cup minced cilantro or parsley
3 tablespoons fresh lime juice
1 tablespoon minced hot pepper or to taste
salt

Combine all ingredients in a serving bowl, seasoning with hot pepper and salt to taste. Cover and let stand at least 30 minutes to give the flavors a chance to fully develop. If prepared more than a few hours ahead, chill. If the salad has been chilled, return to room temperature to serve.

YIELD: 3 1/2 CUPS; 4 SERVINGS

Rice Salad

Rice Salad can be made many different ways. Here's a model to guide you. Decorating with brightly colored tomatoes or orange sections (depending on the nature of the dressing) creates visual appeal.

3 cups cooked brown rice
1 cup Orange-Parsley Dressing (page 188), Piquant Mustard-Tomato Dressing (page 189), or Tomato-Basil Dressing (page 188)

Garnishes of choice: sunflower seeds or toasted pumpkin seeds; capers; radishes; halved cherry tomatoes; peeled orange segments

Have the rice warm or at room temperature. If made with precooked rice, remove from the refrigerator several hours ahead or warm gently in a pot.

Combine the rice and dressing of choice in a serving bowl. Mix well. Let marinate 30 minutes to 2 hours at room temperature.

Just before serving, decorate with seeds, capers, radishes, cherry tomatoes, orange segments, or other colorful condiments of choice.

YIELD: 4 TO 6 SERVINGS

Warm Bulgur Salad

To serve, place in a shallow serving bowl and let diners scoop the salad up with lettuce leaves.

1¹/₂ cups strong peppermint tea
1 cup bulgur (cracked wheat)
¹/₄ cup sunflower seeds
¹/₃ cup chopped red, Vidalia, Maui, or other sweet onion

¹/₂ cup lightly packed chopped parsley
2 tablespoons chopped capers
2 tablespoons lemon juice
salt

Combine the tea, bulgur, and sunflower seeds in a pot. Bring to a boil, cover, and cook over low heat for 10 minutes. Remove from the heat, stir in the onion, and let sit, uncovered, for about 10 minutes. By this time all the liquid should be absorbed. Transfer to a serving bowl.

Using a fork, mix the parsley, capers, and lemon juice into the grain. Season with salt to taste. Serve warm or at room temperature. Just before serving, fluff the salad with a fork to separate the grains.

YIELD: 3 CUPS; 4 TO 6 SERVINGS

VARIATION: For *Cinnamon-scented Cracked Wheat Salad*, omit the capers and add 2 tablespoons currants or chopped raisins to the pot along with the onion. Season with ¹/₂ teaspoon cinnamon when adding the parsley and lemon juice.

Tomato-Basil Dressing

~

A tasty fat-free dressing for green salads, or to pour over thick slices of fresh summer tomatoes, hot steamed potatoes, green beans, or cauliflower, or to use for dressing cooked beans (see Basil-Bean Salad).

1 cup loosely packed fresh basil
  leaves
1 clove garlic
1 tablespoon balsamic vinegar

1 teaspoon French-style or grainy
  mustard
1/2 cup tomato or V-8 juice

Combine all ingredients in a blender or food processor. Puree until the basil is finely chopped and the dressing is emulsified.

If prepared in advance, beat with a fork or shake to recombine before pouring.

YIELD: 3/4 CUP

Orange-Parsley Dressing

~

Two tablespoons of this dressing furnish 3.5 grams of fat with the proportion of specific fatty acids determined by your choice of hemp, flaxseed, or olive oil (see Chapter 2). A typical 2-tablespoon serving of bottled dressing ranges from 12 to 16 grams of fat.

1/2 cup orange juice
1/4 cup red wine vinegar
1 cup loosely packed parsley leaves
1/4 teaspoon salt

1/4 teaspoon cayenne
2 tablespoons hemp, flaxseed, or
  olive oil

Combine all ingredients in a blender or food processor. Puree until the parsley is finely chopped and the dressing is emulsified.

If prepared in advance, beat with a fork or shake to recombine before pouring.

YIELD: 1 CUP

*The
Healthiest
Diet in
the World*

Piquant Mustard-Tomato Dressing

~

As the name implies, this is a tangy dressing. For something more mellow and creamy, try the variation that follows.

1/2 cup cider vinegar
1/4 cup unsweetened or fruit juice–sweetened (natural) ketchup
1 teaspoon prepared mustard

3 tablespoons orange juice
1 teaspoon maple syrup
1 clove garlic, minced
1/2 teaspoon paprika

Combine all ingredients, beating with a fork or whisk until blended. Shake or beat again just prior to serving.

YIELD: 3/4 CUP

VARIATION: For *Creamy Mustard-Tomato Dressing*, beat the dressing gradually into 3 tablespoons yogurt cheese (to prevent curdling).

Creamy Italian Dressing

~

In addition to good taste, you get about 2 grams of largely monounsaturated oleic acid in each 2-tablespoon serving versus 15.5 grams of fat in a standard bottled creamy Italian dressing.

1/3 cup red wine vinegar
2 scallions, thinly sliced
1/3 cup water
1 clove garlic, split
1/2 teaspoon dried basil

1/2 teaspoon dried oregano
1 teaspoon honey
4 canned artichoke hearts, drained
1 tablespoon olive oil
freshly ground pepper

Combine all ingredients except the pepper in a blender or food processor. Puree until smooth. Add freshly ground pepper to taste.

YIELD: 3/4 CUP

189

In Nikki's Kitchen

Yogonaise

~

Yogonaise can be used as a salad dressing or as a dipping sauce for steamed artichokes, asparagus, broccoli, or cauliflower; for binding potatoes in potato salad; and for general use in place of traditional mayonnaise. In return, when made with nonfat yogurt and compared to mayonnaise you receive about seven times the protein (about 1 gram per tablespoon), thirteen times more calcium (about 30 mg per tablespoon), less than half the sodium, and one-third the fat and calories (less than 35 per tablespoon).

1/2 cup yogurt
1 tablespoon grainy mustard

2 tablespoons flaxseed or hemp seed oil

Using a fork, beat the yogurt together with the mustard until evenly blended. Beat in the oil.

YIELD: ABOUT 2/3 CUP

Tofu Mayonnaise

~

Soft tofu makes a surprisingly creamy and tasty "mayonnaise." Each tablespoon also offers more than a gram of protein, a mere 0.5 grams fat, and 20 mg calcium within just 10 calories.

8 ounces soft tofu
2 tablespoons lemon juice
1 tablespoon cider vinegar

2 teaspoons prepared mustard
2 teaspoons light miso
pinch of salt

Combine all ingredients in a blender or food processor. Puree until creamy. Store in the refrigerator and use within 1 week.

YIELD: 1 CUP

Creamy Tofu Russian Dressing

Due to variations in texture between different brands of tofu, the amount of soy milk in this recipe may need adjustment to reach the desired pourable dressing consistency. While the flavor and texture of soft tofu is preferred, the dressing can be made with firmer tofu. If so, additional soy milk will be needed.

8 ounces soft tofu
2 tablespoons lemon juice
1 tablespoon cider vinegar
1 teaspoon prepared mustard
2 teaspoons dark miso
1/2 cup diced peeled cucumber

1/2 cup soy milk
1/2 cup fruit juice–sweetened or unsweetened ketchup
1/4 teaspoon hot pepper sauce or to taste

Combine the tofu, lemon juice, cider vinegar, mustard, miso, and cucumber in a blender or food processor. Puree until evenly blended. Gradually add the soy milk and process to a smooth consistency. Add the ketchup and hot sauce and blend briefly to incorporate. Add additional soy milk, if necessary, to obtain a rich, pourable consistency.

YIELD: 2 CUPS

Creamy Tofu Ranch Dressing

As with Creamy Tofu Russian Dressing, the exact amount of soy milk needed for a rich but pourable consistency may vary depending on the density of the tofu used.

8 ounces soft tofu
2 tablespoons lemon juice
1 tablespoon cider vinegar
1 tablespoon prepared mustard
2 teaspoons light miso

1/2 teaspoon turmeric
1 clove garlic
1/2 cup peeled diced cucumber
1/2 cup soy milk

Combine all ingredients except the soy milk in a blender or food processor. Puree until evenly blended. Gradually add the soy milk and process to a smooth, creamy, pourable consistency.

YIELD: 1 3/4 CUPS

*In
Nikki's
Kitchen*

Cucumber-Yogurt Dressing

This cool and refreshing dressing adds a protein and calcium boost to salads.

1/2 cup diced peeled cucumber
1 clove garlic, sliced
1 tablespoon fresh dill
1/4 teaspoon salt
1 tablespoon lemon juice

1 tablespoon tahini
1 tablespoon flaxseed, hemp, or
   olive oil
3/4 cup yogurt

Combine the cucumber, garlic, dill, salt, lemon juice, tahini, oil, and 1/4 cup yogurt in a blender or food processor. Puree until smooth. Beat in the remaining 1/2 cup yogurt with a fork.

Store in the refrigerator until serving time.

YIELD: ABOUT 1 CUP

Lemon-Tahini Dressing

This fundamental dressing can be modified in a number of ways. For example, for seasoning you can add 1 tablespoon minced fresh dill, parsley, and/or 1 clove chopped garlic. Or, you can add a few vegetables and prepare it in a blender or food processor.

1/4 cup lemon juice
1/4 cup tahini
1/4 cup water

1 teaspoon soy sauce
1/4 teaspoon salt
1/3 cup yogurt

Using a fork or wire whisk, beat the lemon juice into the tahini. Gradually beat in the water until creamy. Stir in the soy sauce, salt, and yogurt.

YIELD: 1 CUP

VARIATION: To add vegetables to the dressing, combine all ingredients except the yogurt in a blender or food processor; add 1 cut-up scallion or a slice of onion, 1 small celery stalk with leaves, and 1 wedge green pepper. Process until the vegetables are integrated into the dressing. Stir in the yogurt.

The Healthiest Diet in the World

Creamy Miso-Mustard Dressing

A good dressing for a mixed salad, coleslaw, or a creamy bean salad.

$1/3$ cup tahini
1 tablespoon prepared mustard
1 tablespoon dark miso

3 tablespoons cider vinegar
$1/4$ to $1/3$ cup water

Using a fork, combine the tahini, mustard, and miso. Beat in the cider vinegar. Gradually beat in the water to make a creamy, pourable dressing.

YIELD: 3/4 CUP

Sauces and Toppings

Sauces and toppings are what cooks all over the world rely on to make foods especially inviting. Almost any unadorned food—plain grains, simple steamed vegetables, basic beans, timid tofu or tempeh—can be brought to life by a shot of sauce or a tablespoon (or two) of topping. Sauces also make spirited dips for vegetables or bread.

In this section you'll find some favorite sauces that offer more than just good taste. Each mouthful adds valuable nutrient helpers, phytochemicals, and sometimes even protein to the meal. Moreover, these sauces help improve the ratio of overall fats, the right fats, and compatible carbohydrates in your daily diet.

Because of their positive nature, we encourage you to indulge. Give grains plenty of gravy. Blanket those beans. Smother your vegetables. And sop up all the sauce.

Portobello Mushroom Topping

The complex sweet-tangy flavor of balsamic vinegar melds with the earthiness of the mushrooms, creating a dynamic topping for polenta, brown rice, or other cooked grains, baked potatoes, pasta, or just a hearty slice of bread. If you want to economize, replace up to half the portobello mushrooms with another variety of exotic or even cultivated mushroom.

4 cups sliced portobello mushrooms (3/4 pound)
1/2 cup chopped shallots or red onion
2 large cloves garlic, minced

2 tablespoons soy sauce
1/4 cup water
1/4 cup balsamic vinegar
1/4 cup canned crushed tomatoes
1/2 cup chopped parsley

Combine the mushrooms, shallots, garlic, soy sauce, and water in a large skillet. Cover and cook over medium-low heat for 10 to 15 minutes, until the mushrooms are tender. Add the vinegar, crushed tomatoes, and parsley. Cook, uncovered, for about 5 minutes, stirring several times, until heated through and the flavor of the vinegar infuses the mushrooms.

YIELD: **4** TO **6** SERVINGS

Sea Vegetable Topping

Arame and hijiki are both mild-tasting seaweeds and good choices for introducing nutritious sea vegetables to the table. (Novices may prefer the less briny taste and tender texture of arame.) Among their many mineral attributes, seaweeds are rich in natural fluoride and iodine, and these particular varieties are good sources of calcium. Use this Sea Vegetable Topping to garnish salads, vegetables, and bean and grain dishes, or add to soups and sandwiches for flavor and nutrition. It can be used immediately and will keep for a week or two in the refrigerator. (For mail order sources see "Resources.")

1/2 cup arame or hijiki
warm water
1/4 cup reserved soaking water

1 tablespoon soy sauce
1 teaspoon toasted sesame oil

Place the seaweed in a bowl and pour on warm water to cover. Let soak for 5 to 10 minutes, until it swells and softens. Drain, reserving 1/4 cup soaking water.

In a small saucepan, combine the seaweed, reserved soaking water, and soy sauce. Simmer, uncovered, for 3 to 5 minutes, or until tender; hijiki may require an additional few minutes.

Remove from the heat and stir in the oil.

YIELD: 3/4 CUP

Chickpea Pesto

Chickpea Pesto can be served in the traditional manner of pesto by simply stirring this entire recipe into 12 ounces of warm pasta immediately after cooking. It will suffice for 4 as an entrée or 6 as an accompaniment. Serve with grated parmesan on the side for cheese eaters to add to taste. Chickpea Pesto is also an ideal garnish for grilled eggplant slices, warm boiled potatoes, or Wine-Simmered Vegetables, and a favorite filling for mushrooms, as in Pesto-Stuffed Mushrooms.

2 tablespoons pine nuts
1/2 cup cooked chickpeas, drained
2 cups lightly packed basil leaves or
   a mixture of basil and parsley
2 cloves garlic, chopped

2 tablespoons chickpea cooking
   liquid
1 tablespoon olive oil
salt to taste

Toast the pine nuts in a dry skillet until aromatic and lightly colored. Be careful not to overcook.

Combine the pine nuts and chickpeas in a food processor and grind. Add the herbs and garlic and puree to a thick paste. Add the chickpea cooking liquid and process until evenly blended. Add the oil and process until completely incorporated. Adjust salt to taste; need will vary according to the saltiness of the beans and whether cheese is served on the side (as for pasta with pesto).

YIELD: 7/8 CUP; 4 SERVINGS

Creamy Walnut Pesto

Serve this Creamy Walnut Pesto on a baked potato; mix with hot steamed green beans, carrots, broccoli, or cauliflower; stir into a combination of hot steamed vegetables and cooked chickpeas or white beans to create a main dish; or spoon into raw mushroom caps or spread on sliced tomato, raw zucchini rounds, or bread for hors d'oeuvres. It's also the pesto of choice for Two Beans with Creamy Walnut Pesto and White Beans and Carrots with Creamy Walnut Pesto. The proportion below is adequate for 4 to 6 servings; for example, 6 baked potatoes, or 1 1/2 pounds cooked vegetables, or up to 1 pound vegetables mixed with 3 to 4 cups cooked beans.

The Healthiest Diet in the World

1/4 cup walnuts
2 cups lightly packed herbs or greens of choice, alone or in combination (basil, parsley, arugula, spinach)

2 cloves garlic, chopped
1/4 teaspoon salt
1 tablespoon light miso
1/4 cup Yogurt Cheese (page 244)

Grind the walnuts in a food processor. Add the herbs or greens, garlic, and salt and puree to a thick paste. Add the miso and Yogurt Cheese and blend once more to a smooth thick sauce.

YIELD: 3/4 CUP; 4 TO 6 SERVINGS

Tomato-Almond Pesto

Spoon this pesto over cooked brown rice and mixed steamed vegetables (carrots, cauliflower, zucchini, green beans), mixing well to incorporate. For an interesting taste variation, replace the basil with cilantro.

1/2 cup almonds
2 cloves garlic, chopped
1/2 cup lightly packed basil leaves
1/2 cup lightly packed parsley

1 cup chopped drained tomatoes
1/2 teaspoon salt
1 tablespoon olive oil

Grind the almonds in a food processor. Add the garlic, basil, parsley, tomato, and salt. Process until the garlic and herbs are finely minced and the ingredients are evenly blended. Add the olive oil and process until incorporated.

YIELD: 1 1/4 CUPS; 4 SERVINGS

In Nikki's Kitchen

Spicy Orange-Nut Sauce

This mildly sweet and spicy sauce can be made with your choice of nut butter. Pour while still warm over steamed, Grilled, or Oven-Roasted Vegetables, tofu, tempeh, pasta, or grains, or serve as a dipping sauce.

<table>
<tr><td>1/2 cup unsalted, unsweetened almond, cashew, or peanut butter</td><td>1/2 teaspoon crushed red pepper flakes</td></tr>
<tr><td>1 3/4 cups orange juice</td><td>2 tablespoons lemon juice</td></tr>
<tr><td>1 teaspoon minced fresh garlic</td><td>1 tablespoon molasses</td></tr>
<tr><td>1 teaspoon minced fresh ginger</td><td>2 teaspoons soy sauce</td></tr>
</table>

In a small saucepan, combine the nut butter, about half of the orange juice, and the remaining ingredients. Place over moderate heat and cook, stirring continuously, until the nut butter softens and melts into the juice. Stir in the remaining juice and continue to cook and stir until the sauce starts to simmer. Continue to stir and simmer gently for 1 to 2 minutes, until the sauce is thick and creamy.

YIELD: ABOUT 1 1/2 CUPS; 4 TO 6 SERVINGS

Creamy Tomato Topping

An ideal garnish for beans, Sunflower Rice Patties, or Millet Polenta Patties. Sprinkle a little chopped fresh parsley, cilantro, or basil on top for appearance.

<table>
<tr><td>1/2 cup Yogurt Cheese (page 244)</td><td>1/4 cup finely chopped rehydrated dried tomatoes</td></tr>
<tr><td>1/4 cup canned crushed tomatoes</td><td>hot pepper sauce to taste</td></tr>
</table>

Combine the Yogurt Cheese and tomatoes in a bowl. Mix until evenly blended. Add the hot sauce to taste.

YIELD: ABOUT 3/4 CUP; 4 SERVINGS

★ TOMATO TIP #3 ★

To rehydrate dried tomatoes, run quickly under cold water, then let sit for about 5 minutes to soften before chopping.

Curry-Yogurt Cream

~

A flavorful topping for beans, grains, baked potatoes or beets, or other simple vegetable dishes.

1 teaspoon curry powder   1/2 cup Yogurt Cream (page 244)

Mix 1/2 teaspoon curry powder into the Yogurt Cream and let sit for 5 minutes. Taste. If not flavorful enough, add the remaining 1/2 teaspoon curry powder, mix, and let sit at least 5 minutes longer before serving. If not used immediately, refrigerate.

YIELD: 1/2 CUP; 4 SERVINGS

Better Than Ketchup

~

Low in sodium, rich in lycopene. For burgers, Baked Tofu Sticks, eggs, or anything else you put ketchup on.

1/2 cup tomato paste   2 teaspoons minced fresh ginger
2 teaspoons maple syrup   1/2 cup apple juice
1/4 cup lemon juice or cider vinegar   pinch cayenne

Using a fork, beat together all ingredients to form a smooth sauce, just a bit thinner than ketchup and seasoned with cayenne to taste. Use at once or store in the refrigerator for long-term use.

YIELD: 3/4 CUP

In Nikki's Kitchen

Salsa Cruda

A very hot salsa. If a more temperate salsa is preferred, use a serrano or other milder pepper, or reduce the jalapeño by half. If cilantro isn't available, or not to your taste, use parsley and cumin in its place.

2 large ripe tomatoes
2 scallions, thinly sliced
1 clove garlic, minced
1 jalapeño pepper, minced
  (2 tablespoons)

2 tablespoons cilantro or
  2 tablespoons flat-leaf parsley plus
  1/2 teaspoon cumin
2 tablespoons fresh lime juice

Chop the tomatoes and place in a serving bowl along with the juice released during chopping. Add the remaining ingredients and mix well. Cover and chill until serving time.

YIELD: 1 1/2 CUPS; 4 SERVINGS

Pineapple Salsa

Serve with grilled tofu or tempeh, Vegetable-Corn Cakes, or Chickpea Roast. Select the hot pepper variety and adjust the amount according to taste preferences. In general, jalapeño tends to be hotter than generic chile peppers and scotch bonnet is the hottest of all. However, even peppers of the same type tend to vary in spiciness due to growing conditions. It's best to start with less and add more after tasting if you're concerned about making a dish too spicy. If the salsa isn't fiery enough, it can be remedied at the last minute by adding cayenne, crushed red pepper flakes (pizza pepper), or hot pepper sauce.

1 cup chopped fresh or drained
  pineapple chunks canned in juice
  (16-ounce can)
1/2 cup chopped sweet red pepper
2 tablespoons minced fresh hot
  pepper

1/4 cup chopped onion (regular, red,
  or a sweet variety like Vidalia)
2 tablespoons chopped fresh mint
1 teaspoon lemon juice

Combine all ingredients. Refrigerate until serving time.

YIELD: 2 CUPS; 6 SERVINGS

Quick Spicy Mexican Tomato Sauce

When you need a Mexican-style tomato sauce, this one will be ready in just 15 minutes.

1 1/2 tablespoons dry red wine or
   cooking sherry
1 small onion, chopped
2 cloves garlic, chopped
2 tablespoons minced hot pepper or
   1/4 teaspoon cayenne

1 tablespoon chili powder
1 teaspoon cumin
4 cups tomato juice

In a saucepan, combine the wine or sherry, onion, garlic, and hot pepper, if using. Cook over medium heat for 2 minutes to soften the onion. Stir in the chili powder, cumin, and cayenne, if using instead of the hot pepper, and cook briefly. Add the tomato juice, bring to a boil, and simmer, uncovered, for about 10 minutes, until the sauce is slightly thickened.

YIELD: **4** CUPS

15-Minute Italian Tomato Sauce

A quickly made red sauce for pasta, Soy Balls, and other Italian applications.

1½ tablespoons dry red wine or
   cooking sherry
2 cloves garlic, chopped
1 medium green pepper, cut into
   thin 1-inch-long strips

3 cups tomato juice
2 tablespoons tomato paste
1 teaspoon oregano
1 tablespoon fresh or
   1 teaspoon dried basil

In a saucepan, combine the wine or sherry, garlic, and green pepper. Cook over medium heat for about 5 minutes, stirring several times, to soften the pepper slightly. Add the remaining ingredients, bring to a boil, and simmer, uncovered, for about 10 minutes, until the sauce is slightly thickened.

YIELD: 3 CUPS

Puttanesca Sauce

A rich, thick, hearty tomato sauce with a lot of flavor. In addition to its nutritional contribution, the miso softens the harshness that's characteristic of some canned tomato products. Puttanesca is excellent on cheese- or tofu-filled ravioli or tortellini, Eggplant Rollatini, as well as on plain pasta. The sauce can also be spooned over other grains, tempeh, or cooked vegetables such as potatoes, cauliflower, green beans, mushrooms, and squash. Two cups sauce is enough for 1 pound ravioli, tortellini, or plain pasta. Those who prefer a looser sauce can stir in a few tablespoons of the water used to cook pasta before serving. For a lighter sauce, replace canned crushed tomatoes with lightly drained and chopped canned whole tomatoes or tomato pieces.

2 cups canned crushed tomatoes
4 cloves garlic, sliced
¼ cup chopped imported black or
   green olives
2 tablespoons capers
½ teaspoon crushed red pepper
   flakes or to taste

1 tablespoon fresh or ½ teaspoon
   dried basil
½ teaspoon oregano
2 tablespoons light miso
2 tablespoons chopped parsley
2 tablespoons toasted pine nuts,
   optional (page 241)

Combine the tomatoes, garlic, olives, capers, red pepper flakes, basil, and oregano in a saucepan. Bring to a boil over medium heat, stirring occasionally. Reduce the heat and simmer gently for 10 minutes. Remove from the heat.

In a small bowl, mix the miso with a little hot tomato sauce. Stir until the miso melts into the sauce. Mix into the pot of hot tomato sauce along with the parsley. Cover and let sit 5 minutes before using. If the sauce needs reheating, place over low heat and cook, stirring, until hot; try not to boil as this diminishes the value of the miso.

If desired, sprinkle toasted pine nuts on top of the sauced dish at serving time.

YIELD: 2 CUPS; 4 SERVINGS

Greek Garlic Sauce

~

Greek Garlic Sauce resembles a garlicky mayonnaise, without the egg and with a minimal amount of oil. It can be put to numerous imaginative uses; for example, spread on raw tomato or cucumber slices, as an appetizer on toast rounds, spooned on top of grilled eggplant slices or beans, as a sauce for steamed vegetables, or lathered on thin slices of toast and floated in a bowl of soup. For a lighter dip for raw vegetables, add some yogurt cheese.

2 small new or red potatoes (6 ounces), quartered
1 cup water
1/2 teaspoon salt
2 cloves garlic

1/4 cup finely chopped parsley or in combination with dill
2 tablespoons lemon juice
2 tablespoons olive oil

Place the potatoes in a small saucepan with the water. Bring to a boil, add 1/4 teaspoon salt, cover, and simmer gently for about 15 minutes, or until the potatoes are quite tender. Drain, reserving the liquid. Remove the peels from the potatoes.

In a bowl, combine the garlic with the remaining 1/4 teaspoon salt and mash completely, using a mortar or the back of a spoon. Add the drained potatoes and mash into the garlic, using a potato masher or fork, until no lumps remain. Beat in the parsley, lemon juice, and 1/3 to 1/2 cup reserved cooking liquid, or as needed, to produce a sauce a little thicker than mayonnaise. Beat in the oil. Served at once at room temperature or chill.

YIELD: 1 CUP

Agliata

Rich garlic sauces are popular in many cultures, with numerous variations. The French have a mayonnaise-based sauce they call aioli. In Turkey, a creamy garlic sauce called tarator is often flavored with chopped parsley and combined with thick yogurt as a dip. The Greeks use a base of potatoes for their garlic sauce. Agliata is the Italian name for the sauce that inspired this recipe. Serve on Tofu-stuffed Artichokes, Tofu-stuffed Sweet Red Peppers, Alan's Curry Tofu Cubes, or cooked rice, or use as a dipping sauce for steamed artichokes.

1 to 2 slices whole-grain bread
1/2 cup soy milk
1/4 cup walnuts
1 large clove garlic, coarsely
  chopped

1 1/2 tablespoons lemon juice
1 tablespoon olive oil
1/8 teaspoon salt

Trim the crusts from the bread and tear the remainder into small pieces to make 1/2 cup crumbs (lightly packed). Combine the bread crumbs and soy milk in a blender and let sit for a few minutes, until the bread absorbs the liquid and becomes soft. Add the walnuts, garlic, lemon juice, olive oil, and salt. Process to a smooth sauce with the consistency of thick heavy cream.

YIELD: 3/4 CUP; 4 SERVINGS

Sweet Onion Gravy

The gentle stewing of the onions for this gravy gives them a rich velvety texture and sweet mellow taste.

2 cups coarsely chopped red onion
  or sweet white onion
2 tablespoons cooking sherry
1/4 cup whole wheat flour

2 cups soy milk
2 tablespoons light miso
freshly ground pepper
salt

In a saucepan, combine the onions and sherry. Cover and cook over low heat for 8 to 10 minutes, until the onions are quite tender. Sprinkle the flour over the onions and stir until evenly mixed. Gradually stir in the soy milk and continue cooking over moderate heat, stirring continuously, until the gravy thickens and begins to boil. Reduce the heat and simmer gently for 1 minute.

Remove from the heat and stir in the miso until thoroughly melted. Season with a generous amount of freshly ground pepper and salt to taste, if desired.

If the gravy needs reheating, place over low heat and cook gently, while stirring, until warm. Do not boil.

YIELD: ABOUT 2 CUPS

Creamy Mushroom Gravy

~

Creamy Mushroom Gravy is delicious made with cultivated white mushrooms. However, for a more pronounced earthy taste, up to half the mushrooms can be exotic varieties such as chanterelles, creminis, shiitakes, or portobellos. Although the flavor is rich, the color of this gravy is dull; if desired, the appearance of a dish can be perked up with a generous garnish of chopped fresh parsley.

<table>
<tr><td>1/2 pound thinly sliced mushrooms (2 1/2 cups)</td><td>2 cups soy milk</td></tr>
<tr><td>2 tablespoons cooking sherry or dry white wine</td><td>2 tablespoons light miso
freshly ground pepper
salt</td></tr>
<tr><td>5 tablespoons whole wheat flour</td><td></td></tr>
</table>

In a saucepan, combine the mushrooms and sherry or wine. Cook over moderate heat, stirring occasionally, for 5 to 8 minutes, until the mushrooms are tender and release their juices. Sprinkle the flour over the mushrooms and stir until evenly blended.

Gradually stir in the soy milk and continue cooking over moderate heat, stirring continuously, until the gravy thickens and begins to boil. Reduce the heat and simmer gently for 1 minute.

Remove from the heat and stir in the miso until thoroughly dissolved. Season with a generous amount of freshly ground pepper and salt to taste, if desired.

If the gravy needs reheating, place over low heat and cook gently, while stirring, until warm. Do not boil.

YIELD: ABOUT 3 CUPS

*In
Nikki's
Kitchen*

Tahini-Mushroom Gravy

This rich creamy gravy is excellent on cooked grains, tofu, tempeh, or chick-peas. Note: If the sauce curdles during cooking (which can happen if it gets too hot), simply remove from the heat and stir vigorously with a fork to recombine.

1/2 cup dried porcini mushrooms	1/2 cup cold water
2/3 cup hot water	1 tablespoon dark miso
1/4 cup tahini	1 lemon wedge

Place the dried mushrooms in a bowl, cover with the hot water, and let stand about 15 minutes to soften. Drain the mushrooms through a strainer, reserving the liquid. Tear the mushrooms into pieces.

In a small saucepan, gradually beat the reserved mushroom liquid into the tahini with a fork. Beat in the cold water until smooth. Add the mushrooms, place over low heat, and cook, stirring continuously, until the sauce just starts to boil.

Stir a little of the hot sauce into the miso to melt. Mix back into the sauce along with the juice from the lemon wedge and heat briefly without boiling.

If reheating is necessary, place over very low heat and cook, stirring gently, until warm, but do not boil.

YIELD: 1 1/2 CUPS; 4 SERVINGS

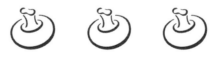

Artichoke-Cheese Sauce

〜

This thick creamy sauce is designed to just coat the surface of hot pasta or vegetables. It can be employed in a number of ways. Our favorite is to steam an assortment of vegetables (for example, cauliflower, potatoes, green beans, carrots), add some cooked chickpeas, and mix the sauce and hot vegetables together. It's also delicious combined with steamed cauliflorets or a simple pasta. The amount here is enough for 4 cups cooked vegetables and chickpeas, or a good-size head of cauliflower, or 3/4 pound pasta. Be sure to cook the sauce over very low heat and stir continuously. It takes only a few minutes to cook, but requires your constant attention during this time.

1 can (14 ounces) artichoke hearts in water
1 cup Yogurt Cheese (page 244)
1/2 cup grated cheese (parmesan, provolone, cheddar, jack, feta, or other natural cheese individually or mixed)

2 tablespoons sun-dried tomatoes, optional
1/8 teaspoon hot pepper sauce
1/4 cup chopped parsley

Drain the artichokes, reserving the liquid. Chop the artichokes into small pieces.

In a saucepan, combine the artichokes with the remaining ingredients except the parsley. Stir in 3 tablespoons reserved liquid. Place over the lowest heat your stove allows and cook, stirring continuously, for about 5 minutes, until the cheese melts and the sauce is hot. If needed, gradually stir in another tablespoon of reserved liquid or water to create a sauce that is quite thick but not stiff. Do not boil. When the sauce is hot and creamy, remove from the heat and stir in the parsley.

To serve, combine with freshly steamed vegetables or hot pasta; mix gently until the sauce is evenly distributed.

YIELD: 2 1/4 CUPS; 4 SERVINGS

*In
Nikki's
Kitchen*

Spicy Marinade

⁓

This recipe makes enough marinade for 1 pound of tofu or tempeh (4 servings) or 1/2 pound of soy product, plus 6 to 8 mushroom caps and enough broccoli, eggplant, cauliflower, sweet potato slices, and the like to serve 2 people. Therefore, if you're marinating only tofu or tempeh, it will accommodate 4 people. But if you intend to use it for tofu or tempeh plus vegetables, double the recipe to feed 4.

1/2 cup white wine
1/4 cup soy sauce
2 cloves garlic, minced

1 hot pepper, minced, or
  1/4 teaspoon crushed red pepper
  flakes or to taste
1 tablespoon toasted sesame oil

Combine the marinade ingredients in a pan (or 2) large enough to hold the chosen food in a single layer. (For directions on preparing foods for grilling, see Asian Grill in "Main Dishes" and Guidelines for Grilling Vegetables (and Fruit) in "Accompaniments.")

Marinate the food 1 to 2 hours at room temperature or longer in the refrigerator. Turn the food several times. While grilling, spoon any remaining marinade over the food.

YIELD: 3/4 CUP MARINADE; 2 TO 4 SERVINGS

Sweet Mustard Basting Sauce

⁓

Use this basting sauce when barbecuing sweet potato or winter squash slices, eggplant, or sliced onion. Enough for 2 large sweet potatoes or 1 eggplant, plus 1 large onion (serves 4 people).

4 tablespoons prepared mustard   2 tablespoons molasses

Combine the ingredients. Brush on one side of the vegetable and place on the grill. When the bottom is cooked, baste the top, turn, and finish grilling.

YIELD: 6 TABLESPOONS

The Healthiest Diet in the World

Spreads

If you want to use more of the right fats, here is an assortment of spreads to use instead of butter, margarine, and cream cheese. In addition to these, Yogonaise and Tofu Mayonnaise, found in "Salads and Salad Dressings," provide alternatives to commercial mayonnaise.

Herb-Cheese Spread

There are many ways to flavor yogurt cheese. The seasonings suggested below can be augmented or replaced by fresh parsley, cilantro, minced garlic, and numerous dried herbs and spices, including cumin, basil, oregano, rosemary, curry spices, and other personal favorites.

$^1\!/_2$ cup Yogurt Cheese (page 244)
1 tablespoon minced scallion or
   chives

1 tablespoon fresh dill or
   1 teaspoon dried dill seeds
pinch salt, optional

Combine all ingredients. Refrigerate several hours to stiffen.

YIELD: $^1\!/_2$ CUP

Soy Butter

~

This basic spread can be jazzed up by adding crushed garlic, minced fresh herbs, or light miso to taste. Compared with butter, it has less than half the calories (45 vs. 100 per tablespoon) and one-third the fat (3.5 grams vs. 11). While more than 40 percent of the fat in butter is in the form of palmitic acid, which is implicated in heart disease, almost 70 percent of the fat in this Soy Butter is polyunsaturated. Moreover, the polyunsaturated omega-3 linolenic acid (LNA) slightly predominates, with a ratio of linoleic LA:LNA of 1:1.3 (see Chapter 2). Of additional note is the presence of 2.5 grams of protein in each tablespoon of Soy Butter, a nutrient that's insignificant in butter.

1/2 cup cooked soybeans, drained   1 tablespoon flaxseed oil

Puree soybeans in a food processor until well ground. Add oil and continue to puree until creamy. Store in refrigerator.

YIELD: **6** TABLESPOONS

Toasted Soy Spread

~

Use as a spread on bread or crackers as you would peanut or other nut butters. Keeps for weeks if refrigerated. When compared with nut butters, Toasted Soy Spread has about half the calories (56 vs. 94 per tablespoon) and half the fat (4 grams vs. 8). In addition, although the total amount of polyunsaturated fatty acid is comparable, in most nut butters they are almost exclusively omega-6 linolenic acid (LA); in Toasted Soy Spread made with flaxseed oil, omega-3 linolenic acid (LNA) is slightly higher than LA, and when hemp oil is used the ratio of LA:LNA is 4:1, or just about ideal (see Chapter 2).

1 cup soy flour   2 teaspoons light miso
2 tablespoons flaxseed or   2 teaspoons honey
  hemp oil   6 tablespoons water

Place the soy flour in a dry heavy skillet and toast over low heat, stirring continuously, until the flour begins to lightly color. This will take about 5 minutes.

Remove from the heat and immediately stir in the oil. Add the miso, honey, and water. Mix until smooth and spreadable, adding a little more water if needed.

YIELD: 3/4 CUP

Tahini-Garlic Spread

~

Tahini is the paste—or butter—derived from grinding sesame seeds. You can read about the distinctive nutritional components in sesame in Chapter 2 to discover why this spread is recommended. Stored in the refrigerator, it keeps for about a week.

1/2 cup tahini
1 tablespoon soy sauce
2 tablespoons lemon juice

1 large clove garlic, crushed
water

Using a fork, beat together the tahini, soy sauce, lemon juice, and garlic to make a thick paste. Gradually beat in a little water to make a smooth spread.

YIELD: 1/2 CUP

Tahini-Miso Spread

~

This basic spread can be made with any variety of miso. A tablespoon of Tahini-Miso Spread furnishes 70 calories, just under 3 grams of protein, and about 6 grams of fat. The presence of miso adds some unique phytochemicals not found in conventional spreads (see Chapter 5).

1/2 cup tahini
1/4 cup miso

about 6 tablespoons water

Combine the tahini and miso. Using a fork, gradually beat in the water until you have a smooth spread. Store in the refrigerator.

YIELD: ABOUT 3/4 CUP

In Nikki's Kitchen

Onion Butter

Mildly sweet and mellow, and packed with good nutrition.

1 tablespoon wine or cooking sherry
1/2 pound onions, thinly sliced into
  half-rings (about 1 1/2 cups)

1 teaspoon soy sauce
1 tablespoon soy flour
2 tablespoons water

Heat the wine or sherry in a skillet. When warm, add the onions and soy sauce. Cover and cook over very low heat for about 20 minutes, stirring occasionally, until the onions are soft enough to mash with a fork. When they reach this stage, mash with a fork or potato masher until pulpy.

Dilute the soy flour in the water. Stir into the onions and cook, continuing to stir for 3 to 5 minutes, until the mixture is thick and creamy, and the soy flavor mellows.

Chill before serving. Store in the refrigerator.

YIELD: 1/2 CUP

Roasted Sweet Red Pepper Puree

Use this delicious and versatile fat-free spread by itself on crackers or bread, or on sandwiches as you would mayonnaise, mustard, ketchup, or other flavoring mediums. It keeps for a couple of weeks in the refrigerator.

1 large or 2 medium red peppers
  (about 10 ounces)
1 clove garlic, sliced

1/8 teaspoon salt
1 teaspoon wine vinegar

Place the red pepper on a baking sheet and broil 4 to 6 inches beneath the heat for about 15 minutes, until the skin is blistered. Turn several times to cook evenly. Alternatively, hold the pepper over a gas flame using tongs and brown on all sides. When the skin is completely blistered, wrap the pepper in a clean cloth to steam for a few minutes. When cool enough to handle, peel off the skin, cut the pepper open, and remove the seeds, stem, and any thick ribs. Cut the pepper into several pieces.

Combine the roasted pepper, garlic, salt, and wine vinegar in a blender or food processor. Puree until smooth.

Use at once or refrigerate.

YIELD: ABOUT 3/4 CUP

Spicy Green Pepper Puree

Depending on the "heat" of the hot pepper, this can be a quite spicy spread. It keeps for a couple of weeks in the refrigerator.

1 large or 2 small to medium green
  peppers (about 8 ounces)
1 small hot pepper
1 clove garlic, sliced

2 tablespoons lightly packed
  cilantro
1 teaspoon lemon juice
$1/8$ teaspoon salt

Place the peppers on a baking sheet and bake in an oven at 450°F. until the skins begin to brown. This will take about 20 minutes for the hot pepper and about 30 minutes for the green pepper. When adequately cooked, the green pepper skin will be a bit crisp and start to pull away from the flesh. Alternatively, broil the peppers 4 to 6 inches below the heat for about 15 minutes, or until the skin of the hot pepper is just browned and the skin of the green pepper is blistered. With either method, turn the peppers several times to cook evenly.

When the skin is roasted, wrap the peppers in a clean cloth to steam for a few minutes. When cool enough to handle, peel off the skin, cut the peppers open, and remove the seeds, stem, and any thick ribs. Be especially careful handling the hot pepper. You may want to wear surgical gloves and proceed as directed on page 181. Cut the peppers into several pieces.

Combine the roasted peppers, garlic, cilantro, lemon juice, and salt in a blender or food processor. Puree until smooth.

Use at once or refrigerate.

YIELD: $1/2$ CUP

Roasted Green Pepper
and Avocado Mayonnaise

~

This recipe is a variation of Spicy Green Pepper Puree. The addition of avocado to the mixture gives it the creaminess of mayonnaise, without the egg or oil. In fact, it's essentially a reduced-fat guacamole that can be used on sandwiches or as a dip for raw vegetables. Depending on the "heat" of the hot pepper, it can be quite spicy. For a mild "mayonnaise," the hot pepper can be omitted.

1 large or 2 small to medium green
   peppers (about 8 ounces)
1 small hot pepper
1 clove garlic, sliced
2 tablespoons lightly packed
   cilantro

1 teaspoon lemon juice
1/4 teaspoon salt
1/2 small ripe California avocado

Place the peppers on a baking sheet and bake in an oven at 450°F. until the skins begin to brown. This will take about 20 minutes for the hot pepper and about 30 minutes for the green pepper. When adequately cooked, the green pepper skin will be a bit crisp and start to pull away from the flesh. Alternatively, broil the peppers 4 to 6 inches below the heat for about 15 minutes, or until the skin of the hot pepper is just browned and the skin of the green pepper is blistered. With either method, turn the peppers several times to cook evenly.

When the skin is roasted, wrap the peppers in a clean cloth to steam for a few minutes. When cool enough to handle, peel off the skin, cut the peppers open, and remove the seeds, stem, and any thick ribs. Be especially careful handling the hot pepper following the guidelines on page 181. Cut the peppers into several pieces.

Combine the roasted peppers, garlic, cilantro, lemon juice, and salt in a blender or food processor. Puree until smooth. Remove the peel from the avocado half and dice. Add to the puree and process until smooth.

Use at once or refrigerate.

YIELD: 3/4 CUP

Simple Baking

You'll find the recipes for baked goods in this section somewhat different from standard recipes, for in addition to being made exclusively with whole grains, they're carefully designed to provide maximum Golden Guideline value along with pleasure. Very little concentrated fat is employed, if any. Instead, the native fats in flaxseed, wheat germ, soy, and nuts, which are intrinsically balanced with other supporting nutrients, are responsible for the main source of fat. This strategy results in a lower overall fat content compared with traditional counterparts and a better balance of fatty acids. Moreover, it adds important fiber, lignans, and resistant starches that can improve the G-Force, or blood sugar response (see Chapter 1). The use of yogurt to help counterbalance the mineral-binding capacity of phytates found in whole grains is another intentional part of the plan.

Golden Biscuits

Homemade biscuits are surprisingly easy to make, and when you compare the nutritional makeup of these Golden Biscuits to ones from a mix or packet of refrigerated dough, the incentive is even greater. For example, each Golden Biscuit (weighing 2.25 ounces) furnishes 134 calories, 6.5 grams protein, 23 grams carbohydrate, 4.5 grams fiber, 2.7 grams fat, and 279 mg sodium. In contrast, a 2-ounce biscuit made from a brand-name mix or refrigerated dough ranges from 180 to 190 calories, supplies just 3 to 4 grams protein, and while comparable in carbohydrates contains only 1 gram of fiber or less. Fat content is more likely to be 7 to 10 grams per biscuit, and sodium runs as high as 540 mg or more. Of course, Golden Biscuits also provide the vitamins and minerals associated with whole grains and apples, the phytochemicals found in soy and flaxseed, and the beneficial factors in yogurt, as well.

1³/₄ cups whole wheat flour
¹/₄ cup soy flour
¹/₄ cup flaxseed meal (page 239)
1 teaspoon baking powder

¹/₂ teaspoon baking soda
¹/₂ teaspoon salt
¹/₄ cup unsweetened applesauce
³/₄ cup nonfat yogurt

Preheat the oven to 425°F.

Combine the dry ingredients. Make a well in the center and add the applesauce and yogurt. Mix until all ingredients are moistened. Begin with a spoon, then use your hands to knead gently in the bowl until you have a soft dough.

Transfer the dough to a cutting board and pat into a 1-inch-thick square. Cut into eight 2-inch squares. Place about 1 inch apart on an oiled baking sheet. Bake for 15 minutes, or until golden.

YIELD: 8 2-INCH BISCUITS

Savory Oat Biscuits

By using oats as half of the grain component, each biscuit provides one-eighth of the daily suggested intake of the important soluble fiber that makes oats so popular (see Chapter 1). Along with this you receive 135 calories, 4.5 grams protein, 16.5 grams carbohydrate, 2.4 grams total fiber, 6 grams fat, 187 mg sodium, and some important vitamins and minerals, including as much calcium as found in half a cup of milk. To put a few more vegetables into your diet, you can embellish the recipe by adding ¹/₄ cup chopped green pepper and/or ¹/₂ cup fresh or frozen corn kernels to the dough. The final product is a rough-textured biscuit that gets dropped onto the baking sheet rather than rolled. Best eaten while still warm, although reheating or toasting leftovers is quite satisfactory.

1 cup oats
1 cup whole wheat flour
1 tablespoon baking powder
¹/₄ teaspoon salt
¹/₈ teaspoon pepper

¹/₂ teaspoon dried dill or basil
¹/₄ cup canola oil
¹/₄ cup sliced scallions
1 cup yogurt

Preheat the oven to 400°F.

Combine the dry ingredients. Stir in the oil until the mixture resembles coarse crumbs. Add the scallions and yogurt and mix just until the dry ingredients are evenly moistened.

Mound the biscuits by 1/4 cupfuls onto an oiled baking sheet. Bake for 20 minutes, or until the biscuits are nicely browned.

YIELD: **10** BISCUITS

Appleberry-Corn Muffins

~

A hearty muffin (each just over 3 ounces) with an excellent texture and flavor. These muffins aren't very sweet, but if preferred, the maple syrup can be increased to 1/4 cup. For those considering the nutritional contribution of their baked goods, each muffin provides 142 calories, 4 grams protein, 27 grams carbohydrate, 3.5 grams fiber, 8 grams sugar, and 2.5 grams fat. This is at least 100 fewer calories than comparable commercial corn muffins, which have substantially more carbohydrate and less fiber, about twice the sugar, and from two to four times the fat.

1 cup whole wheat flour
1 cup cornmeal
1/4 cup flaxseed meal (page 239)
2 teaspoons baking powder
1/2 teaspoon baking soda
1/2 teaspoon salt
1/2 teaspoon cinnamon

1 teaspoon minced orange rind
1/2 cup fresh or thawed frozen
  berries (blueberries, raspberries,
  sliced strawberries)
1 cup unsweetened applesauce
1 cup soy milk
3 tablespoons maple syrup

Preheat the oven to 375°F.

In a mixing bowl, combine the flour, cornmeal, flaxseed meal, leavening agents, salt, cinnamon, orange rind, and berries. Make a well in the center and add the applesauce, soy milk, and maple syrup. Mix gently, but thoroughly, until all ingredients are completely moistened.

Spoon the batter into the cups of a muffin tin that have been wiped with oil or lined with paper muffin cups; fill almost to the top. Bake for 20 minutes. Remove from the oven, let the muffins sit for 5 minutes, then remove from the baking pan and transfer to a wire rack to cool.

YIELD: **10** MUFFINS

★ FLAX FACTS ★

Grinding flaxseed in a blender or spice mill produces a reddish brown meal that's also referred to as flaxseed flour. In the right proportion, flaxseed meal adds a delicate nutlike flavor to baked goods and substantially reduces the need for fat in the recipe. In addition, the soluble fiber and lignans in flaxseed slow the rise in blood sugar that normally follows the eating of carbohydrate-rich foods such as muffins. (For more on flaxseed meal, see "Gold Star Basics.")

Banana–Oat Bran Muffins

~

Each lightly sweetened muffin weighs in at just under 3 ounces, with 185 calories, 5.5 grams protein, 33 grams carbohydrate, 4 grams fiber, 12 grams sugar, and 5 grams fat. It tastes more of banana than honey and isn't very sweet. If a sweeter muffin is desired, increase the honey to 4 tablespoons.

2 cups whole wheat flour
1/4 cup oat bran
2 teaspoons baking powder
1/2 teaspoon baking soda
1/2 teaspoon salt
1/3 cup walnut pieces

1 cup mashed banana (2 medium bananas)
1 cup soy milk
1 tablespoon canola oil
3 tablespoons honey

Preheat the oven to 375°F.

In a mixing bowl, combine the flour, oat bran, leavening agents, salt, and walnuts. Make a well in the center and add the mashed banana, soy milk, oil, and honey. Mix gently, but thoroughly, until all ingredients are completely moistened.

Spoon the batter into the cups of a muffin tin that have been wiped with oil or lined with paper muffin cups; fill almost to the top. Bake for 20 minutes. Remove from the oven, let the muffins sit for 5 minutes, then remove from the baking pan and transfer to a wire rack to cool.

YIELD: 10 MUFFINS

VARIATION: To turn these into *Banana–Wheat Germ Muffins*, replace the oat bran with 1/4 cup wheat germ.

★ MOIST MUFFINS ★

When baking muffins, if there isn't enough batter to fill all the cups in the muffin tin, add about 1/2 inch water to each empty cup to prevent the pan from scorching. This also helps keep the muffins moist.

Honey-Yogurt Muffins

~

These muffins are especially tender, and yet dispense more than 6 grams of protein apiece. Overall, each one delivers 164 calories, 28 grams carbohydrate, 3 grams fiber, 9 grams sugar, and 4 grams fat. Like other baked goods made with yogurt, they're a good source of calcium.

2½ cups whole wheat flour
1 teaspoon baking powder
1 teaspoon baking soda
½ teaspoon salt

2 tablespoons wheat germ
3 tablespoons canola oil
¼ cup honey
2 cups yogurt

Preheat the oven to 400°F.

In a mixing bowl, combine the flour, leavening agents, salt, and wheat germ. Make a well in the center and add the oil, honey, and yogurt. Stir gently with a fork just until the dry ingredients are completely moistened.

Spoon the batter into the cups of a muffin tin that have been wiped with oil or lined with paper muffin cups; fill each two-thirds full. Bake for 20 minutes. Remove from the oven, let muffins sit for 5 minutes, then remove from the baking pan and transfer to a wire rack to cool.

YIELD: 12 MUFFINS

3-Grain Polenta Bread

~

This dense, moist bread that resembles baked polenta provides a perfect bed for heavily sauced tempeh, tofu, beans, or vegetables (for example, Tofu Chili, White Beans with Swiss Chard, Quick Mixed Vegetables in Tomato Juice, Chiles Rellenos). To serve in this manner as an underlayer, cut into fourths. For a breadstuff, cut into eight or nine pieces. Can be eaten while still warm or prepared well in advance.

¾ cup cornmeal
2 tablespoons soy flour
2 tablespoons flaxseed meal
  (page 239)
½ teaspoon baking soda

¼ teaspoon salt
1½ cups yogurt
1 tablespoon maple syrup
1 teaspoon canola oil

Preheat the oven to 400°F.

Combine the dry ingredients in a mixing bowl. Add the yogurt and maple syrup. Mix gently, but thoroughly, until the dry ingredients are completely moistened.

Pour the oil into an 8-inch-square baking pan. Place in the oven for 2 to 3 minutes, until hot. Spread the batter in the prepared hot baking pan. Bake for 30 minutes, until the edges are lightly browned.

YIELD: 4 SERVINGS

In Nikki's Kitchen

Desserts

A wedge of sweet watermelon, a bowl of ripe berries, a juicy peach, a crisp apple . . . these are nature's most simple and delectable dessert offerings. A serving of fruit can be made more enticing as a dessert by presentation; you don't have to be an experienced cook to put together simple platters like these:

- Cut the fruit into wedges and set on a plate surrounded by pecan halves and dates.
- Cut pineapple pieces into triangles and attach toothpicks holding red grapes.
- Place wedges of lime around cantaloupe and honeydew slices. (Lime juice brings out the flavor even in lackluster fruit.)
- Combine peeled kiwi rounds with sweet fresh cherries.

In this section you'll find some additional ideas for embellishing fruit, as well as a few baked goods you can serve with confidence.

Maple-Orange Nectarines

Sweet poached nectarines in maple-orange syrup make an excellent dessert whether they're served warm, at room temperature, or chilled. They can be garnished with Whipped Yogurt "Cream" or Whipped Tofu Topping. You can also enjoy them on top of pancakes, simple un-iced cakes, and mixed with plain yogurt for a meal or snack.

4 firm but ripe nectarines
1/2 cup orange juice

2 tablespoons maple syrup
2 tablespoons slivered almonds

Divide the nectarines into slices. There are two ways to do this. You can cut the fruit from stem to blossom end, gently twist to pry the halves apart, remove the pit, and cut into wedges; or, using a small paring knife, you can cut the whole fruit into wedges from stem to blossom end and gently pry the pieces off of the pit.

Combine the juice and maple syrup in a skillet. Bring to a boil over medium heat. Add the nectarines and cook, stirring occasionally, for 5 minutes.

Transfer the nectarines to a bowl, using a slotted spoon so that the liquid remains in the skillet. Simmer the liquid left in the pan for 3 to 5 minutes, until lightly thickened. Pour over the nectarines and let sit at room temperature for at least 15 minutes.

Serve while still warm, at room temperature, or chilled. When ready to serve, spoon into individual dishes and top each with some of the slivered almonds.

YIELD: 4 SERVINGS

Asian Melon

⌐

Gently spiced ginger syrup imparts an Asian flavor to this simple melon dessert.

1 orange
3/4 cup water
1/4 cup honey
1-inch knob of fresh ginger, peeled
  and thinly sliced

4 cups sliced or cubed honeydew,
  cantaloupe, or other muskmelon
fresh mint leaves, if available

Using a vegetable peeler, remove 2 long strips of peel from the orange. Combine the peel in a small saucepan with the water, honey, and slices of ginger. Bring to a boil. Simmer, uncovered, over moderate heat for 15 minutes, until the syrup thickens slightly and is reduced to about 1/2 cup.

Pour the syrup into a bowl large enough to accommodate the fruit. Let cool to room temperature. When cool, remove the orange peel and ginger. Squeeze the orange and add 1/4 cup juice to the syrup. Add the melon to the syrup and chill until serving time.

To serve, spoon into serving dishes and garnish with fresh mint leaves, if available.

YIELD: 6 SERVINGS

In Nikki's Kitchen

Marinated Figs

⁓

Figs are one of the sweetest fruits. Marinated in juice, they produce a dessert of elegant simplicity. Although this dish takes only a few minutes to prepare, it should be done ahead of time since at least 8 hours of marination are needed.

12 dried golden figs
2 tablespoons raisins

1¼ cups apple juice
2 tablespoons lemon juice

Combine the figs, raisins, and apple juice in a small saucepan. Bring to a boil and simmer for just 1 minute. Remove from the heat and add the lemon juice.

Transfer to a bowl and let marinate in the refrigerator for at least 8 hours before serving.

YIELD: 4 TO 6 SERVINGS

Favorite Fruit Salad

⁓

Almost any combination of fruit can be included in fruit salad, but to make it extra special we have two tips: include walnuts and dates.

2 apples, diced
2 bananas, sliced
other fruit in season, as desired

juice of 3 oranges
8 to 12 dried dates
generous amount of walnut pieces

Combine the apples, bananas, and other fruit in season in a bowl. You will want at least 4 cups for 4 servings. Add the orange juice to preserve the color and provide a syrup. Cut the dates into small pieces and add. Mix to coat all the fruit with juice and distribute the dates. Top with an impressive amount of walnuts.

YIELD: 4 SERVINGS

★ THE BEST ANTIOXIDANT FRUITS ★

In a scientific ranking by the U.S. Department of Agriculture of the antioxidant capability of 12 fruits, strawberries ranked highest, followed in descending order by plums, oranges, red grapes, kiwi, pink grapefruit, white grapes, bananas, apples, tomatoes, pears, and honeydew melon. The antioxidant activity of strawberries was twice the capacity measured in oranges and red grapes, seven times higher than in bananas and apples, 11 times that of pears, and 16 times more potent than the melon.

The Healthiest Diet in the World

Banana Soft Serve

All it takes is frozen bananas and a food processor to produce one of the creamiest desserts around. People are amazed when they find out there's no cream and no sweetening in this well-liked treat.

1 banana per serving

Peel the bananas and wrap in airtight, freezer-proof packaging. Freeze at least 24 hours or up to 3 months.

Just before serving, remove the bananas from the freezer, break into chunks, and place in a food processor fitted with the steel blade. Process until the banana breaks up, passes through the icy stage, and becomes creamy and whipped with air. The consistency will be that of soft-serve ice cream. Serve at once.

Strawberry Frozen Yogurt

By blending Yogurt Cheese with fruit you can produce a tantalizing frozen dessert. Using the pattern below, try your hand with other fruit flavors.

2 cups fresh strawberries	1 cup Yogurt Cheese (page 244)
3 tablespoons fruit juice–sweetened berry preserves	1/2 teaspoon vanilla extract
	1 to 2 tablespoons maple syrup

Combine the berries and preserves in a blender or food processor and puree. Remove from the work bowl and beat in the Yogurt Cheese, vanilla, and maple syrup until evenly combined. The amount of maple syrup needed will depend on the sweetness of the berries and individual taste; begin with 1 tablespoon, taste, and adjust if needed.

Transfer to a shallow metal pan or freezer container. Freeze for 2 to 3 hours, until firm. Return the mixture to a processor (or blender if you don't have a food processor), breaking into chunks. Process at high speed until smooth. This may require a little stopping and scraping the sides until the frozen yogurt begins to soften. Continue until the mixture is the consistency of soft-serve ice cream. At this point you can eat the frozen yogurt or return it to a freezer container and freeze solid. Remove from the freezer about 10 minutes before serving to soften slightly.

YIELD: 1 PINT

223

In Nikki's Kitchen

★ NUTRITIOUS TOPPINGS FOR FRUIT AND BAKED GOODS ★

Instead of high-fat whipped cream or chemical-laden imitations, try one of these alternatives. You may want to adjust the sweetening slightly according to taste and use: For capping something very sweet, a subdued selection is preferable; on top of plain cakes, baked apples, or tart fruit, a sweeter taste may be desired. One cup of topping will serve 4 generously, but with these recipes—which provide 4.5 grams protein, 85 to 115 mg calcium, and 2 grams fat or less per 1/4 cup—there's no reason to stop people from taking extra.

Whipped Yogurt "Cream"

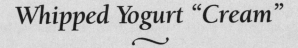

1 cup Yogurt Cheese (page 244)   1 teaspoon vanilla extract
1 tablespoon honey or maple syrup

Using a fork or wire whip, beat the ingredients together until creamy. Use at once or refrigerate.

YIELD: 1 CUP

Orange-Yogurt Cream

1 cup Yogurt Cheese (page 244)   2 to 3 teaspoons honey
2 tablespoons orange juice   1/2 teaspoon grated orange rind

Using a fork or wire whip, beat the ingredients together until creamy. Use at once or refrigerate.

YIELD: 1 CUP

Whipped Tofu Topping

8 ounces soft tofu (1 cup mashed)   1 1/2 tablespoons maple syrup
3 tablespoons apple juice   1/2 teaspoon almond or vanilla extract

Combine all ingredients in a blender or food processor. Puree until creamy.

YIELD: SCANT 1 CUP

Gold Chip Cookies

Gold Chip Cookies are an enhanced version of a traditional favorite.

1½ cups oats
1 cup whole wheat flour
¼ teaspoon salt
¼ teaspoon baking soda
½ cup chopped almonds, hazelnuts, or filberts

¾ cup chocolate or carob chips
½ cup maple syrup
⅓ cup unsweetened applesauce
2 tablespoons canola oil
1 teaspoon vanilla extract

Preheat the oven to 375°F.

In a blender or food processor, grind the oats to a coarse flour. In a large bowl, combine the oat flour, whole wheat flour, salt, and baking soda. Mix well. Add the nuts and chips and mix again. In a separate bowl, whisk together the maple syrup, applesauce, oil, and vanilla extract. Stir the wet ingredients into the dry, mixing until thoroughly moistened.

Drop the dough by the tablespoonful onto oiled baking sheets, leaving about 1 inch between cookies. Flatten gently with your hands or the prongs of a fork. Bake 15 to 20 minutes, until the cookies are lightly browned on the bottom. Transfer to a wire rack to cool.

YIELD: **28** 2-INCH COOKIES

*In
Nikki's
Kitchen*

Chewy Oat Cookies

~

This lowfat cookie has a great texture and flavor without being cloyingly sweet like most commercial lowfat baked goods.

1½ cups whole wheat flour	1 teaspoon minced orange rind
½ cup oats	¼ cup chopped raisins
3 tablespoons flaxseed meal (page 239), wheat germ, or a mixture	½ cup chopped walnuts
	⅔ cup unsweetened applesauce
¾ teaspoon baking soda	½ cup honey
½ teaspoon baking powder	2 tablespoons maple syrup

Preheat the oven to 325°F.

Combine the flour, oats, flaxseed meal or wheat germ, leavening agents, orange rind, raisins, and walnuts in a mixing bowl. Add the applesauce, honey, and maple syrup. Stir until evenly blended and the dry ingredients are thoroughly moistened.

Drop the dough by the tablespoonful onto oiled or nonstick baking sheets. Flatten gently with the prongs of a fork. Bake for 20 minutes, until golden. Transfer to a wire rack to cool.

YIELD: 30 2-INCH COOKIES

A scissors is a handy tool for "chopping" raisins or other dried fruit.

Oat Nut Clusters

~

Appealingly crunchy, with a subtle sweetness that develops in your mouth.

6 tablespoons tahini	¼ cup sliced Brazil nuts or almonds
¼ cup honey	1 cup oats
½ teaspoon cinnamon	

Preheat the oven to 350°F.

In a mixing bowl, beat the tahini with the honey until smooth. Work in the remaining ingredients to form a stiff dough. (You can use your hands to do this.)

Using a teaspoonful of dough at a time, shape into compact balls and place on an oiled baking sheet. Flatten by pressing gently with the palm of your hand.

Bake for 12 to 15 minutes, until golden. Remove from the oven and let cool for a minute or two before transferring to a wire rack to cool completely.

YIELD: 20 1-INCH COOKIES

Nutty Cheesecake Bars

A custardlike topping on a nut-crumb base. Easier to eat if chilled after baking.

1/2 cup whole wheat flour	2 tablespoons chopped sunflower
2 tablespoons flaxseed meal	seeds
(page 239)	1 cup Yogurt Cheese (page 244)
1/4 teaspoon nutmeg	1 egg
1 tablespoon maple syrup	3 tablespoons honey
2 tablespoons chopped walnuts or	1 tablespoon orange or apple juice
pecans	

Preheat the oven to 350°F.

In a mixing bowl, combine the flour, flaxseed meal, and nutmeg. Stir in the maple syrup and then work together with your hands until crumbly. Add the chopped nuts and seeds. Press into the bottom of an oiled 8-inch-square baking pan. Bake for 12 minutes.

Meanwhile, beat together the Yogurt Cheese, egg, honey, and juice.

Spread the Yogurt Cheese mixture over the partially baked crust. Return to the oven for 30 minutes, until the surface is set and just beginning to lightly color. Cool to room temperature, then chill for at least half an hour before serving.

To serve, cut into 12 bars, each 1 inch wide and 4 inches long. Store in the refrigerator.

YIELD: 12 1 x 4-INCH BARS

Brownies

These brownies are lean and mean, with just 3.5 grams of fat each, yet rich in texture and taste.

³/4 cup whole wheat pastry flour
1 teaspoon baking powder
¹/4 teaspoon salt
¹/2 cup chopped walnuts or pecans
¹/2 cup mashed tofu (4 ounces)
2 tablespoons canola oil

2 tablespoons honey
¹/3 cup maple syrup
1 teaspoon vanilla extract
¹/4 cup unsweetened cocoa or carob powder

Preheat the oven to 350°F.

Combine the flour, baking powder, salt, and nuts in a bowl.

Combine the tofu, oil, honey, maple syrup, vanilla, and cocoa or carob powder in a blender or food processor and process until completely smooth. Stir into a bowl with the flour mixture until completely blended. If too thick to blend together, add a tablespoon or so of water, as needed.

Spread the batter into an oiled 8-inch-square baking pan. Bake 20 to 25 minutes, until firm. Don't overbake. Let cool in the pan at least 15 minutes before cutting.

YIELD: 16 2-INCH SQUARE BROWNIES

Very Berry Shortcakes

Each component of these fruit-topped cakes—the base, the fruit, and the whipped topping—can be made separately, either just prior to serving or ahead of time. The fruit and topping can be held in the refrigerator. The base can be served warm from the oven or at room temperature, or it can even be assembled and kept in the refrigerator for last-minute baking. When shopping for the berries, figure on using 1 pound or 1 dry pint strawberries, and ¹/2 pound (a little less than 1 dry pint) blueberries.

Base:

²/3 cup whole wheat flour
¹/3 cup cornmeal
2 tablespoons wheat germ
1 teaspoon baking powder

¹/4 teaspoon baking soda
2 tablespoons canola oil
¹/3 cup nonfat yogurt
1 tablespoon maple syrup or honey

Fruit:

2¹/₂ cups sliced strawberries
¹/₄ cup orange juice

1 tablespoon maple syrup or honey
1¹/₂ cups blueberries

Topping:

1 cup Whipped Yogurt "Cream"
(page 224), Orange-Yogurt Cream
(page 224), or Whipped Tofu
Topping (page 224)

Preheat the oven to 425°F.

To prepare the base, combine the dry ingredients in a mixing bowl. Stir in the oil and mix with a fork, wire whip, or pastry blender until completely incorporated. Add the yogurt and honey and mix until all ingredients are well combined into a ball of dough. Toward the end, kneading gently with your hands will work best.

Oil a baking sheet or the removable bottom of a 9-inch tart pan. Pat the dough into an 8- to 9-inch circle, ¹/₄ inch high. Using the prongs of a fork, divide into 6 pie-shaped wedges. Do not separate. Bake for 15 minutes, until golden.

The filling can be prepared while the base bakes or ahead of time. Combine 2 cups strawberries, the orange juice, and sweetener in a blender or food processor. Process quickly to a coarse puree. Transfer to a bowl and stir in the blueberries and remaining ¹/₂ cup sliced strawberries. If prepared in advance, chill until serving time.

To serve, separate the base into 6 wedges and split each one open by piercing through the center with a fork. Lay the top and bottom pieces of the wedge soft side up on each serving plate. Top generously with fruit and a dollop (2 generous tablespoons) of the topping of choice.

YIELD: **6** SERVINGS

*In
Nikki's
Kitchen*

Applesauce-Date Cake

~

A dense cake with a moist, puddinglike texture. Fine as is; excellent topped with Whipped Yogurt "Cream."

1 cup unsweetened applesauce	1/4 teaspoon salt
1/2 cup yogurt	2 cups whole wheat flour
3/4 cup honey	1/4 cup soy flour
1 teaspoon vanilla extract	1 teaspoon baking powder
1/2 teaspoon cinnamon	1 teaspoon baking soda
1 teaspoon minced orange rind	1/2 cup cut-up dates

Preheat the oven to 350°F.

In a large bowl, beat together the applesauce, yogurt, and honey. Beat in the vanilla, cinnamon, orange rind, and salt.

In a separate bowl, combine the flours, baking powder, baking soda, and dates.

Gradually add the dry ingredients to the wet ingredients, mixing gently but thoroughly until evenly blended and the dry ingredients are completely moistened.

Spread the batter into an oiled, floured 8-inch baking pan. Bake about 35 minutes, until the center is firm and the cake tests done. Cool in the pan.

YIELD: 16 2-INCH SQUARES

Fresh Fruit Tart with Cheese Filling

~

This elegant tart tastes as impressive as it looks. To facilitate preparation of the 3 components—crust, filling, and fruit topping—begin with the cheese filling and refrigerate while you make the crust and prepare the fruit. The whole operation should be completed from several hours to as much as a day in advance so the tart has a chance to chill.

Crust:

1/2 cup whole wheat flour	1/4 teaspoon baking soda
1/3 cup cornmeal	2 tablespoons canola oil
1 tablespoon flaxseed meal (page 239)	1/4 cup yogurt
1/2 teaspoon baking powder	1 tablespoon honey

Cheese Filling:

1½ cups Yogurt Cheese (page 244)
2 tablespoons honey

1 teaspoon vanilla extract

Fruit Glaze:

3 cups fresh peeled peaches,
  nectarines, strawberry halves,
  blueberries, or raspberries,
  individually or in combination

2 tablespoons honey
1 tablespoon cornstarch or
  arrowroot
2 tablespoons lemon juice

To prepare the crust, preheat the oven to 425°F. In a mixing bowl, combine the dry ingredients. Stir in the oil and mix with a pastry blender, wire whip, or fork until completely incorporated and crumbly. Stir in the yogurt and honey. Mix until all ingredients are well blended, kneading gently in the bowl with your hands at the end to form a ball of dough. Oil a 9-inch tart pan or pie pan with a removable bottom. Press the dough over the bottom and up the sides of the pan to make a thin shell. Prick the surface liberally with a fork. Bake for 10 minutes, until golden. Cool before filling.

To make the filling, using a fork, beat together the Yogurt Cheese, honey, and vanilla. Refrigerate if not used right away.

To make the fruit glaze, place 1 cup of the fruit in a small saucepan and mash with a fork or potato masher. Add the honey, cornstarch, and lemon juice. Set over low heat and cook, stirring continuously, until the mixture is thick and translucent and no longer has a milky appearance. Remove from the heat and let cool for a few minutes.

When the crust is at room temperature, fill with the sweetened Yogurt Cheese. Arrange the remaining 2 cups fruit on top of the filling. Using a spoon, gently spread with the glaze to completely cover. Chill for several hours before serving.

YIELD: 9-INCH TART; 8 TO 10 SERVINGS

*In
Nikki's
Kitchen*

Fruit and Tofu Pie

~

If you've never tried tofu pie, or did and were disappointed, this creamy version with its fresh fruit topping is sure to win you over.

Crust:

1¼ cups crumbs made from whole-grain cookies and/or whole-grain ready-to-eat cereal

¼ cup wheat germ
2 to 4 tablespoons orange juice

Filling:

1 pound firm tofu
¼ cup honey
2 to 4 tablespoons orange juice

½ teaspoon almond extract
1 teaspoon vanilla extract

Topping:

¼ cup fruit juice–sweetened orange marmalade
1 teaspoon honey
⅓ cup orange juice
1½ teaspoons arrowroot or cornstarch

1 tablespoon lemon juice
2 cups peeled orange segments, thin kiwi wedges, sliced banana, and/or strawberries

Preheat the oven to 350°F.

Prepare the crumbs for the crust by grinding the cookies and/or cereal in a blender or food processor. Combine with the wheat germ and just enough juice to keep the mixture together when pressed between your fingers. The amount of juice will vary depending on how soft or crisp the crumbs are. Press over the bottom and sides of a 9-inch pie pan. Bake for 8 minutes. Remove from the oven and cool at least 5 minutes before filling.

To make the filling, pat the tofu dry and crumble into a blender or food processor. Add the remaining filling ingredients, using 2 tablespoons of juice initially. Puree until completely smooth and creamy, adding additional juice if necessary. (The firmness of the tofu will influence how much juice is needed.) Spread the filling evenly into the cooled crust. Bake 20 to 25 minutes, until set and barely colored. Cool to room temperature.

To make the topping, combine the marmalade, honey, and all but 1 tablespoon of the orange juice in a small saucepan. Cook over low heat until melted. Mix the remaining tablespoon orange juice into the arrowroot or cornstarch until dissolved. Add to the hot marmalade and cook, stirring constantly, until thick and translucent. Remove from the heat, stir in the lemon juice, and fold together with the fruit. Let cool to room temperature, then spread over the cooled pie. Chill several hours before serving.

YIELD: 9-INCH PIE

Drinks

Water is the beverage of choice; since it doesn't need much preparation, this section is brief. As we suggest in Golden Guideline #8: Liquids of Life, you can encourage water drinking by making it readily accessible. Here are some ways to accomplish this:

- Keep containers of water in the refrigerator.
- Set water out on the table at mealtime.
- Use bottled still or sparkling water if this is more appealing than tap water.
- Give everyone in your household a personal water bottle to carry with them.
- When company comes to visit, bring out a tray of pretty glasses filled with still or sparkling water. This is a customary act of welcome in many cultures.

To make water even more refreshing, add some lemon, lime, or orange slices. Another strategy is to dilute juices by about one-half with sparkling or still water to create a tasty thirst-quencher with substantially fewer calories and a lower G-Force than juice.

Herbal teas, as well as green, oolong, and black teas, all make additional suitable hot and cold beverages. Tea can be brewed weak or strong, according to taste, by varying the ratio of herb or tea leaves to water and adjusting the brewing time. The usual approach for both black and green teas is outlined below. Oolong is prepared in the same manner as black tea. Herbal tea is also brewed in this way. (Note that since most herbal teas are free of caffeine and oxalate, the upcoming notes in Basic Black Tea pertaining to these compounds aren't relevant.)

Another beverage to include is soy milk, which can be consumed as is or turned into hot drinks and shakes to garner the benefits of soy (see Chapter 5).

Basic Black Tea

⁓

The volume of tea leaves needed per cup and steeping time are ultimately a matter of personal taste. The following information will help you determine appropriate parameters. Note that the finer the leaves, the less you need and the shorter the brewing. (On the other hand, tea aficionados report that larger leaves render a better-tasting beverage.)

The longer tea leaves steep and the hotter the water, the higher the levels of caffeine and oxalates, until maximum extraction is reached after about 5 minutes. Brewing longer than this turns tea bitter. Naturally, the more leaves used per cup, the higher the caffeine and oxalate potential. In addition, vigorous stirring dramatically increases oxalates. Oxalates are a concern primarily to people prone to kidney stones. As noted in Chapter 8, drinking tea in combination with calcium diminishes the oxalate effect. Thus, one obvious way to avert problems is to add dairy milk or calcium-fortified soy milk.

For each mug or 2 small teacups:

tea leaves (see table below for amount)   6 to 8 ounces freshly boiled water

Place a strainer with tea leaves in a cup or pot. Pour in the hot water. Steep to desired strength, which is typically 3 to 5 minutes (see table). Remove the tea leaves and serve. You can generally brew leaves a second time.

TEA BREWING TABLE

Tea Type	Leaf Volume (teaspoons)	Steeping Time (minutes)
very fine leaves, as in tea bags	1/2 to 1	3
small whole-leaf tea; most Darjeelings and broken orange pekoe	1	3 to 4
medium-size whole-leaf teas, as in most common loose varieties	1 rounded	4 to 5
scented and fruit-flavored teas, including jasmine and Earl Grey	1/2 to 1	2 to 3
Oolong (traditional Chinese method)	2	5 to 6

In Nikki's Kitchen

Basic Green Tea

Properly prepared green tea is made using water that has cooled to 165 to 185°F. and is steeped for only 1 to 3 minutes. When made according to these guidelines, green tea contains less caffeine and oxalates than black tea.

For each mug or 2 small teacups:

1 flat to rounded teaspoon tea leaves

6 to 8 ounces water

Place the tea leaves in a strainer. Place the strainer in a cup or pot.

Bring the water to a boil. Turn the heat off and let the water sit for 2 minutes before pouring over the tea leaves. Steep 1 to 3 minutes. Remove the tea leaves and serve. You can generally brew leaves a second time.

Iced Tea

There are several ways to brew iced tea, whether black, green, or herbal. One is to prepare the tea as directed above or according to taste and chill it. If serving over ice, the preferred approach is to make an extra-strength brew by using twice the regular volume of leaves per cup. A third method, which results in excellent flavor and the least caffeine and oxalates, is the cold-water technique presented below. No matter which you choose, if sweetening is desired try diluting the tea by up to one-half with orange, apple, or other pure fruit juice. Another strategy to use with iced black tea is to add calcium-fortified soy milk (vanilla or plain).

Cold-Water Brewing:

double the quantity of tea suggested per cup in the Tea Brewing Table (page 235)

1 quart cold water

Place the tea leaves directly in a 1-quart or larger jar or in a large tea ball. Cover with cold water. Refrigerate for at least 6 hours. Remove the tea ball, or if the leaves are loose strain the tea into a second container. If desired, the leaves can be used again to make hot tea.

YIELD: 1 QUART

Hot Spiced Tea

A good pick-me-up for the morning or during the day. The recipe below fills an 8-ounce mug. For larger mugs or multiple servings, increase the tea and soy milk in equal proportions. If you like a slightly sweeter tea, use vanilla soy milk instead of plain.

1/2 cup strong black tea
1/2 cup soy milk, calcium-fortified
  brand preferred

piece of cinnamon stick
freshly ground pepper

Prepare the tea according to the instructions for Basic Black Tea (page 235). Simultaneously, in a small saucepan, heat the soy milk with the cinnamon stick to just below boiling.

Fill the mug halfway with tea. Pour the milk into the mug, discarding the cinnamon. Grind some fresh pepper on top of the tea and serve.

YIELD: 8-OUNCE MUG

VARIATION: For *White Ginger Tea*, replace the cinnamon with 1/2 teaspoon grated fresh ginger per serving. Strain the hot milk into the tea if you want to remove the ginger. Omit the pepper.

Hot Wheat Drink

When you're finished drinking this soothing hot soy beverage, eat the softened cereal at the bottom of the cup with a spoon.

1 cup soy milk
1 1/2 teaspoons honey
1 teaspoon vanilla extract

1-inch stick cinnamon
1 tablespoon wheat germ

Combine all ingredients in a small pot and heat gently, until just below the boiling point. Serve at once.

YIELD: 1 AMPLE OR 2 SMALL SERVINGS

237

Banana-Soy Shake

~

Blend soy milk and fruit for a variety of refreshing shakes. The banana used in this version can be combined or replaced with strawberries, sliced peaches, kiwi, papaya, mango, or other tender fruit of choice, using about 1 cup fruit for each cup of soy milk. To enhance the perception of sweetness, sprinkle freshly grated nutmeg or cinnamon on top of each serving. Depending on the sweetness of fruit, you may want to add a teaspoon of maple syrup or honey as well.

1 cup soy milk	**4 ice cubes**
1 banana	

Combine all ingredients in a blender and process until the ice is completely melted. Serve at once.

YIELD: **2** 8-OUNCE SERVINGS

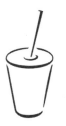

The Healthiest Diet in the World

Gold Star Basics

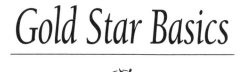

Flaxseed Meal

To improve the body's assimilation of the elements in flaxseed, the seeds should be ground in a blender or spice mill. This transforms them into a reddish brown powder, referred to as flaxseed meal. Flaxseed meal, which has a delicate nutty flavor, can be sprinkled on cereal, added to spreads, toppings, and casseroles, or used in baking to replace some of the flour. Because of its natural oil content, incorporating flaxseed meal into the recipe for baked goods substantially reduces the need for added fats. In addition, the soluble fiber in flaxseed slows down the rise in blood sugar that normally follows the consumption of carbohydrate-rich foods. (For more on flaxseeds, see Chapters 1 and 2.)

When ground, flaxseeds produce a little less than twice as much meal as the original measure of seeds. Thus, 1/2 cup flaxseeds will yield a scant cup of flaxseed meal. Grinding can be done as needed, or you can prepare a modest quantity in advance and store it in the refrigerator for use over the coming week or two.

To prepare, place the flaxseeds in a blender or spice mill. Grind at high speed until reduced to a soft powder. Use immediately, or store in a tightly covered container in the refrigerator.

Fresh Tomato Puree for Cooking

To recapture the flavor of fresh tomatoes after the season is over, we prepare this handy cooking medium when tomatoes are at their peak. It can be stored in the refrigerator for several days or frozen for future use. Fresh tomato puree can be used in any recipe calling for tomato juice.

Method #1: Cut the tomatoes into wedges and place in a saucepan. Bring to a boil over medium heat and simmer about 10 minutes, or until all the pieces are softened. Puree in a food mill to remove the skins.

Method #2: When a food mill isn't available, bring a large pot of water to a boil. Plunge the tomatoes into boiling water for a minute or two, until the skins break. Transfer from the hot water to a colander to drain and cool. When the tomatoes are cool enough to handle, peel them. Place the peeled tomatoes in a blender or food processor and puree. Transfer the puree to a pot and simmer 5 minutes.

Method #3: Here is what to do with the inside of a tomato when making stuffed tomatoes. Slice the top from the tomato. Remove the tomato pulp with the aid of a curved grapefruit knife and serrated grapefruit spoon. Place the pulp and all the liquid you can capture in a blender or food processor. Puree. Transfer the puree to a pot and simmer 5 minutes.

NOTE: Be sure to taste for seasoning when using Fresh Tomato Puree instead of canned tomato juice in a recipe; canned tomato juice is presalted and thus additional salt may be needed in the finished dish.

★ TIPS FOR STORING TOMATO PRODUCTS ★

When using a prepared tomato product such as tomato paste, tomato juice, tomato puree, or canned crushed tomatoes in a recipe, you may need only part of the contents. What's left can be transferred to a nonreactive container (glass, plastic, or stainless steel) and refrigerated for a few days. Or, for long-term keeping, these tomato products all freeze well. If you use only small amounts at a time (as a flavoring agent, for example), ice cube trays make a convenient freezing container; place 2 tablespoons tomato product in each small compartment. When frozen solid, remove from the trays, transfer to a plastic bag, and return to the freezer. In choosing other containers, try to gauge a suitable amount for recipes so you can easily defrost only what you need. If drained canned tomatoes are called for in cooking, the canning liquid can be similarly reserved. It makes a great soup base or substitute for stock.

Spiced Sherry

～

To zip up the flavor of dishes that call for cooking sherry, use Spiced Sherry in its place.

1 hot pepper   **cooking sherry**

Roast the hot pepper over an open flame or in a broiler, turning to char all sides. Wrap in a clean cloth towel for a few minutes. Scrape off the charred skin with a small paring knife. Place the pepper in a glass jar and mash gently with a fork to break up into pieces and release the seeds. Pour in enough cooking sherry to generously cover. Cover and refrigerate. Let steep several hours before using.

Strain off the sherry as desired for cooking. Replenish by pouring more sherry over the pepper to maintain a good cover. Pieces of the pepper can also be used in cooking as desired. Spiced Sherry keeps for several weeks in the refrigerator.

Toasted Pine Nuts and Pumpkin Seeds

～

Toasted pine nuts and pumpkin seeds can be used to garnish salads, vegetables, and cooked grains. Plan on toasting 1 tablespoon for every 2 servings.

To toast, place in a dry skillet over moderate heat and cook, shaking the pan frequently, until the pine nuts are just golden or until the pumpkin seeds are lightly colored and most of them have "popped." This takes just a few minutes, but requires constant attention to avoid burning.

*In
Nikki's
Kitchen*

Roasted Garlic Heads

Roasted garlic pulp is great for seasoning or mashed on bread as a spread. We've seen various methods for preparing the whole heads. Some recipes call for cutting off the top third of the head and rubbing it with oil. Others wrap the head in foil. The approach described below is the simplest and has always given good results. Cooking can be done in a toaster oven to conserve energy.

whole head(s) of garlic, as needed

Preheat the oven to 400°F.

Place the whole head(s) of garlic on a baking sheet. Bake for 40 minutes, or until the head yields easily when gently pressed.

Remove from the oven. When cool enough to handle, remove the outer papery layers, slice off the top or cut with scissors to expose the pulp, separate into individual cloves, and hold each one at the bottom and squeeze to force out the creamy interior.

Roasted Garlic Cloves

Use this technique when you need only a few cloves. A toaster oven can be used to conserve energy.

garlic cloves, as needed

Preheat the oven to 400°F.

Place the unpeeled cloves of garlic in a baking pan in a single layer. Bake for 20 to 25 minutes, or until soft and very lightly colored. Remove each clove as it's done. Don't allow the garlic cloves to become too brown or they'll be bitter.

When cool enough to handle, peel or simply squeeze out the pulp.

Roasted Peppers

sweet or hot peppers, as needed

Broiler method: This approach is convenient for roasting just 1 or a number of peppers. Arrange the peppers on a baking sheet. Place 4 to 6 inches below the heat. Broil for about 15 minutes, turning several times during cooking, until the skin is charred and blistered all over. When the skin is completely blistered, remove from the broiler and wrap the peppers in a clean cloth for a few minutes to steam. When cool enough to handle, scrape off the skin using a small paring knife, cut open, and remove the seeds.

Open flame method: This approach is most convenient when roasting just 1 or 2 peppers. Place the peppers over a gas flame using tongs. Brown on all sides. When the skin is completely blistered, proceed as in the Broiler Method.

Oven method: This approach takes longer than the other two, but requires less monitoring; it's most suited for roasting a number of peppers at one time or when the oven is being used for other dishes as well. Preheat the oven to 450°F. Arrange the peppers on a baking sheet. Bake for 30 minutes, until the pepper skin is a bit crisp and pulls away from the flesh. Turn several times to promote even cooking. When done cooking, wrap the peppers in a clean cloth and proceed as in the Broiler Method.

Using Dried Porcini Mushrooms

Dried porcini mushrooms are a terrific flavor enhancer.

Take a handful of dried mushrooms, place in a bowl, and pour on enough warm water to cover. Let soak for about 10 minutes, until tender. Use as follows:

1. Gently squeeze the moisture from the uncooked, soaked mushrooms back into the bowl. Add the mushrooms to casseroles, vegetable dishes, grains, soups, and sauces. Strain the liquid through a coffee filter or fine mesh strainer to remove any sediment and use in broths, sauces, and when a liquid is called for in salad dressings.

2. Transfer the mushrooms and strained liquid to a small pot. Add a pinch of salt and simmer for 2 minutes. Use as a topping on grains or pasta. Or, remove the mushrooms from the liquid and place on salads. Use the remaining cooking medium to flavor sauces, in broths, and in recipes that call for a little simmering liquid.

3. As a seasoning ingredient, grind dried (unsoaked) porcinis in a coffee grinder or miniprocessor to a powdery consistency. Use a generous pinch to flavor broths, soups, salad dressings, and yogurt cheese.

*In
Nikki's
Kitchen*

Yogurt Cheese

~

Yogurt Cheese, made by draining the liquid whey off yogurt to create a thick, mild-tasting cheese, is featured in Golden Guideline #7. This versatile food can be used in dips, spreads, toppings, baking, sauces, soups, fillings, and more, as our recipes and Nikki's dialogue box on page 444, Things to Do with Yogurt Cheese, demonstrate.

In the countries where yogurt cheese originated, yogurt is commonly hung in a linen bag to drain. Lining a strainer with cheesecloth or using a drip coffee filter are others ways to accomplish the job. But far simpler is to utilize a reusable yogurt cheese funnel designed specifically for this purpose (see "Resources").

Yogurt Cheese can be made with any unflavored or flavored yogurt, so long as it doesn't contain gelatin or modified food starch, which hold the liquid whey in suspension so it can't drain off. The time it takes to drain the liquid and the final yield vary slightly from brand to brand. On average, it takes about 4 hours to reach sour cream consistency, and 12 hours until a soft spreadable cheese is achieved. Two cups of yogurt will yield about 1 cup Yogurt Cheese. There is always some in process in our refrigerator.

> ### ★ STEP-BY-STEP YOGURT CHEESE ★
> 1. Set the yogurt cheese funnel or other device of choice on a stable container large enough to hold the liquid that drains off.
> 2. Fill the selected strainer with yogurt. Cover with a suitable-size plastic lid, plate, or waxed paper for hygiene.
> 3. Place in the refrigerator to drain. You can leave the cheese in the strainer as long as you like, but after about 20 hours it won't get any thicker. Therefore, you might want to transfer it to a container, rinse the strainer, and prepare another batch.

Yogurt Cream

~

Richer than regular yogurt, but not spreadable like Yogurt Cheese, this is an ideal topping for baked potatoes, chili, soups, and stews. The yield varies according to the original yogurt; expect to end up with about half the amount of yogurt you begin with.

plain yogurt

Prepare as for Yogurt Cheese, but drain for only 2 hours.

Basic Bean Cooking

Beans can be purchased dried or canned. Home-cooked dried beans provide the best flavor and texture, and are also less expensive than buying precooked canned beans. For convenience, cook extras, as beans can be refrigerated for a week or so or frozen for the future. Canned beans are good pinch hitters in recipes that call for precooked beans; if salted, you'll need to reduce the salt called for in recipes.

Dried beans last almost indefinitely if stored in dry, airtight containers at room temperature. For best eating, however, try to use them as fresh as possible, or at least within a year of purchase. Beans toughen with age and this increases their cooking time.

Begin preparation by rinsing and discarding any beans that are shriveled or severely discolored or damaged. Also look for the occasional stone.

Most dried beans require soaking prior to cooking to replace the water lost in drying, to hasten cooking, and to increase digestibility; exceptions are lentils (red, green, and French), split peas (green and yellow), and baby lima beans (although limas cook more quickly if presoaked). Whether you choose the traditional or quick-soak method, be sure to select a pot that will accommodate the beans once they expand (some as much as three times their dried volume). Note that with a pressure cooker, you can get around this step.

Traditional soak: A general rule is to use 3 cups of water for each cup of dried beans. Soaking can be done up to 8 hours at room temperature or longer in the refrigerator.

Quick soak: Combine the rinsed beans with three times their volume of water. Bring to a boil for 2 minutes. Cover, remove from the heat, and let stand 1 to 2 hours. Then proceed with cooking.

Some people prefer to discard the soaking water, rinse the beans, and cook them in fresh water to get rid of some of the hard-to-digest sugars (and the resulting gas). This is a matter of preference. Certain herbs and spices, including caraway seed, dill, fennel, coriander, ginger, epazote, as well as the seaweed kombu, are also reputed to decrease flatulence. (For more on this subject, see Chapter 6.)

Cooking is the same after either soaking method, as well as for beans that don't require soaking. If replacing the water, use about two times more water than beans. Beans should be allowed to boil vigorously for 5 to 10 minutes at the onset of cooking. This helps destroy any potentially noxious constituents. (The heat of pressure cooking is similarly effective. However, if a slow cooker is used, the beans should be boiled for the prerequisite 10 minutes first; otherwise, temperatures won't be high enough to destroy nutrient-compromising components.) After this brief boiling period, add gas-reducing seasonings or a strip of kombu, if desired, cover the pot, and simmer gently, keeping the heat as low as possible. Low heat conserves the liquid and also helps keep the beans from splitting. It's a good idea to check progress occasionally, stirring to promote even cooking and adding more liquid if needed. Don't salt until cooking is almost completed, as salt toughens their skin. Figure on about $1/2$ teaspoon salt per cup of dried beans. Because acid also toughens the skin, ingredients such as tomatoes, wine, lemon juice, and vinegar shouldn't be added until the last half hour of cooking.

Use the timetable that follows as a guide and cook beans until completely tender. When done, beans will have an even creamy texture throughout; if the center is still hard, they require longer cooking. Beans shouldn't be eaten raw or undercooked. However, if beans are to be cooked again in a recipe, cook until just tender.

To dramatically decrease cooking time, beans can be prepared in a pressure cooker (see Pressure Cooking in Cooking Techniques, on page 249).

Beans can usually be interchanged in recipes if you want to experiment or have run out of one kind, as long as you take into account their different cooking times.

Once cooked, beans can be kept about a week in the refrigerator. To freeze, pack in a moisture-proof container. For best flavor and texture, use within six months.

★ TIMETABLE FOR COOKING DRIED BEANS ★

Most dried beans measure 2 to $2^{1}/_{2}$ cups per pound. In general, 1 cup dried beans yields $2^{1}/_{2}$ to 3 cups cooked. Timing varies somewhat depending on the age of the beans and the total volume in the pot.

Bean (presoaked)	Cooking time
adzuki beans	1 hour
black beans	$1^{1}/_{2}$ to 2 hours
black-eyed peas	$1^{1}/_{2}$ hours
garbanzo beans (chickpeas)	2 to 3 hours
great northern (cannellini)	$1^{1}/_{2}$ to 2 hours
kidney beans	$1^{1}/_{2}$ to 2 hours
lentils (unsoaked)	30 to 45 minutes
lima beans	45 minutes to $1^{1}/_{2}$ hours
navy and pea beans	1 to $1^{1}/_{2}$ hours
pinto beans	$1^{1}/_{2}$ to 2 hours
soybeans	3 to $3^{1}/_{2}$ hours
split peas (unsoaked)	30 to 45 minutes

Canned Beans

Where time is a factor, canned beans can generally be used in recipes calling for precooked beans. Organic canned beans with very little added salt have the best flavor. Avoid brands that are seasoned or have sweeteners added.

Canned beans should be stored in a cool, dry place and used within a year of purchase for best flavor and texture. In recipes calling for bean cooking liquid, the liquid surrounding the canned beans can be used as a cooking medium, thinned or extended with water if necessary; if salted, be sure to reduce (or omit) the salt in a recipe. If beans are surrounded by congealed liquid, rinse well under cold running water before using.

The heat of processing makes canned beans mushier than home-cooked beans, although garbanzos and soybeans are two varieties that hold up quite well. This may somewhat alter the texture of dishes, unless mashing or pureeing are indicated. When using canned beans, keep cooking time to a minimum to avoid making them even softer.

Basic Grain Cooking

The preparation of whole grains is almost effortless. It merely involves combining the grain with a suitable amount of liquid and simmering gently for an appropriate length of time. How much liquid and how much time are outlined below. The liquid can be plain water, broth, diluted tomato juice, or some other flavorful medium according to recipes. No matter what the proportion, either of two basic approaches can be followed.

Boiling water method: Bring a measured amount of liquid to a boil in a pot and sprinkle the grain in slowly. Once all the grain is introduced, cover and set the heat to low so that the liquid barely simmers. Cook until the grain is tender and the liquid absorbed. With this technique the grains swell rapidly, causing them to remain separate when done.

Cold water method: Rinse the grain through a strainer under cold water to remove surface starch. Place in a pot with the specified amount of cold liquid and bring to a boil. Cover, turn the heat to low so that the liquid barely simmers, and cook until tender. With this approach the grain may be just a bit more sticky.

Regardless of the method, during cooking the liquid should barely simmer. Furious boiling causes grains to burst, making them gummy rather than fluffy. Don't stir during cooking, unless directed in the recipe, as this loosens the starch on the outer surface and also alters the texture. (In dishes like risotto and polenta, stirring is called for to create the characteristic creaminess.)

The need for salt will vary with the flavor of the cooking medium and personal preferences. A general guideline is 1/2 teaspoon salt per cup of dry grain. This can be added during cooking or afterward. For rice and millet, the addition of salt tends to harden the grain and adds to the cooking time. Thus, it's best to wait at least 15 minutes into cooking before salting.

To determine doneness, when the cooking time is almost over, insert a chopstick or poke the grain with a fork to see if all the liquid has been absorbed at the bottom of the pot. Chew a few top grains to check tenderness. If not done, continue to cook, adding a little more liquid, if needed, to prevent scorching. If the grains are tender but a little liquid still remains, uncover partially and cook a little longer, until dry. When cooking is completed, remove from the heat and, if possible, let sit in the covered pot for 10 to 15 minutes before serving.

Other convenient ways to cook grains include pressure cooking (see Pressure

One cup of dry grain produces two to three times as much cooked, or enough for four servings as an accompaniment. For a featured dish, or large appetites, plan on 1 to 1½ cups cooked grain per serving. Timing will vary somewhat with the total volume in the pot, the size of the flame, and the fit of the lid.

Grain (1 cup dry)	Liquid (cups)	Cooking time (minutes)
barley, hulled (whole grain)	2⅔	75 to 90
brown rice	2 to 2¼	45 to 50
couscous (whole wheat)	1½	10
cracked wheat (bulgur)	2	15 to 20
kamut	2½	75
kasha (buckwheat)	2	20
millet	3	30
oat groats	2	45
quinoa*	2	15
rye berries	2	50
wheat berries	2	50
wild rice	2½	50

*Rinse quinoa thoroughly in cold water before cooking to remove the bitter residue that coats the seeds.

Cooking in Cooking Techniques, on page 249) or using a rice cooker, an electric appliance suitable for cooking most grains.

Basic Cooking Techniques

To conserve nutrients and minimize the need for adding concentrated fats (that is, butter and oil), we rely on several favorite cooking techniques.

Steaming

Steaming is one of the simplest ways to prepare vegetables without adding fat. The process involves placing cut-up or whole vegetables in a steamer basket set above rapidly boiling water. The pot is then covered, allowing the steam to penetrate and cook the vegetables.

For even cooking, keep the size of the pieces uniform and spread them out over the bottom of the steamer, rather than piling them too deeply. If using a collapsible steaming basket, choose a broad pot that allows the bed to fully expand.

Note: Tofu and tempeh can also be cubed and steamed.

Step-by-Step Steaming

1. Fill the pot with one to two inches of water and bring to a boil over high heat.
2. Insert the steamer with food, cover, and reduce the heat low enough to maintain a boil.
3. Cook as directed in the recipe or to taste. Keep in mind that the smaller the pieces, the faster they'll cook. If a range of time is given in a recipe, test by piercing with a fork after the minimum suggested time. Continue cooking, if necessary, until the food reaches the desired doneness.

Seasoning Suggestions

If you're steaming vegetables as an accompaniment:

- Season after cooking (and while still hot) with a splash of soy sauce, freshly squeezed lemon juice, or a flavorful vinegar
- Sprinkle with herbs, minced lemon rind, and/or freshly ground pepper
- Drizzle with a bit of olive, flaxseed, or hemp oil, or toss with a favorite salad dressing

Stir-Steaming

Stir-steaming refers to a technique of cooking food quickly in a wok or skillet, stirring almost constantly until the vegetables begin to wilt. The food is then finished off by tightly covering the pot and letting it steam in its natural juices or a bit of added liquid to just cook through. If a heavy, well-seasoned wok or cast-iron or high-quality stainless-steel skillet is used, food won't stick. If needed, a bit of liquid such as wine, cooking sherry, diluted soy sauce, vegetable broth, lemon juice, bean cooking liquid, or even water can be added during the stirring phase to prevent sticking.

Stewing

Foods that are inherently moist, such as onions, mushrooms, and peppers, can be cooked under cover in a high-quality stainless-steel or cast-iron pot, allowing them to stew in their own juices. For additional flavor, or where a food's own juices are insufficient, a few spoonfuls of broth, bean cooking liquid, diluted soy sauce, wine, cooking sherry, mild vinegar, or even water can be included.

Pressure Cooking

The pressure cooker is one of our most prized utensils. If you want whole-foods with fast-food convenience, nothing beats the pressure cooker. Most foods cook in about 70 percent less time, and flavor and nutrients are well conserved. Although a pressure cooker may be intimidating at first, it's really a very easy tool to use, especially if you get a model with a quick-pressure-release valve. A

6-quart pressure cooker is suitable for most households; if cooking for more than six, however, an 8-quart cooker may be preferred.

When using a pressure cooker, be sure to follow the manufacturer's instructions for assembling and operating. Some basic principles that can be applied to all units follow.

Basic Principles of Pressure Cooking

Pressure cooking depends on liquid to produce the necessary steam. Use a recipe designed for the pressure cooker or manufacturer's guidelines for the proper ratio of water to solid matter. As a general guideline:

1. Load the cooker with the prepared ingredients and required amount of liquid. Never fill more than two-thirds the height of the pot.
2. Close the cooker and place on high heat. Be sure the steam-release valve is properly aligned to prevent steam from escaping.
3. Once full pressure is achieved (as indicated in the operating manual), reduce the heat to just maintain pressure. Begin timing at this point.
4. When the recommended cooking time is over, remove the cooker from the heat. Reduce the pressure by carefully and slowly opening the pressure-release valve (if applicable), until steam no longer escapes and the safety lock recedes. For models without a pressure-release valve, the cooker can be cooled down under cold water.
5. When pressure cooking in the steaming basket, add ½ cup water for up to 5 minutes of pressure cooking, 1 cup water for 6 to 10 minutes, and another 1 cup water for each additional 10 minutes.

Timing

Timing is crucial to the success of pressure cooking. Begin as soon as pressure is reached. Use a kitchen timer to avoid miscalculation. If uncertain as to timing, it's best to underestimate. If you've guessed wrong, you can always bring the pressure up again and cook a bit longer.

Selecting a Pressure Cooker

There are many different pressure cookers on the market. Older models feature a weight balanced loosely on top. The weight jiggles as it releases bursts of steam. When cooking is completed, you must wait for the pressure to reduce naturally or carry the loaded pot to the sink and run it under cold water. This type of pressure cooker is the most temperamental to use.

Newer pressure cookers use a spring valve to set specific pressure, or rely on a concealed weight that can be regulated somewhat by listening to the pot hiss. Both of these designs are easy to use, and although the latter isn't always as precise in timing, this cooker usually costs less. We have used this less-expensive model with great success. Since just a little steam is released during cooking, these newer cookers are also relatively quiet. Moreover, most new pressure cookers have several built-in safety mechanisms, as well as a button for quickly releasing the steam, which is a very worthwhile convenience.

Whatever model you choose, make it stainless steel, not aluminum.

Cooking Under Pressure

Vegetables Vegetables cook quite quickly under pressure. The preferred technique is to place the prepared vegetables on the steaming basket above boiling water. As a general guideline, add 1/2 cup water for up to 5 minutes of pressure cooking, 1 cup water for 6 to 10 minutes, and another 1 cup water for each additional 10 minutes.

Where pressure cooking time is given as "0," remove the cooker from the stove as soon as the full pressure is achieved and reduce pressure quickly. When a range is given, variations are due to size and age (for example, larger and older vegetables require more cooking.)

Vegetable	Preparation	Water (cups)	Time (minutes)
artichokes	whole	1 1/2	11
asparagus	end trimmed	1/2	1 to 2
beets	whole, small whole, medium	1 1 1/2	10 12 to 16
broccoli	full stalks florets	1/2 1/2	2 1
brussels sprouts	whole	1/2	3
cabbage	quartered cut into strips	1/2 1	5 to 6 2
carrots	1/2-inch-thick coins large chunks whole	1/2 1/2 1	1 2 4 to 7
cauliflower	whole florets	1 1/2	5 2
green beans	whole, ends trimmed 1-inch lengths	1/2 1/2	1 to 2 0 to 1
leeks	3-inch pieces	1/2	3
onions	wedges	1/2	1
parsnips	whole 1-inch chunks	1 1/2	8 to 10 3 to 4

In Nikki's Kitchen

Vegetable	Preparation	Water (cups)	Time (minutes)
peppers	halved, stuffed with precooked filling	1/2	3
potatoes	new, whole whole, small (3 oz) whole, medium (5 oz) whole, large (8 oz) 3-inch cubes 1 1/2-inch cubes 1/2-inch-thick slices	1/2 1 1 1/2 2 1/2 1 1/2 1 1/2	5 10 15 25 12 6 2
pumpkin	large wedges	1	8 to 10
squash, acorn	halved, seeds removed	1	7
squash, yellow	halved, stuffed with precooked filling	1/2	3
sweet potato	whole halved	1 1/2	6 to 8 3 to 4
turnips	1-inch cubes or 1/2-inch-thick slices	1/2	3 to 4
zucchini	1/2-inch rounds	1/2	1

Dried Beans Beans may be soaked or not prior to pressure cooking. Unsoaked beans need longer cooking and more water, but also froth less and hold their shape better. To reduce the froth and foam that develop when cooking beans:

- Never fill the cooker more than halfway.
- Don't use less than 1 1/2 cups water.
- Wipe the inside of the pressure cooker lid with a little oil.

Whether cooking soaked or unsoaked beans, the procedure is the same. Combine the beans and water as recommended below. You can alter the amounts proportionately. Bring to a boil and skim off any surface froth. Close the cooker, bring the pressure up over medium-high heat, reduce the heat to just maintain pressure, and cook for the time indicated. At the end of cooking time, reduce the pressure either by waiting 5 minutes and then slowly turning the steam-release valve to allow gas to escape gradually (don't open all at once), by waiting 5 minutes and running the pot under cold water, or by letting the pot cool down on its own. If the beans aren't completely cooked, return to pressure and cook another 5 minutes. This can be repeated as many times as necessary. Don't add salt until after cooking.

Bean	Volume (cups)	Presoaked (water/cups)	Time (minutes)	Unsoaked (water/cups)	Time (minutes)
adzuki	2	3	10	4	15
black beans	2	3	6	5	25
black-eyed peas	2	3	5	4	15
garbanzos (chickpeas)	2	2	18	5	48
great northern (cannellini)	2	4	7	5	35
kidney beans	2	4	8 to 10	5	35 to 40
lentils	2	do not soak	NA	4½	10
lima beans	2	3	5	5	15 to 18
navy beans or pea beans	2	3	7	5	30
pintos	2	3	7 to 8	5	35
soybeans	2	4	16 to 18	5	45

Grains The volume of grains more than doubles with cooking. As with dried beans, they shouldn't exceed the halfway point in the pressure cooker initially. Wash and drain well prior to cooking. Combine with two times their volume of water, unless otherwise directed. Close the cooker and bring to pressure over high heat. Lower the heat to just maintain pressure and cook for the specified time. Remove from the heat and let sit 5 minutes. Then gradually open the pressure-release valve (don't open all at once) or reduce the pressure under cold water.

If the grains aren't tender at the end of the designated time, return to pressure and cook for an additional 5 minutes. This can be repeated as many times as necessary. When cooking is completed, if a little liquid remains, stir well and it will probably be absorbed in a few minutes. If too much to absorb, drain. (Some people prefer to cook grains in a large volume of water and drain off the excess. This causes a small loss of nutrients, but the liquid can be reserved for broth or a cooking medium.) Don't salt until after cooking.

Caution: Small grains such as millet, quinoa, kasha, and cracked wheat shouldn't be pressure cooked, as they can clog the valve.

In Nikki's Kitchen

Grain	Time (minutes)
barley, whole	30
barley, pearled	20
brown rice*	15
kamut	45
rye berries†	35
wheat berries†	35
wild rice	25

*For brown rice, use an equal volume of grain and liquid.
†For a drier texture, reduce the liquid to 1¹/₂ cups per 1 cup of these grains.

*The
Healthiest
Diet in
the World*

The Golden Pantry

To use the Golden Guidelines effectively, the appropriate foods must be available. "The Golden Pantry" provides a comprehensive list of things to keep in your cupboard, refrigerator, and freezer. With these items routinely on hand, you'll have no trouble following our recipes and devising similarly nourishing meals and snacks.

Many pantry staples can be found in the supermarket. However, for a larger selection, the natural food store is your best bet. Whenever possible, choose organic products.

The Grain Pantry

Grains are the predominant ingredient in flours, hot and ready-to-eat cereals, pasta, breadstuffs, crackers, cookies, and cakes. Grains that are left intact—which means most of the bran and all of the germ remain—have the most to offer. They contain the full potential of vitamins and minerals, unlike refined grains, which are missing the bran and germ. The bran is the source of fiber; thus, to reap the real benefits of grains, the word "whole" must precede "wheat," brown rice takes priority over white rice, and whole-grain cornmeal (sometimes called stone-ground or unbolted) is preferred to the more typical "degermed" cornmeal. The roster of grains has been expanded in the last few years; many choices that have been used historically in other parts of the world and are enjoying a resurgence in North America.

Storage: Grains should be stored in airtight containers in a cool, dark, dry place. Heat and light lessen their quality and moisture encourages mold. Properly stored, whole grains last for years, although it's best to use them within six to nine months. Whole grains that are ground into flour or meal should be refrigerated and preferably used within two to three months.

Amaranth	Oats
Barley (hulled)	Quinoa
Buckwheat (kasha)	Rice (brown)
Cornmeal (whole grain, unbolted; not degermed)	Rye
	Spelt
Cracked wheat (bulgur)	Wheat germ
Flaxseed meal	Whole wheat
Kamut	Wild rice
Millet	

The Bean Pantry

The common bean varieties are listed below. A more adventurous assortment is available through specialty mail-order sources (see "Resources"). The names alone are intriguing enough to tempt you to try them: appaloosas, calypsos, whippoorwills, tongues of fire, baccacia beans, winged beans, soldier beans, black turtles, Jacob's cattle, rattlesnake beans.

Cooked dried beans have a better texture and flavor than canned beans, but the convenience of a can is a big selling point. Canned beans suffer from two culinary limitations—their tendency to be mushy and salty. Consequently, they work best in recipes that call for pureeing or mashing, or where texture isn't critical. Brands geared to the health food market tend to be unsalted or relatively low in salt; otherwise, be sure to reduce the salt in recipes. Rinsing canned beans for a few minutes under cold water will wash away a substantial amount of salt, but then you lose the surrounding liquid, which can serve as a useful cooking medium. Avoid brands that are sweetened. (For those whose bean use may be constricted by time, the pressure cooker is another option. Pressure cooking directions are found on page 249.)

Bean varieties can be interchanged in recipes if you want to experiment or have run out of the specified kind. However, if uncooked dried beans are called for, you may have to make adjustments for variations in cooking time.

Storage: Dried beans keep practically forever if maintained in a dry, airtight container, preferably away from heat and light. However, the sooner they're eaten, the better they taste. Legumes toughen with storage and as they age they take longer to cook.

Cooked beans can be preserved in the refrigerator for about a week, or frozen up to six months.

Bean Selections

Adzuki beans (aduki)	Cannellini beans
Black beans	Chickpeas (garbanzos)
Black-eyed peas (cowpeas)	Cranberry beans (Roman beans)

Fava beans	Pigeon peas
Great northern	Pink beans
Kidney beans	Pinto beans
Lentils (red, green, and French)	Red beans
Lima beans	Soybeans
Mung beans	Split peas
Navy beans	White beans
Pea beans	Whole dried peas

The Soy Foods Pantry

Soy foods that are included in "In Nikki's Kitchen" are listed below, along with storage recommendations.

Soybeans, dried: Stored in an airtight container, they'll keep practically forever. Canned cooked dried soybeans are available in natural food stores.

Soy flour: Available both full fat and defatted (we prefer the former). Refrigerate.

Tofu: Comes in soft, regular, firm, extra firm, and silken varieties, and preseasoned forms as well. If recipes don't specify, firm is always a safe choice, but regular or extra firm will generally also work.

Unless aseptically packaged (sold in shelf-stable boxes), tofu should be kept cold. Sealed containers are usually dated. Once opened, keep submerged in water and refrigerated for up to a week. Changing the water daily keeps the tofu fresh. Tofu sold loose from bulk containers should be handled the same way. Tofu can be frozen for up to six months (see the directions on page 89). Freezing dramatically changes the texture, making it the preferred form for some recipes, but not interchangeable with fresh tofu in others.

Tempeh: Tempeh can be made with soybeans only, or combined with grains. Sometimes vegetables or seasonings are added as well. For the most protein and soy constituents, all-soy tempeh is suggested. However, some people prefer the milder flavor of grain-containing tempeh.

Refrigerate up to ten days or freeze for three to six months. White or gray patches on the surface are normal, but avoid tempeh covered with black patches or showing mold of any other color. When spoiled, tempeh has an ammonia-like odor.

Soy milk: Select full-fat soy milk; whether or not it's fortified with calcium and vitamins is your choice. Shelf-stable varieties of soy milk are dated. Refrigerate after opening. Fresh soy dairy milk and reconstituted powders require refrigeration. Treat as you would dairy counterparts.

Soy sauce: Use only genuine (traditional) soy sauce. Real soy sauce (sometimes referred to as shoyu) is prepared by aging soy beans along with cracked roasted wheat, salt, and water, then squeezing the resulting cake to produce the characteristic brown liquid. The soy sauce known as tamari is made without adding wheat. Sometimes alcohol is added to these products to preserve them. Commercial soy sauce production in the United States relies on a chemical process using hydrolyzed soy protein, corn syrup, and caramel coloring; no aging or fermentation take place. This kind of soy sauce should be avoided.

Soy sauce keeps indefinitely at room temperature.

Miso: Miso can be made with soy alone, or a combination of soy and grain. The darker the miso, the stronger the flavor. Lighter miso is a bit sweet. All miso is salty.

Miso keeps for a long time, but should be refrigerated. The white mold that sometimes forms on the surface is harmless. It can be scraped off or mixed in.

The Vegetable Pantry

Variety and abundance is the goal when it comes to vegetables. A comprehensive list of vegetables to sample is included in Chapter 4 under Picking Vegetables.

Fresh vegetables are almost always the preference. Buy organic whenever you can, particularly when it comes to vegetables you eat frequently.

Although we don't use them often, frozen vegetables can be a great convenience and add to seasonal variety. For example, frozen corn and peas can be added to grains, soups, and mixed vegetable dishes at the last minute for color, flavor, and a nutrition boost. And frozen spinach is very handy when chopped spinach is called for in a filling mixture (as for Eggplant Rollatini).

The only canned vegetables we use are canned tomato products (including whole and crushed tomatoes, tomato puree, tomato paste, and tomato juice) and canned artichoke hearts or bottoms.

In the dried vegetable category, mushrooms (of all varieties) are quite useful for intensifying the flavor of numerous dishes, as are dried tomatoes. When dried tomatoes are referred to in our recipes, we mean the leathery moisture-free product, not the kind swimming in oil. With one or more varieties of dried seaweed in the pantry you will be able to make our Sea Vegetable Topping, Orange-Arame Salad, and do some experimenting on your own. Seaweeds can be found in natural food stores, Asian markets, or ordered by mail (see "Resources").

The Fruit Pantry

A broad assortment of fruit to pick from is found in Picking Fruit, which is part of Chapter 4.

As with vegetables, fresh organic fruit is the best choice. When orange or lemon peel is included in a recipe, buying an organic specimen is even more important. Other useful fruit items include dried fruits, unsweetened applesauce (for baking), canned unsweetened pineapple, unsweetened fruit juices (especially orange and apple for use as cooking mediums), and frozen berries.

The Nut/Seed Pantry

Choose unsalted nuts and seeds that are either raw or dry roasted, preferably organic. Nuts in the shell keep longer, but shelled nuts are more convenient, especially for cooking. Small quantities can be kept in airtight containers at room temperature for snacking. However, to preserve for more than a few weeks, the refrigerator is better.

Many nuts and seeds are also available ground as nut "butters." Choose brands that contain nothing but the nut. Never buy a nut butter that has hydrogenated oil listed in the ingredients. Store nut butters in the refrigerator.

Nut/Seed Varieties

Almonds
Brazil nuts
Butternuts
Cashews
Filberts (hazelnuts)
Peanuts
Pecans

Pine nuts (pignolia)
Pistachios
Pumpkin seeds
Sesame seeds (tahini is the "butter" form)
Sunflower seeds
Walnuts

Concentrated Fats

Since the majority of fats in *The Healthiest Diet in the World* come from intact foods (nuts, seeds, grains), rather than concentrated extracts such as oils and butter, you'll only need a limited supply of items in this category. The discussion of Edible Oils in Chapter 2 will acquaint you with the various choices and their characteristics. For some of these products, the natural food store is your primary source. We suggest you have the following on hand:

Olive oil: Virgin or extra virgin. The preferred all-around choice for cooking and salads. Store at cool room temperature in opaque containers or a dark cupboard.

Canola oil: Purchase a brand that is cold-pressed (specified on the label), rather than expeller-pressed (which is what the majority of commercial products are). Use in limited amounts, mainly for baked goods. Store in the refrigerator.

Flaxseed oil: As a nutritional booster, where appropriate (as explained in Chapter 2), and a flavoring element in certain recipes. This isn't a cooking oil and should be used only on raw or already cooked foods. Keep in the refrigerator, preferably in an opaque bottle. Use within two months.

Hemp oil: If you're interested in using hemp oil, mail order may be necessary (see "Resources"). Can be used wherever flaxseed oil is appropriate and should be handled similarly.

Sesame oil: Sesame oil (and particularly toasted sesame oil) can be used in small amounts as a flavoring agent. It keeps well at cool room temperature, but refrigeration maintains quality longer.

The Dairy

The principal dairy items you need to fulfill *The Healthiest Diet in the World* are yogurt and homemade yogurt cheese (page 244). Also useful are eggs. A few recipes call for cheese (mainly feta or parmesan), but it isn't essential to any.

Miscellaneous

Flaxseeds: Flaxseeds are sold in natural food stores. Buy whole seeds and grind in small batches as needed. Store whole seeds and ground meal in the refrigerator.

Vinegars: There is an incredible selection of vinegars on the market, both flavored and unflavored and they make great seasoning agents, if not overdone. To keep our recipes usable for everyone, we have restricted our choices to balsamic, wine, and cider vinegar. In a pinch, white vinegar can replace wine or cider vinegar, but it is somewhat harsher. If you enjoy other exotic vinegars, feel free to experiment with them in cooking, as well as on salads and as a seasoning for simple cooked vegetables.

Cooking wines: Cooking sherry and Chinese cooking wine (marketed for this purpose and not suitable for drinking) make excellent cooking mediums. They keep indefinitely at room temperature. Dry red and white drinking wines are also included in some recipes. If you enjoy a glass of wine, conserve the rest of the bottle in the refrigerator for cooking. Nondrinkers needn't purchase a high-price wine for cooking, but be sure to pick a dry (not sweet) variety.

Sweeteners: When sweeteners are called for in "In Nikki's Kitchen," they are either honey, molasses, or pure maple syrup. As they keep for a very long time (honey and molasses in the food cabinet, maple syrup in the refrigerator), we stock them all.

Mustard: Prepared mustard is a handy flavoring agent. There are many tasty types on the market, some smooth and creamy, some grainy, others sweet, and some creatively spiced. Stored in the refrigerator, mustard will keep for a long time.

Herbs and spices: The possibilities here are numerous. As preground herbs and spices don't keep their vibrant flavor forever, try to buy only what you think you'll use within three to six months. Store in airtight containers, and not where it's overly warm. The dried seasonings we use most often are listed below. In addition, we suggest you make frequent use of fresh garlic, fresh gingerroot, and fresh parsley. Fresh cilantro, basil, and dill are also recommended in some dishes. Prepared hot pepper sauce is another good seasoning/condiment (for those so inclined).

Herb/Spice Varieties

Basil
Bay leaf
Cayenne
Chili powder
Cinnamon (both sticks and ground)
Crushed red pepper flakes
Cumin
Curry powder (we recommend
   imported varieties from India)

Mint
Mustard (dry)
Nutmeg (we recommend buying the
   whole nut and a grater)
Oregano
Paprika
Pepper (freshly ground)
Turmeric

Baking soda and baking powder: If you bake, you will want these in the cabinet. If not, they're unnecessary.

Cooking Implements

The Healthiest Diet in the World doesn't require any exotic cooking equipment, just the basics—pots and pans, knives, a blender and/or food processor. However, there are a few tools that make certain tasks so much easier they deserve special mention.

Yogurt cheese funnel: A strainer specially designed to drain the liquid whey off of yogurt, leaving a thick, rich cheese (see "Resources").

Pressure cooker: If time is a factor, the pressure cooker is a tool you'll love. Cuts cooking time for beans, grains, soups, and more by at least half (see "Resources").

Salad spinner: Daily salads are more likely to become a reality if you have a salad spinner to remove the moisture from freshly washed greens. In households with children, this is a safe tool kids love to operate.

Collapsible steaming basket: This practical device, which fits inside an ordinary pot, is still the best tool for steaming vegetables.

Potato masher: A handy tool not only for potatoes, but for mashing beans, tofu, avocado, and sauces to a rough, homey consistency.

PART III

Mentor

CHAPTER 1

Controversial Carbohydrates

❧

The position of carbohydrates in our diet is the subject of a great deal of attention. The 1995 Dietary Guidelines issued by the U.S. Department of Agriculture recommend choosing "most of your foods from the grain products group (6–11 servings), the vegetable group (3–5 servings), and the fruit group (2–3 servings)." The 1996 guidelines developed by the American Cancer Society counsel you to "choose most of the foods you eat from plant sources," including "five or more servings of fruits and vegetables each day," and "other foods from plant sources, such as breads, cereals, grain products, rice, pasta, or beans several times each day."

Unfortunately, several major points haven't been taken into account by these sweeping recommendations, and what they have overlooked is significant: These include the properties of individual carbohydrate-containing foods, the varying nature of carbohydrates themselves, and the differences in how we each process them. All of these factors can have a profound impact on your well-being.

Many health professionals counsel a high-carbohydrate diet for weight management, to control blood sugar levels in non-insulin-dependent (type II) diabetes, and to prevent heart disease, diverticulosis, and certain cancers. Other health professionals contend that carbohydrates elevate blood levels of insulin, which in turn can inhibit fat breakdown, promote storage of body fat, increase levels of circulating triglycerides (fat), and trigger low blood sugar levels. These practitioners believe that as a result, excess carbohydrates promote obesity, heart disease, diabetes, and hypoglycemia.

As you are about to discover, people's individual biochemistry probably makes both camps right to some degree. Therefore, it is imperative that you know how carbohydrates act within the body in order to determine how they fit into your individual diet. Some of the things that can help you make that determination are understanding (1) how carbohydrates are used to produce energy, as well as the long-term results of increased carbohydrate intake; (2) the influence of carbohydrates on fat storage and fat breakdown; (3) the part carbohydrates play in controlling total food intake; and (4) the other nutritional elements found in carbohydrate-containing foods.

A Brief History of Carbohydrates

Carbohydrates are one of the three main components in food, along with protein and fat. They are the body's primary source of energy. During digestion they're converted into glucose and absorbed into the bloodstream. This glucose is what the more familiar term "blood sugar" refers to.

Every cell in the body uses glucose to function. The cells absorb glucose from the bloodstream and transform it into energy via a complex oxidation process that many people refer to as "burning calories." While energy can also be generated by the oxidation of fats and proteins, the brain, the central nervous system, and a few other specialized cells depend entirely on glucose.

In order to adapt to the lifestyle changes that have taken place over the course of human history, the body has developed regulatory mechanisms that control the ratio of carbohydrate burning to carbohydrate intake. It is assumed that in the early days of hunting and gathering, carbohydrates were less common in the diet than they became once people settled down and began growing grains and cultivating plants. This shift in the diet presumably required considerable transformation within body chemistry, as the human system went from relying on an inconsistent food supply (predominantly protein and fat) to having a continually available reserve of food (with more carbohydrates). This condition of "food on demand" is compounded by the fact that since the beginning of the industrial revolution there has been an almost limitless offering of sweet (and fatty) foods.

Where Carbohydrates Come From

Carbohydrates occur in two basic forms: starches and sugars.

Commonly eaten foods high in starch are:
- Wheat, rice, and other grains
- Cereal and pasta
- Bread and other baked goods
- Root vegetables such as potatoes, rutabagas, and turnips
- Legumes (dried beans)

Other vegetables contain lesser amounts of starch, and much of this is in a form known as fiber that isn't readily converted to energy.

Commonly eaten foods high in sugar are:
- Fruit
- Certain vegetables (for example, corn, sweet peas, beets, carrots, parsnips, and winter squash)
- Milk

- Concentrated sweeteners such as table sugar, corn syrup, honey, molasses, maple syrup, and the like

Depending on which foods are chosen to supply the body with carbohydrates, they can concurrently furnish essential vitamins, minerals, and other biologically active substances such as fiber and phytochemicals. Or, they can be nutritionally empty—that is, devoid of these elements.

NIKKI'S DIALOGUE BOX

Complex Carbohydrates DO NOT Mean High Fiber

"The term 'complex carbohydrates' is often used as a synonym for starch. Some people interpret this to mean 'high fiber,' or think complex carbohydrates affect blood sugar differently or are a more desirable kind of starch. These beliefs aren't necessarily true. Complex carbohydrates *are* starches: they can be either high or low in fiber and, depending on many different factors, can have varying effects on blood sugar levels."

What the Body Does with Carbohydrates

There has probably never been a time in human history when dietary practices changed as much as during the past 150 years. This makes it easier to understand how the body's inability to keep up with these changes, and our individual biochemistry, might substantially alter the way any one person utilizes carbohydrates. And this is why knowing how the body uses carbohydrates can help you find a compatible place for them in your diet.

In order for carbohydrates to be absorbed they must first be broken down into simple sugars. This is accomplished in the stomach and intestines by the action of specific enzymes that convert most of the carbohydrate into glucose (blood sugar). Depending on the source, however, some of the carbohydrates may not be completely digested and are subject to bacterial fermentation. These are appropriately named *resistant starches*.

As glucose forms it passes into the bloodstream for delivery throughout the body. The body's regulatory mechanisms strive to keep the level of glucose in the blood within a narrow range. To preserve this status, most of the glucose produced during the digestion of food must be absorbed rapidly into the cells. There it is either turned into immediate energy (calories) or stored for later use.

The body stores energy for the future in two forms. The first way is by converting it into what is known as glycogen. This glycogen is stored in the liver and in muscle tissue and can vary considerably over the course of a day in response to food intake and exertion. Moreover, it can be maximized by eating a lot of carbohydrates—a tactic called "carbohydrate loading" that many athletes employ in order to store energy for endurance while performing. In any case, the overall capacity to store glycogen is quite small. Any additional remaining glucose is preserved for later use by transforming it into fat and depositing it in what is known as adipose tissue—what most of us think of as body fat.

All three of these processes—glucose absorption, glycogen synthesis, and fat storage—are stimulated by insulin, a hormone produced by the pancreas. Insulin production responds directly to the amount of glucose in the blood: When blood sugar concentrations rise, so does insulin secretion. When blood sugar levels fall, insulin secretion diminishes and a signal is sent to the liver to release hormones that transform glycogen back into glucose. When blood glucose concentrations are again adequate, insulin provides the signal to quit releasing glycogen.

Before the body resorts to using stored glycogen for fuel, however, a more powerful system may intervene: hunger, the primitive force that arouses us to seek food and consume it. (We will look at the effect of blood sugar and insulin on hunger a little later on.)

Although fat is an additional dietary source of energy, carbohydrates are used preferentially by the body if they're available. What this means is that when large amounts of carbohydrates are eaten there is less need to use fat as fuel. This influences the long-term outcome of how the body processes the fats we consume.

High or Low: Which Way to Go?

Scientific interest as to whether the overall amount of carbohydrate in the diet influences how the body handles carbohydrate itself has spawned a number of experiments. The goal of this research has been to measure if calorie needs are changed by altering carbohydrate intake. The conclusion, thus far, is that a wide range of carbohydrate intake can be tolerated by so-called "normal" individuals. This means they can eat more or less without appreciable weight fluctuations. However, the *total volume* of carbohydrate does make a difference in the way the body manages various other nutrients:

• For example, the fate of fats you eat is controlled to a great extent by the amount of carbohydrate you eat. When carbohydrate intake is habitually low, only a small amount of stored glycogen is created. To maintain energy levels, as blood sugar drops, fat is used as the energy source. This fat can be supplied by food or stored tissue fats.

• On the other hand, as carbohydrate intake rises, glycogen stores increase. Because the body prefers to get its energy from carbohydrates, when glycogen storage is ample, if recently eaten carbohydrates don't provide enough glucose to meet immediate needs, the abundant glycogen stores are mobilized. When this happens, dietary fats aren't used for energy. The fate of these fats influences fat levels in the blood and in body cells.

Some people's systems control these variables quite comfortably. But many others encounter trouble due to genetic predisposition or poor diet, which reduces their ability to handle carbohydrates efficiently.

To create a long-term balance between food intake and energy output, the body may "readjust" itself by increasing the number and size of individual fat cells. Studies confirm a direct relationship between carbohydrate intake, the accumulation of body fat, and the blood level of circulating fats (known as triglycerides). As you will read in the upcoming section Hyperinsulinemia and Heart Disease, elevated triglycerides are linked with several coronary risk factors. There is also evidence that as fat cells expand due to accumulated fat deposits, they become "insulin resistant." This, in part, explains why body weight is often associated with impaired glucose tolerance and diabetes. In fact, insulin resistance, which is discussed in depth in the following section, is a pivotal concern for each of us as we strive to discover our most compatible carbohydrate choices.

Understandably, it can be distressing to learn that as we eat less fat and more carbohydrates there is a tendency to spontaneously produce more circulating and stored fats. What is even more troublesome to some people is the discovery that sugars have a more pronounced impact on this phenomenon than starches. As you continue to read this chapter, you will see how profound this association between carbohydrates, fats, and ultimately your health can be.

Upon hearing that eating too much carbohydrate can lead to weight gain, insulin resistance, and unhealthy levels of fat in the bloodstream, many people assume avoiding carbohydrates would be better. But this, too, takes its toll. When carbohydrate intake is restricted, fat and protein must provide the body with the energy it demands. This isn't the most favorable choice for the central nervous system, including the brain, for these cells function best when glucose is readily available to them.

Furthermore, if carbohydrates are restricted, in order to turn fat and protein into energy, the body has to work harder. This places a burden on the kidneys and liver and is a potential threat to health. When the diet is simultaneously low in calories, another concern arises. Ordinarily, the role of protein is to provide raw materials for building enzymes, hormones, antibodies, and numerous other vital substances. If protein must be sacrificed for energy, all bodily systems suffer. Another task that depends on protein is the growth and repair of muscle tissues. If protein must be relinquished for energy, new muscle tissue can't develop. In fact, if this situation persists, over time all muscles (including the major organs) may be compromised.

Most people can tolerate at least 40 percent of their calories from carbohydrate. Those who handle carbohydrates well should be able to go as high as 60 percent. Since carbohydrates are normally measured in grams, you can use the following table to determine a reasonable carbohydrate intake for yourself.

Calorie Intake	Grams Carbohydrate at 40% Calories	Grams Carbohydrate at 50% Calories	Grams Carbohydrate at 60% Calories
800	80	100	120
1,000	100	125	150
1,200	120	150	180
1,500	150	188	225
1,800	180	225	270
2,000	200	250	300
2,200	220	275	330
2,400	240	300	360
2,800	280	350	420
3,000	300	375	450

*To compute carbohydrates at any calorie level: calories × desired percent ÷ 4 = target level carbohydrates in grams
Example: Target level of carbohydrates for 1,650 calorie intake at 45 percent calories = 1,650 × .45 (742.5) ÷ 4 = 185 grams
Note: Preference should always be given to the carbohydrates in whole grains, legumes, and vegetables.

The Delicate Carbohydrate-Insulin Balance

As we have already said, most of the carbohydrate we eat is digested and converted into glucose. This glucose is absorbed into the bloodstream and transported to the cells with the help of insulin. There it's converted into energy. If there's more than enough glucose to meet immediate energy needs, the excess is stored in the liver, muscles, and fat cells for use at some other time.

Insulin is one of several hormones that regulate this energy-generating and storage process. The job of these hormones is to keep blood glucose levels fairly constant at all times. If this system fails, the body can suffer in many ways.

When everything is working properly, as glucose levels rise a corresponding amount of insulin is produced. In addition to regulating the amount of glucose that remains in the blood, insulin also directs how much glucose is used for immediate energy and how much will be stored in muscles and body fat. Insulin indirectly influences the fate of the fats we eat as well, by signaling the body as to when it should release glycogen stores to produce energy, rather than burning dietary fats.

Given this intricate balance, a reasonable objective is to minimize stress on the system that regulates it. This can be done, to a large extent, through food selection. Foods that release glucose gradually, rather than in quick intense spurts, afford the greatest protection (see G-Force: A New Perspective on Carbohydrates, on page 280). Additionally, it helps to have a continuously available supply of glucose, rather than running down blood sugar and glycogen reserves by going for long stretches without eating.

High-carbohydrate diets have been used experimentally to treat diabetes and heart disease. Results have been mixed. Some people are able to control blood sugar and reduce blood cholesterol by eating a lot of carbohydrate. For others, carbohydrates have the exact opposite effect, elevating blood sugar and triglycerides and creating ratios of cholesterol markers that are believed to indicate an unhealthy situation. The controlling factor, in all probability, is how people match their sources of carbohydrates to their unique biochemical disposition. Using the information in this chapter will help you maintain a good balance.

Insulin Resistance and Health

For numerous reasons, the insulin response and this delicate insulin-glucose balance can become impaired. If too little insulin is released, glucose accumulates in the blood and the cells don't receive adequate nourishment. This condition is known as elevated blood sugar, or hyperglycemia.

If too much insulin is released, blood sugar may drop below normal levels. This condition is called hypoglycemia.

A third scenario is also possible. In this case, the insulin-receptor sites in the cells are "inhospitable," and the effectiveness of insulin is dulled, causing a condition known as "insulin resistance." To overcome this and coax the receptors to let glucose enter the cells, the body may unleash more insulin than it would normally need. Often this tactic successfully keeps blood sugar within a normal range, but a side effect is elevated levels of insulin in the blood. This is called hyperinsulinemia and it's far more common than was ever before recognized.

Insulin resistance is technically known as "resistance to insulin-stimulated glucose uptake." This is just a cumbersome way of saying that the cells don't allow glucose to enter, even though the insulin that should facilitate this is available. This condition is present in the majority of people who have impaired glucose tolerance or non-insulin-dependent diabetes. Despite a boosted production of insulin, their cells still don't allow glucose to enter and their blood sugar levels remain high. In addition, an estimated 25 percent of people who have normal glucose levels are believed to be insulin resistant; they just aren't aware of it because the extra insulin they produce is enough to force the passage of glucose into the cells.

The possible consequences of blood sugar–insulin imbalance include:

- Weight gain
- Diabetes

271

- Heart disease
- Immune dysfunction
- Hypoglycemia

The causes of insulin resistance are not clear. It is presumed to be genetically determined to some degree. However, it is also clearly modified by environmental influences such as diet and exercise. If we eat too much carbohydrate the body preferentially stores fat. This leads to a change in body mass, which is one of the factors that cause cells to become insulin resistant. Insulin-resistant cells have trouble handling carbohydrates efficiently. The end result may be mild carbohydrate intolerance or more pronounced diabetes. A vicious circle, if ever there was one.

NIKKI'S DIALOGUE BOX

What to Do About Carbohydrates If You Suspect Problems

"The best advice for anyone who thinks they may be insulin resistant is to design a diet around carbohydrates that improve the insulin–blood sugar connection. Once again, foods that release glucose gradually, rather than in quick intense spurts, minimize the effects of insulin resistance. Those foods are described in G-Force: A New Perspective on Carbohydrates, on page 280. Likewise, it's best to have a continuously available supply of glucose, which is why it may be unhealthy for some people to go for long stretches without eating, and why consuming frequent small meals is recommended."

The Weight Connection

When an insulin-resistant person eats carbohydrates, the glucose that emerges in the bloodstream may be accommodated by releasing more insulin than is normally needed.

Too much insulin in the blood:

- Increases hunger and the desire for carbohydrate-rich food
- Increases the number and size of fat cells
- Prevents the body from removing stored energy from muscle and fat tissues

In other words, with too much insulin in the bloodstream you gain weight.

While the majority of people aren't insulin resistant, those who are experience an increase in appetite rather than satisfaction following carbohydrate-rich meals, a tendency to gain weight even with a modest calorie intake, and difficulty shedding unwanted pounds. In the long run, in addition to its influence on appetite and weight, insulin resistance may provoke other, more serious side effects, as the following sections confirm.

For Women Only. A factor of special interest to women is the counterinfluence of other hormones on insulin's effectiveness. One of these hormones has the unwieldy name *glucocorticosteroids*. Glucocorticosteroids block insulin from doing its job. Since estrogen helps counter the insulin-depressing effects of glucocorticosteroids, menopausal and postmenopausal women are most affected. In younger women, estrogen may protect against insulin resistance. However, when estrogen levels decline, women become more prone to insulin resistance. This is a possible explanation of why some women gain weight when they reach menopause, even though their food patterns haven't changed.

Non-Insulin-Dependent Diabetes

Non-insulin-dependent diabetes (sometimes called type II diabetes) is a condition of hyperglycemia. It develops when the pancreas loses its ability to produce enough insulin to overcome the severity of insulin resistance. As a result, glucose builds up in the blood.

Some of the problems that occur when glucose is abnormally elevated are well recognized. They include increased susceptibility to infection, greater incidence of heart and kidney diseases, and vision disturbances that can lead to blindness. Despite the prevalence of diabetes and an enormous amount of research into its causes, consequences, and control, there are still a surprising number of unanswered questions.

The complications of diabetes are probably due to more than one factor. Because of the body's impaired ability to absorb glucose, the energy needs of many cells may not be met. At the same time, due to elevated levels of glucose circulating in the blood, some cells—such as those in the brain, kidney, and eye lens—may be hit with an unsuitable amount of glucose.

In addition to the difficulties that arise directly from having too much sugar in the bloodstream, some of the cardiovascular disturbances associated with diabetes appear to be a result of too much circulating insulin.

NIKKI'S DIALOGUE BOX

Does eating sugar cause diabetes?

"The medical-nutrition community has insisted for years that eating sugar and refined carbohydrates *does not* cause diabetes, while health activists have continued to challenge this. Now, a study by Harvard researchers supports the latter view. Based on a six-year follow-up of over 65,000 disease-free, forty- to sixty-five-year-old U.S. women who participated in the Nurses' Health Study, their conclusion is that 'diets with a high glycemic load [see G-Force, on page 280] and a low cereal fiber content increase risk of diabetes in women.' Cola drinks, jams, refined breadstuffs, white rice, and potatoes were among the foods associated with diabetes incidence. To counter this, they suggest that 'grains be consumed in a minimally refined form.' In other words, eat whole grains."

Hyperinsulinemia and Heart Disease

As we have already said, hyperinsulinemia—or extra insulin in the blood—is a concern not only for diabetics. Hyperinsulinemia also occurs in many people who don't have diabetes.

The relationship of hyperinsulinemia to heart disease hasn't received much attention until recently. When there is excess insulin in the bloodstream, blood pressure has a tendency to rise to unhealthy levels. Moreover, in experimental animals, a high intake of simple carbohydrates (sugars) causes blood pressure to become more sensitive to dietary salt. High blood pressure, or what is clinically named hypertension, is strongly associated with an increased risk of strokes and heart attacks.

Circulating fats, called serum triglycerides, also increase when insulin remains in the bloodstream. There has been some dispute over whether or not the elevated triglyceride levels associated with high-carbohydrate diets are a risk factor for heart disease. What has been observed is that when abnormally high triglyceride levels are the result of insulin resistance, cholesterol-containing HDL lipoproteins are reduced, while very-low-density lipoproteins (VLDLs) rise. In blood chemistry reports, these are considered markers for heart disease.

High concentrations of blood triglycerides may affect heart disease in yet another way. The hormone plasminogen helps thin the blood, preventing dangerous clots from forming. There is a strong association between blood triglycerides and a substance that inhibits plasminogen.

Is insulin itself a direct promoter of heart disease, or does it influence heart disease by altering other risk factors? We don't have the answer yet to that question, but the result is the same: *Unless the amount of insulin in the blood is within a normal range, your heart may be at risk.*

Syndrome X. Syndrome X is the name given to a frequently observed cluster of health problems that simultaneously includes:

- High blood pressure
- Cholesterol abnormalities
- Elevated triglyceride levels
- A concentration of fat around the abdomen

People with this syndrome are more prone to strokes and heart attacks. Although these disorders have been linked together for years, the common thread wasn't recognized. It's now believed that hyperinsulinemia is the underlying cause.

Blood pressure, cholesterol, and triglyceride levels are the three most targeted areas for reducing the risk of heart disease. Trying to control these factors without addressing the possibility of insulin resistance as the basis may merely mask the symptoms, while prolonging the real problem. Some evidence is the fact that researchers haven't been able to demonstrate that reducing hypertension via drug treatment, even when done successfully, decreases either incidence or death from heart disease. This isn't surprising; if hypertension is complicated by insulin resistance, the overflow of insulin into the blood must be remedied before heart disease can be minimized.

Treating hypertension with drugs doesn't reduce insulin resistance or alleviate hyperinsulinemia. In some cases drug-induced blood pressure management is actually accompanied by a worse blood lipid profile; that is, higher triglycerides, a higher concentration of damaging very-low-density lipoproteins (VLDLs), and lower protective high-density lipoproteins (HDLs). On the other hand, interventions that reduce insulin to normal levels often correct high blood pressure, along with improving blood lipids. It's interesting to note that in addition to diet, exercise changes how the body uses carbohydrates and improves insulin resistance. Not surprisingly, exercise is also recommended to control blood pressure, and is one of the few ways to improve the HDL ratio.

Syndrome X Indicators

Resistance to insulin-stimulated glucose uptake
Glucose intolerance
Hyperinsulinemia
Increased very-low-density lipoprotein (VLDL) cholesterol
Decreased high-density lipoprotein (HDL) cholesterol
Elevated triglycerides
Hypertension

Cancer Link

In their extensive "Harvard Report on Cancer Prevention" (1997), Harvard School of Public Health researchers cite a number of dietary links. One topic of particular relevance is the connection they propose between insulinlike growth factors (IGFs), which are triggered by insulin, and the development and proliferation of cells. IGFs have been identified as growth factors for cells lining the colon and have a role in the development of colon cancer cells. They're also involved in mammary tissue development. Studies show that the estrogen derivative estradiol works together with IGF in the development of certain types of breast cancer. These experts conclude that chronic exposure to insulin (hyperinsulinemia) may play a role in cancer at these sites, and specifically implicate insulin resistance as a cause.

Immune Dysfunction

The interaction between insulin and fats can have an indirect effect on the immune system. Dietary fats are broken down in the body into fatty acids, which in turn are transformed into a variety of regulatory substances (discussed in Chapter 2). A critical element in this process is an enzyme stimulated by insulin. Too little insulin suppresses fatty acid transformation and thereby inhibits the production of infection- and inflammation-fighting agents. Too much insulin may overstimulate the transformation of particular fatty acids, creating an imbalance that sets off a chain of events that depresses immune function and promotes inflammation, tumor growth, and several related pathologies. Chapter 2 discusses the consequences of underavailability and overavailability of specific fatty acids in more detail.

In addition, because hyperinsulinemia blocks the release of fatty acids from adipose (fatty) tissue, it can induce a deficiency of essential fatty acids, especially in a diet that's low in fat and certain fats in particular. Without these fatty acids, production of the regulatory substances mentioned above and examined closely in Chapter 2 are curtailed. As a result, the immune system becomes impaired. This sequence of events has been confirmed in experiments with rats.

Hypoglycemia

Clinical diagnosis of hypoglycemia, or low blood sugar, is made when blood glucose falls below normal levels. Hypoglycemia is frequently accompanied by such physical symptoms as shakiness, extreme hunger, lightheadedness, dizziness, sweating, confusion, headache, fatigue, irritability, agitation, depression, anxiety, hyperactivity, and muscle twitches and tremors. Many more people believe they suffer from hypoglycemia than medical tests corroborate and, indeed, the symptoms can occur even without significantly lowered blood sugar levels.

This is explained by the fact that when blood sugar is falling, as it does after a large influx of insulin, the body reacts by releasing hormones, such as adrenaline, that stimulate glucose production by the liver. The brain is highly sensitive to these hormone changes and displays this in the form of the reactions described above. We interpret these unpleasant sensations as hypoglycemia, and the manifestations are real, even though blood sugar measurements may not actually dip very low.

The symptoms of low blood sugar (as well as genuine hypoglycemia) are triggered by eating foods that cause a rapid rise in blood glucose and a large insulin response. The problem can be prevented in the same way that hyperinsulinemia is handled: by eating foods and food combinations that slowly release glucose into the bloodstream and avoiding foods that cause a glucose rush.

Carbohydrates and Appetite

We noted earlier that although other cells in the body can get the energy they need from fats and to some degree proteins, the brain and central nervous system must be fueled by carbohydrates. Our early hunter-gatherer ancestors had to rely on the most easily available source of carbohydrate, which they found in fruit. This primal diet, rich in sugars, provided a readily available energy supply that encouraged the development of a large central nervous system. The corollary to this is that as the human brain and central nervous system grew, more carbohydrate was required to nourish it. Many researchers believe that this initial dependence on sugars has genetically programmed a fundamental taste for sweets into our food preferences.

The human appetite is extremely complicated. It still isn't clear how food intake is regulated by the body—in other words, how we know when to start eating and when to stop. There are apparently one or more receptors in the brain that receive signals telling us when we are satiated and when we are hungry. Some of these receptors, along with additional receptors in the liver, respond to insulin. Experiments demonstrate that even small declines in blood sugar can prompt people to request food. It follows that if the body's glucose-insulin response is at all impaired, the ability to regulate food intake may suffer.

Research supports the notion that all carbohydrates—both sugars and starches—quickly suppress hunger and boost satiety for a given period. Under ideal conditions, this is true: The body responds by matching insulin levels to the glucose that is released from carbohydrate breakdown and our appetite diminishes. But sometimes this works against us, as when rapidly absorbed carbohydrates (sugars and certain starches) cause insulin to be released very early and more sharply. Depending on how your body handles this situation, two things can occur:

1. This quick insulin reaction will cause satisfaction to be short-lived and hunger will soon return. The natural response is to eat more.
2. Repeated spurts of elevated blood sugar encourage cells to become insulin resistant, setting the stage for the body to increase and preserve its fat reserves.

Weight Woes

An estimated one-third of Americans living in the 1990s are at least 20 percent over their ideal weight. This number is up from the 20 to 25 percent of people deemed to be "too heavy" during the 1950s, '60s, '70s, and '80s. Not surprisingly, many observers have commented how odd it is that, despite the current infatuation with low-fat diets, national weight levels have gone up, not down.

Reducing fat intake is probably a healthy idea for many people. But to attract the burgeoning low-fat market, manufacturers have compensated for reducing fat content by increasing the carbohydrate (sugar) content of their products in order to make them palatable. The proliferation of these low-fat foods, compounded by government-sanctioned dietary recommendations emphasizing pasta, bread, and fruit, has most likely contributed to the weight-gain explosion.

There are several reasons why restricting fats while eating carbohydrates freely undermines many people's attempts to lose weight. When people habitually consume a lot of carbohydrates their muscle tissues become saturated with glycogen. When glycogen storage reaches its maximum, the body turns the excess carbohydrates into fat, expanding its fat mass in order to balance energy input and energy output. This increased fat mass not only causes weight gain, it can slow down weight loss as well.

There is still another weight-related factor to contend with that is exacerbated

★ HYPERRESPONDERS OR THOSE WHO JUST LOOK AT FOOD . . . ★

There is an interesting corollary to the innate ability of the brain to respond to "the first sign of food." By this statement we mean not just the presence of food in the stomach, or even the mouth, but the mere expectation of food.

Perhaps you've heard some people bemoan the fact that they "just look at food and gain weight." This may be more than an imagined event. In her research on appetite control, Judith Rodin, Ph.D., has discovered what she calls "hyperresponders." For these people, sensitivity is so heightened that the sight, smell, or sometimes just the thought of food stimulates insulin release. This external stimulus can create genuine hunger. Thus, hyperresponders must use a great deal of "willpower" to keep from eating. But even if they manage to overpower their hunger, the insulin that is spontaneously released due to their hyperresponse can encourage fat storage and inhibit fat reduction—in effect, just as if they had eaten! These are the people for whom weight gain occurs easily and weight loss can be difficult to achieve.

Some possible signs that you may be hyperresponsive to food are:

1. Even when not hungry, you can't resist snacking while around food.
2. The smell of food is an irresistible temptation to eat.
3. Eating is triggered by environmental cues, such as seeing food, talking about food, thinking about food.
4. You eat as much as you're given, even after you're satisfied.

by carbohydrate-rich foods. The body is designed for glucose to rise following food intake. The brain expects this and, to meet the challenge of keeping blood sugar at a constant level, sends signals to increase insulin production at the first sign of food. Insulin release continues to build as eating progresses. The problem for insulin-resistant people is that their insulin output can be as much as three to eight times higher than that of people considered to be in the normal range. How long this condition lasts varies from person to person. But if it persists, fat storage will be encouraged.

As you already know, repeated spurts of elevated blood sugar (or short-term hyperglycemia) increase insulin resistance. Therefore, foods that raise blood sugar levels rapidly or dramatically have a greater tendency to promote weight gain. As you will discover in the upcoming section, G-Force, foods differ not only in the total amount of glucose they generate, but in the speed of delivery as well. Paradoxically, the foods that have the most immediate impact on the entry of glucose into the blood are sugars and certain starches—precisely the foods people turn to when they reduce fat intake.

How Often Should I Eat?

One question that people frequently ask is "How often should I be eating?" Is it necessary to eat three meals a day? Or can you get by with less? Is eating small meals every few hours better? These are difficult questions to answer, since individual differences in how the body processes food allow some people to go for long stretches without eating, while for others this pattern can be harmful.

Before our ancestors settled down and started cultivating their own food, there were often periods of feasting followed by famine. The sympathetic nervous system, seeking to keep body weight stable, adapted to these events by enabling cells to adjust their rate of energy use to food availability. Thermogenesis is the word that describes this action. When food is provided, thermogenesis increases, speeding up energy production (the burning of calories); when food is withheld, thermogenesis decreases and the body guards its energy reserves. This is what some people mean when they say they have a "fast" or "slow" metabolism.

To defend against the lean times, the body developed an additional means of protection. This was to generate enough insulin when food was abundant to build fat stores for times when food was scarce. When food is constantly available, as it is for most people nowadays, this strategy loses its primary function.

In fact, these safeguards may help explain why people who consume most of their food in a concentrated period—that is, one or two large meals—often have trouble losing weight. When food is routinely withheld for long stretches of time, the body is reminded of its past experience with famine. Thermogenesis decreases and calories are conserved. The body further responds by treating the next meal as it would an ancestral feast; that is, it produces enough insulin to hoard some of the potential energy. It does this by increasing fat mass. Because true stretches of famine are uncommon in most of our lives, these fat stores rarely need to be deployed, and the original intent of skipping meals to lose weight backfires.

The answer to the original question, "How often should I eat?", therefore depends in part on how efficiently your body turns what you eat into energy and how little or much your weight tends to fluctuate. If your weight is pretty steady, chances are you can withstand skipping some meals now and then. But if your weight seesaws up and down, or refuses to let go of stored fat that is realisti-

★ THE SURPRISING NEWS ABOUT ARTIFICIAL SWEETENERS AND WEIGHT ★

Artificial sweeteners, including saccharine, cyclamates, and aspartame, don't turn into glucose and therefore don't raise blood sugar levels. Because of this many people assume they can only help with weight control.

If you look back at our discussion of evolution, however, you may perceive how these sweeteners could actually stimulate weight gain. Remember, when the brain anticipates food, and sweet food in particular, it sends out signals that arouse insulin even before glucose gets to the bloodstream. Since the brain can't detect the absence of calories, insulin is released even if there is no work for it to do (i.e., there is no glucose released for it to escort into the cells). As long as this uncalled-for insulin remains in circulation, the effects of hyperinsulinemia, including fat storage and retention, are set in motion. Moreover, this unsatisfied expectation of calories may manipulate the brain in a way that stimulates hunger. This effect has been demonstrated in experiments on animals.

cally too much for your frame, eating more often can literally "jump-start" your calorie-burning mechanism. Studies have also shown that a "nibbling" feeding pattern, or what some people like to call "grazing," results in flatter blood glucose and insulin responses and lower triglycerides and LDLs than eating the same volume of food in infrequent large meals.

Managing Carbohydrates

Two important attributes that can be used to gain control of carbohydrate-rich foods are the speed of their impact on blood sugar and the kinds and amount of fiber they contain. We conclude this chapter with details on each of these topics, and tables that will help guide your food selection.

G-Force: A New Perspective on Carbohydrates

Although the *total amount* of calories produced by carbohydrates is determined by weight—that is, each gram of carbohydrate equals 4 calories—the *speed* at which foods turn into glucose fluctuates. This relative measure of how fast the carbohydrate in a particular food is converted to glucose and enters the blood is technically known as the glycemic index, or what we call *G-Force*. Foods with a high G-Force raise blood sugar levels quickly; this is usually matched by a rapid rise in insulin. Foods with a low G-Force cause blood sugar levels to rise gradually, in which case insulin is usually released more evenly. What is remarkable about G-Force is that it doesn't necessarily parallel the amount of carbohydrate in a food. In other words, some foods that are high in carbohydrate content have less impact on blood sugar levels and insulin production than foods with fewer carbohydrates.

You will read below about the limitations of G-Force. But even with its limitations, it remains a useful tool for choosing compatible carbohydrates to help stabilize blood sugar and insulin levels. The best way to prevent the aftermath of insulin overload that we have been discussing is to downplay carbohydrates with a high G-Force. At the same time, your diet should include carbohydrates that contribute positively to health by supplying vitamins, minerals, fiber, and other biologically active elements.

In addition, G-Force can influence sports performance and appetite control. Consuming foods with a low G-Force prior to prolonged strenuous exercise has been found to sustain energy and increase endurance. In contrast, eating foods with a high G-Force following exercise leads to faster replenishment of muscle glycogen (the storage form of carbohydrates).

Using G-Force in Food Selection

The G-Force (glycemic index) of foods is determined by controlled laboratory testing. The G-Force Ratings table on page 284 shows the relative influence of common carbohydrate-containing foods on blood sugar. The higher the number, the more the food will disrupt blood sugar levels. The lower the number, the more moderate its impact will be. A food is generally considered to have a high G-Force if it is rated above 69.

The ratings assigned to foods clearly illustrate a wide range in the extent to which different carbohydrate foods raise blood sugar, despite similar carbohydrate amounts. In other words, 50 grams of carbohydrate from 3 slices of bread don't necessarily have the same effect on the body as 50 grams of carbohydrate from 1¼ cups of spaghetti, or 1¼ cups of lentils, or a little over a quart of milk, or 55 grapes.

In general, a diet that moderates blood sugar by taking advantage of G-Force features nonstarchy vegetables, soy products and other legumes, nuts, seeds, eggs, and some dairy products. Meat eaters can also add fish, lean meat, and poultry. Products made from grains (cereals, pasta, baked goods) and starchy vegetables such as root vegetables, peas, and corn, should be consumed in modest amounts and in the proper context (see Curbing G-Force on page 283), as should fruit, since fructose, the predominant sugar in fruit, is handled in a unique manner (see Fruit: A Unique Force, below). Concentrated sweeteners—sugar, honey, maple syrup, molasses, corn syrup, and such—should be limited and combined with foods that can reduce their high G-Force impact.

Fruit: A Unique Force

When you look at the table of G-Force Ratings you'll notice that fruit is surprisingly low considering how sweet it is. Don't be fooled: Eating a lot of fruit, drinking fruit juice, and eating too many fructose-, honey-, and fruit juice–sweetened foods can have a negative impact on glucose, insulin, and triglyceride levels, especially in people who are insulin resistant and diabetic. This means that, like grains and starchy vegetables, fructose-containing foods should be chosen with reserve and within the framework of the entire diet.

The reason for this is that fructose, the principal form of sugar in fruit, is handled differently by the body than other sugars and the technique used to measure glycemic index (G-Force) doesn't account for this. Although people who respond well to most sugars can readily convert fructose into stored glycogen, if insulin levels are already high, as they often are when cells are insulin resistant, fructose stimulates the liver to release glycogen in the form of glucose. This raises blood sugar levels significantly, and the secretion of insulin in response can prolong hyperinsulinemia.

Furthermore, the hormones released in order to process fructose are troublesome. In fact, they increase secretion of very-low-density lipoproteins (VLDLs), which are the precursors to the low-density lipoprotein cholesterol (LDL) that is associated with coronary disease. Fructose can also increase blood triglycerides, especially in a diet that is routinely high in carbohydrates.

An additional concern is that when the body is in a "starved" state, the production of glucose from fructose is more dramatic. Therefore, a pattern of skipping meals and substituting fruit instead can make it more difficult for some people to control blood sugar. On the other hand, when the body is in a "fed" state, the transformation process changes, and the rate of VLDL output is greater. This means that overeaters who consume a lot of fructose-rich foods may be inviting coronary problems.

Many people have been led to believe that because blood sugar levels don't rise as much after eating fruit or fructose-sweetened foods, the consequences are minor. As you can see from the discussion above, this isn't so.

Limits of G-Force Ratings

There are shortcomings to G-Force ratings that you should keep in mind: While predetermined tables of glycemic index can provide an initial basis for food choices, actual glucose responses to foods are highly individual; the manner in which a single food is prepared, as well as combinations of food, can change the results; the volume of a food actually consumed must be taken into account; and many carbohydrate-containing foods aren't listed in any published tables. (Looking at similar foods suggests where they might lie, but this is somewhat speculative.)

Despite these limitations, G-Force is still a useful tool. However, it was never intended to be used in isolation and shouldn't be the sole criterion for food selection. The total amount of carbohydrate consumed in a sitting and the presence of other foods are critical. Moreover, additional considerations, such as fat, protein, fiber, and overall nutritional content, can be just as important.

G-Force is influenced by many things: food processing, preparation techniques, ripeness, genetics. Although these environmental factors can have unexpected outcomes, in general the more a food is tampered with, the higher the G-Force.

Fiber: Disruption of fibers raises G-Force. That is, whole apples have a lower G-Force than apples blended to a puree or apples turned into juice; instant potatoes affect blood sugar more profoundly than fresh cooked potatoes; and when dried beans are ground and processed to make them quick-cooking (as for instant soups and other rehydratable bean products) their G-Force rises compared with whole beans or even beans that are cooked and then ground. When the fiber is removed from grains, their G-Force rises, but surprisingly not by very much.

Particle size: As particle size decreases, G-Force generally increases. For example, the G-Force of wheat kernels increases as you go from the whole berry, to cracked wheat or bulgur, to more finely ground (and refined) couscous, and finally to flour. Similarly, "instant" rice and "instant" oats have a higher G-Force than their slower-cooking counterparts, as do mashed potatoes compared with baked or boiled potatoes.

In foods containing a mixture of ingredients, the particle size of individual components can alter the picture. In bread making, for example, the addition of rye kernels or cracked wheat kernels (a larger-size element) to flour (a smaller-size element) can reduce the G-Force significantly.

Processing techniques: G-Force is elevated by extrusion cooking and explosion puffing of grains to create ready-to-eat cereals and snack foods, and the chemical modification of grains that takes place to expand their potential use for manufacturers. This latter process is described on foods labels as "modified food starch."

Ripeness: The riper the fruit, the greater the G-Force.

Cooking method and time: The cooking of grains, vegetables, and fruit ruptures cell walls, making glucose more available, which often raises G-Force. For some foods, boiling and pressure cooking is reported to raise G-Force more than roasting. While there doesn't seem to be much written about the effect of microwaving food, as the G-Force Ratings table reveals, the G-Force is higher for microwaved potatoes than for boiled, steamed, baked, and even mashed specimens.

Heat also acts on certain elements in food to alter digestibility. For instance, there are enzyme inhibitors in some raw foods that slow down their digestion. Cooking destroys some of these; as a result, digestibility rises, and so does blood sugar (and therefore G-Force).

Genetics: The genetic type of a particular grain can be relevant due to variations in protein content and the structural composition of the starch. This helps explain the wide discrepancies in G-Force among pastas, breads, rice, and the like. As with grains, the specific variety of certain vegetables changes their G-Force.

Curbing G-Force

Foods eaten in combination perform differently than foods eaten singly. If an individual food has a high G-Force, the release of glucose can be tempered and prolonged by combining it with a food that has a low G-Force. The magnitude of response can also be reduced by consuming just a small amount of a food that has a high G-Force. In addition, overall meal size can have power over glucose and insulin responses.

Some but not all studies show that eating a protein-containing food along with a carbohydrate-containing food will lower its G-Force and foster a gradual, sustained release of glucose into the bloodstream. Exemplary combinations include: putting milk on cereal; adding nuts or seeds to cereals and grains; topping a potato with yogurt; eating an apple with cheese; spreading almond butter on a pear. The rise of blood sugar can also be curbed by mixing glucose-sustaining starches in the form of oat bran, flaxseed, and wheat germ with other grains. Similarly, legumes, which have a low G-Force, have a muting effect on grain-based foods.

However, the reverse can occur when foods with a high G-Force are combined, as when you add sweetener to cereal, mix fruit into grain dishes, or put jelly on bread.

These G-Force-curbing principles were applied in designing our recipes. That

Mentor

is why you find wheat germ, flaxseed meal, nuts, beans, tofu, yogurt cheese, and the like in dishes that are predominately grain- or root vegetable–based.

How to Use G-Force

To sum up, balancing foods so they deliver glucose gradually into the bloodstream can have a profound influence on appetite and health. By lowering the G-Force of a meal without any change in calorie content, you may find a difference in how hungry you are an hour or two later, you may find it easier to lose weight if weight loss is indicated, and you may discover that other health markers that are out of line, such as blood pressure and blood lipid measurements, improve.

To accomplish this gradual glucose release, select most of your carbohydrates in the form of foods with a G-Force lower than 69. In addition, combine carbohydrate-containing foods with moderate amounts of fat and protein, rather than eating carbohydrates separately.

G-FORCE RATINGS*

G-Force ratings rank foods according to their short-term effect on blood sugar levels. The higher the number, the more likely it is that a food will cause blood sugar (and insulin levels) to rise. Foods rated above 69 are classified as having a high G-Force. These ratings have been determined in a laboratory setting using measured amounts of individual foods that provide 50 grams of carbohydrate.

The G-Force is meant to serve as a general reference tool, providing a relational measure based on one criterion only. G-Force should not be the sole reason for selecting a food. Moreover, inclusion in the list below isn't an endorsement of an item, while the absence of other foods isn't because they aren't significant, but may be due to a lack of data.

The table is organized by food categories. Foods are listed alphabetically within each category. Sometimes more than one entry is included to reflect differences in variety or preparation.

Food	G-Force
Bakery Products	
Cake	
Angel food	95
Doughnut	108
Pound cake	77
Sponge cake	66
Cookies	
Arrowroot	95
Graham crackers	106

*These ratings are compiled from several published tables and measure the impact of foods using white bread as a reference. In other words, white bread is assigned a rating of 100 and all foods are ranked comparatively. Due to differences in study subjects, as well as variations in method, numbers may vary slightly from study to study.

Food	G-Force
Oatmeal	79
Shortbread	91
Vanilla wafers	110
Crackers	
Melba toast	100
Oatcakes	81
Rice cakes	110
Rye	
Kavli	101
Ryvita	90
Taco Shells	97
Wheat	
Soda crackers	106
Stoned wheat	96
Muffins	
(average of several varieties)	85
Waffles	109
Beverages	
Soda, orange	97
Bread	
Bagel	103
Baguette	136
Hamburger bun	87
Kaiser rolls	104
Oat bran bread	68
Pita (white)	82
Pumpernickel	71
Rye flour bread	92
Rye kernel bread	66
Rye-linseed	78
Tortillas, corn	54
Wheat	
Cracked wheat	75
Gluten-free	129
White	100
Whole wheat	95
Breakfast cereals, ready-to-eat	
All Bran	60
Bran Chex	83
Cheerios	106
Cocopops	110
Corn Chex	118
Cornflakes	119

Mentor

Food	G-Force
Grapenuts	96
Grapenuts Flakes	114
Muesli	80
Nutri-grain	94
Puffed Rice	132
Puffed Wheat	105
Rice Krispies	117
Shredded Wheat	97
Total	109
Breakfast cereals, cooked	
Cream of wheat	
Regular	94
Instant	105
Mixed whole grain	70
Oatmeal	87
Instant	94
Oat bran	78
Rice bran	27
Cereal grains	
Barley	49
Buckwheat (kasha)	78
Bulgur (cracked wheat)	68
Cornmeal	98
Couscous	93
Millet	101
Rice	
Brown	79
Instant	114
White	
Basmati	83
Converted (parboiled)	68
Instant	128
Long grain	81
Short grain	126
Rye berries	48
Wheat berries	59
Wild rice	81
Dairy Foods	
Milk	
Full-fat	39
Skim	46
Yogurt	
Low-fat, plain	20
Low-fat, with fruit	47

Food	G-Force
Frozen Desserts	
Ice cream	87
Tofutti	164
Fruit (see Fruit: A Unique Force, page 281, for full details)	
Apple	54
Apple juice	58
Apricot, canned	91
Apricot, dried	44
Banana	77
Cherries	32
Fruit cocktail, canned	79
Grapefruit	36
Grapefruit juice	69
Grapes	66
Kiwi	75
Mango	80
Orange	63
Orange juice	74
Papaya	83
Peach	60
Canned in juice	67
Canned, light syrup	74
Canned, heavy syrup	83
Pear	51
Canned in juice	63
Pineapple	94
Pineapple juice	66
Plum	55
Raisins	91
Watermelon	103
Legumes	
Black beans	43
Black-eyed peas	59
Chickpeas (garbanzos)	47
Canned	60
Fava beans	110
Green peas, dried	32
Kidney beans	42
Canned	74
Lentils, green	42
Lentils, red	36
Lima beans	50
Navy (white)	54

Food	G-Force
Pinto beans	55
Canned	64
Soybeans	25
Canned	20
Split peas, yellow	45
Pasta	
Gnocchi	95
Linguine, durum wheat	
Thick	65
Thin	78
Macaroni	64
Rice pasta (brown rice)	131
Spaghetti	
White, durum wheat	78
Whole wheat	53
Tortellini, cheese	71
Snack foods	
Chocolate	70
Corn chips	103
Fruit leather	100
Jelly beans	114
Life Savers	100
Mars Bars	97
Muesli bars	87
Peanuts	21
Popcorn	79
Potato chips	77
Pretzels	116
Sugars	
Fructose	32
Glucose	137
Honey	104
Lactose	65
Maltose	150
Sucrose	92
Vegetables (root and other starchy varieties)	
Beets	91
Carrots	101
Corn	78
Parsnips	139
Peas, frozen	68
Potatoes	
Baked (russet)	80

Food	G-Force
Baked (Burbank)	112
Instant	118
New (waxy type)	80
White, nonspecific	
Baked	85
Boiled	80
Mashed	100
Microwaved	117
Steamed	93
Pumpkin	107
Rutabaga	103
Sweet potato	77
Yam	73

Friendly Fiber

Fiber is certainly a familiar dietary term, although when most people hear the word "fiber" they think only of bran. Indeed, the outer layer of grains—which is where bran comes from—is one prominent source of fiber. But the complete story of fiber is much more encompassing and important than just bran. Two new aspects are the presence of plant lignans and resistant starch.

Dietary fiber is the term applied to plant components that can't be fully broken down in the human digestive tract. It is composed of carbohydrate and noncarbohydrate matter. Products of animal origin don't contain any fiber.

In healthy individuals, a diet that is high in fibrous carbohydrates generally benefits blood sugar levels. A high-fiber diet can also help regulate blood sugar in many diabetics.

Fiber-rich carbohydrates lower the risk of certain cancers and can have a positive impact on reducing heart disease. This may seem contradictory after reading about the negative effect carbohydrates can have on blood pressure, triglycerides, and certain cholesterol components, which are all considered risk factors for heart disease. However, if carbohydrates are viewed in the context of a total diet, the picture may be a bit different. For instance, when a panel of Swedish experts convened to discuss the implications of carbohydrate research on nutrition recommendations and product development, they came to the general consensus that high-carbohydrate diets don't increase the risk of hyperlipidemia (elevated blood fats), *so long as the dietary fiber content is also high* (emphasis ours). They also noted that only soluble dietary fiber (discussed below) had blood cholesterol–lowering properties and expressed concern about sugars, particularly fructose and sucrose, raising blood triglyceride levels. The advantage of low-glycemic-index foods (i.e., low G-Force ratings) in relation to blood fat levels was considered significant.

One of the longest ongoing diet projects in the United States is the Health Professionals Follow-up Study conducted by the Harvard School of Public Health.

This research began in 1986 and involved more than 51,000 men aged forty to seventy-five. Among their findings: a decreased incidence of heart attacks as fiber intake increased. While the researchers admitted that the men with high-fiber diets tended to have better overall health habits, after adjusting for this, lower risk was associated with fiber itself.

As the Harvard researchers in the above study concur, it's difficult to isolate the benefits of fiber when reviewing research on the subject, since many fiber-rich foods also contain other protective nutrients. Whether it's the direct presence of fiber, some indirect influence fiber has on other dietary constituents or body mechanisms, or another unmeasured factor in foods that are coincidentally high in fiber (such as plant lignans or resistant starch), most studies point in the same direction: Eating ample amounts of fiber-rich vegetables and legumes, along with modest amounts of whole, unprocessed grains and fruit, results in the best health outcomes. Once again, we can't overemphasize the fact that the majority of studies that support a protective role for fiber do so in the context of wholefoods. No assumption can be made that these findings apply to extracted fiber (i.e., pure bran; fiber supplements).

Types of Fiber

There are two general classifications of fiber: water-insoluble and water-soluble.

Water-insoluble fiber is what people once called "roughage." This fiber facilitates the movement of foods through the digestive tract. By increasing digestive mass in the stomach and small intestine, insoluble fiber enhances satiety and slows down digestion. When accompanied by adequate liquid, insoluble fiber keeps bowels moving smoothly. This explains, in part, how it may lower the risk of colon and rectal cancers; when the removal of potential carcinogens (which end up in stools) is sped up, they have less opportunity to act. Another proposed mechanism is that insoluble fiber directly binds or dilutes carcinogens. In any event, a comprehensive analysis of observational as well as controlled studies supports the notion of a protective effect associated with more frequent consumption of vegetables and high-fiber grains.

Water-soluble fiber absorbs water during digestion, forming a gel-like substance. This results in increased fecal bulk, as well as the ability to activate bacterial fermentation and thereby alter intestinal microflora. These traits may explain some of the health-protective effects attributed to water-soluble fiber. For example, it appears to lower blood cholesterol levels due to the ability of this gel to bind with cholesterol and incorporate it into the increased stool mass. Similarly, water-soluble fiber may offer protection against hormone-induced cancers by incorporating estrogens released by the intestine into the stool in a form that prevents them from being reabsorbed into the bloodstream.

The potential to curb blood glucose depends on fiber type. Soluble fiber (as in beans) has a profound ability to stabilize blood glucose levels; the insoluble fiber in wheat and rice has little effect. The importance of both soluble and insoluble fiber in relation to blood sugar disorders may go beyond glucose regulation, however. In non-insulin-dependent diabetics and others with impaired glucose tolerance, insoluble wheat and rice fibers do help reduce hyperinsulinemia, as well as triglycerides and cholesterol. Triglycerides and cholesterol are also lowered by soluble fibers. This is more evidence supporting the need for a diverse diet.

Oat Fiber. Oat bran has received a lot of attention because of its ability to lower cholesterol. Oats and barley contain a type of soluble fiber called beta-glucan. Experimental diets, in which subjects with elevated blood cholesterol were fed pure oat bran, have reduced overall cholesterol levels without decreasing the good HDLs. When oat bran feeding was discontinued these changes didn't last, indicating that to be of real benefit soluble fiber must become a permanent fixture in the diet. These cholesterol-lowering properties appear to be most effective when cholesterol levels are already elevated, and produce smaller changes (or sometimes none at all) in subjects within normal range.

A composite review done by the Food and Drug Administration of thirty-seven studies estimates that regular consumption of oat bran or oatmeal, in an amount providing 3 grams or more of the soluble fiber beta-glucan, can achieve a 5 percent blood cholesterol reduction. On a daily basis, using uncooked measurements, this amounts to about 1/3 cup oat bran (40 grams dry weight) or 3/4 cup oats (60 grams dry weight). Of course, this can be accomplished by combining equivalent amounts of the two, and by adding barley as well, which has even more beta-glucan than oats. But a more practical approach would be to integrate lesser—and more comfortable—amounts of these grains into a diet plentiful in beans as explained next.

Beans Beat Oats. One criticism of the oat bran experiments is that people were fed larger quantities of oat bran than most diets are likely to include in a day. In one study, daily oat bran intake of a little over 1 cup (100 grams) uncooked measure, during a three-week period, lowered cholesterol by 19 percent. Half this amount (50 grams) lowered it by 12 percent.

Although hardly publicized at all, the same researchers repeated their study using beans. When subjects ate 1 1/2 cups cooked dried beans (115 grams dried) each day, reductions in cholesterol and triglyceride levels were similar to those of the group consuming 100 grams of oat bran. Moreover, by combining these two foods on the daily menu, there was an equally successful outcome using lower, more realistic amounts of oat bran (about 1/3 cup dry weight). Even the daily inclusion of about 1/2 cup canned beans (which have a bit less fiber than their cooked dried counterpart) made a significant difference in cholesterol and triglyceride levels, reducing them by 13 and 12 percent, respectively.

Plant Lignans

Plant lignans are another impressive constituent associated with food fibers. Lignan-forming compounds (classified as precursors) are found in whole grains, predominantly in the bran. They are especially abundant in flaxseed and legumes. Microflora in the digestive tract transform lignan precursors into compounds that have anticancer potential. Called enterolactone and enterodiol, these compounds have a structure that resembles estrogen, but have no actual estrogen activity. In fact, their effect may be just the opposite. By altering the levels of biologically available estrogens, lignans are believed to offer protection against estrogen-related cancers, including colon, breast, ovarian, endometrial, and possibly prostate cancers.

One way this might work is demonstrated in studies in which flaxseed was added to the diets of premenopausal women. These women experienced longer luteal phases (the period between ovulation and menstruation during which progesterone predominates over estrogen) and fewer anovulatory cycles (during which no eggs are released). Because a short luteal phase and chronic anovulation have been linked to an increased risk of breast cancer, the potential for diet to influence sex hormones could be useful. Similarly, lignans are believed to mediate hot flashes and other hormonally triggered discomforts in menopausal women.

In animal experiments, lignan production as a result of feeding flaxseed suppresses the generation and growth of tumors in both the colon and mammaries. Note: The processing of flaxseeds into flaxseed oil removes most of the lignans; therefore, only the seeds and not the oil are a reliable source of lignans.

Gas: Embarrassing but Healthy

People may be troubled (or embarrassed) by digestive gas, but the comforting news is it may signal good health. Resistant starch is a fairly recent classification that refers to undigestible starches that remain in the small intestine. These undigested starches are made up of molecules that are too large to be absorbed into the bloodstream. Instead they enter the colon and are fermented into short-chain fatty acids by microflora. Many people experience this activity as increased flatulence—or gas. It can occur as long as six to ten hours after eating.

There is increasing evidence that the by-products of carbohydrate fermentation serve a vital function in the colon, exerting, for example, anticancer properties. In fact, although many studies investigating the relationship of colon cancer to fiber intake fail to note the distinction between nonstarch components and resistant starches, more precise investigation pinpoints resistant starch as the real key to the apparent protective effect of a fiber-rich diet.

One way resistant starch appears to work is by interfering with the action of potentially harmful by-products of protein fermentation. These by-products (including ammonia and phenols) are especially high in meat eaters. They're associated with skin cancer, as well as tumor growth in the bowel and bladder. Re-

★ FIBER AT A GLANCE ★

More fiber is retained if the peel or skin on produce such as apples, pears, and potatoes is eaten. Juicing fruit and vegetables reduces their fiber content, as can cooking. High heat, especially under pressure as in canning, can disrupt cell walls, which accounts for the lower fiber content of canned vegetables and fruit compared to raw and home-cooked varieties, as well as canned versus cooked dried beans.

Foods containing water-insoluble fibers:
 Fruit
 Vegetables
 Whole grains and products made with whole grains
 Wheat bran
 Wheat germ
 Flaxseeds
 Legumes
 Nuts and seeds*

Foods containing water-soluble fibers:
 Fruit
 Vegetables
 Oats and oat bran
 Barley
 Flaxseeds
 Legumes

Foods containing resistant starch:
 Whole grains
 Legumes
 Flaxseeds
 Tuberous vegetables
 Banana

* Nuts and seeds aren't considered a source of carbohydrates, since very little of their carbohydrate fraction is digestible, and therefore it doesn't turn into glucose; the carbohydrates they contain are mostly in the form of fiber.

searchers also believe that butyrate, one of the short-chain fatty acids generated during the fermentation of resistant starch, helps activate the specific tumor suppressor gene that protects against colon cancer.

Another way in which resistant starch may operate is by raising the acidity in the colon. This in itself may have a beneficial effect although the reason for this is unknown.

The short-chain fatty acids produced during the fermentation of resistant starch presumably play a role in lowering blood cholesterol as well. Moreover, they do this by reducing the more damaging low-density lipoproteins (LDLs) without compromising the protective high-density lipoproteins (HDLs).*

* As with many health mechanisms, there isn't an absolute understanding of how this works. The belief is that short-chain fatty acids, in conjunction with the bile-suppressing action of fiber, reduce the synthesis of cholesterol in the liver. As a result the very-low-density lipoproteins (VLDLs), which are precursors of LDL cholesterol, are kept out of the bloodstream.

The amount of starch that escapes digestion is influenced by the fiber content of a food, food processing, the presence of antinutrients and enzyme inhibitors, and interactions between various starch and protein components. If this sounds familiar, look back at our discussion of G-Force. It appears that the factors that contribute to making starch more resistant are the same factors that decrease G-Force. Likewise, overprocessing of grains not only increases their G-Force, it simultaneously decreases the amount of protective resistant starch. In other words, if you want the carbohydrates in your diet to enhance your health, eat wholefoods.

How Much Fiber?

There is little dispute about the necessity for fiber in the diet, but there are differences of opinion as to how much fiber a healthy diet should provide. The average dietary fiber intake in the United States is estimated to be approximately 12 grams. Although no official recommendation has emerged, this is less than studies suggest is needed for any protective potential to be realized.

One formula that has been proposed is "age + 5"; that is, beginning at the age of two years, the total daily fiber consumption should equal 5 grams added to your age, until the age of twenty years. Thus, a target intake for a two-year-old would be 7 grams of fiber; for a seven-year-old, 12 grams; at age thirteen this would increase to 18 grams; and by the time we get to twenty, 25 grams of fiber daily should continue for a lifetime. Other health practitioners advise 35 grams of fiber a day. Most controlled studies of fiber performance have used from 40 to 50 grams of fiber.

No breakdown has been suggested as to how much of each type of fiber is needed. Cholesterol-reducing trials using soluble oat or bean fiber amount to about 18 grams of soluble fiber per day, although measures as low as 7 grams have produced modest cholesterol-lowering potential. This conforms with a general recommendation suggesting 5 to 13 grams of soluble fiber for every 1,000 calories of food consumed (although on diets containing fewer than 1,000 calories this wouldn't hold up). Since many fiber-rich foods contain soluble and insoluble fibers, eating generously in this area is bound to cover both needs. For some concrete examples, see the table Fiber Content of Some Common Foods, on page 296.

Remember: High-fiber diets must provide adequate fluids; otherwise fiber can be constipating or an irritant. Approximately six to eight 8-ounce cups per day of water or similar liquid are recommended (see Golden Guideline #8).

Fiber's Bad Rap

Antinutrients are substances within foods that limit or inhibit the body's use of other nutritious food constituents. For many years concern has been voiced about the potential for fiber to act in this manner in relation to certain minerals. This can't be easily ignored, since many people don't get enough of some minerals to begin with, and mineral absorption is compromised by many factors. Minerals must withstand the rigors of digestion and absorption, and some studies show that fiber can reduce their availability. This is highly contestable, however; most studies implicate other substances within fibrous foods as the real culprits. The most pivotal of these are termed phytates.

Beans, whole grains, and nuts all contain notable amounts of phytates. On the other hand, these foods are also among the best sources of minerals and this appears to offset the negative impact of phytates on availability. Grains provide a clear example. The removal of the bran and germ during the refining of grains causes both fiber and mineral losses. In comparisons between fiber intake, mineral supplies, and mineral absorption, although the proportion of minerals absorbed may be lower as fiber increases, the actual amount is often greater. In other words, the higher amount of calcium, copper, iron, magnesium, potassium, zinc, and selenium in whole grains more than compensates for reduced availability.

Despite the pessimistic speculation regarding phytates and minerals that is presented in the next few paragraphs, most studies don't indicate any threat. Long-term studies comparing people on low- and high-fiber diets, and studies of vegetarians (who generally eat more fiber than meat eaters), demonstrate an ability to adapt to and tolerate reasonable increases in dietary fiber without developing mineral or other nutrient deficiencies. There is also speculation that phytates confer protection against colon and breast cancers and kidney stones, and are somehow involved in tempering the negative effects of insulin (which may be a clue as to why whole grains and beans are effective in mediating blood sugar disorders). Their interaction with iron, described below, may lower the risk of coronary heart disease as well.

Minerals that are most likely to be compromised by the presence of phytates are iron and calcium. In the case of iron, this could have surprising benefits. To put this in a favorable light, phytates may reduce the risk of cancer and heart disease by preventing the formation of iron-generated free radicals, highly unstable substances within the body that can activate harmful oxidation (see Chapter 3). Furthermore, when vitamin C intake is ample, iron absorption increases dramatically (and free-radical formation is curtailed), overcoming the consequences of phytates.

The most serious repercussion of phytate-mineral interference is on calcium. This can be offset by consuming ample calcium-containing foods.

Because there are no reliable tests to measure zinc status, the effect of phytates on zinc absorption is difficult to determine. Vegetable fiber doesn't appear to have any adverse effect, but grain fiber remains a concern. Interestingly, zinc absorption can be improved by adding animal protein to a grain-rich meal. Since zinc is essential for normal growth, wound healing, and a responsive immune system, perhaps the classic combinations of cereal and milk, pasta and cheese, and similar grain-dairy traditions are actually a legacy of survival rather than sheer whim.

There is no indication that copper, selenium, or chromium are displaced by consuming high-fiber foods.

Mentor

The manner in which food is prepared can, to some extent, influence the presence of phytates. For example, cooking legumes and grains decreases phytate levels, and this is magnified by pressure cooking. Likewise, sprouting beans and grains significantly reduces phytate content. In the case of baked goods, yeast and sourdough fermentation lower phytate levels compared with unleavened breadstuffs or quick breads raised with baking powder and baking soda. Moreover, while the addition of milk to flour preparations appears to inhibit the breakdown of phytates, the use of fermented dairy—such as yogurt and yogurt cheese—doesn't interfere in this process, presumably due to the presence of lactic acid, which creates a more acidic environment. The conclusions to be drawn from this are that pressure cooking beans and grains and eating bean sprouts, fermented soy products such as tempeh, miso, and natto, sourdough breads, and baked goods prepared with yogurt may all encourage optimal mineral absorption.

FIBER CONTENT OF SOME COMMON FOODS

Food Item	Amount	Total fiber (grams)	Soluble (grams)	Insoluble (grams)
Beans, cooked				
black beans	1 cup	15	4	11
black-eyed peas	1 cup	6	1	5
chickpeas	1 cup	12	4	8
lentils	1 cup	18	3	15
lima beans	1 cup	13	3	10
navy beans	1 cup	11	3	8
red kidney	1 cup	13	5	8
soybeans	1 cup	11	4.5	6.5
soybeans, dry roasted	1/2 cup	7	3	4
soy tempeh	4 ounces	7	—	—
split peas	1 cup	16	5	11
white beans	1 cup	11	3	8
Grains				
barley, whole	1 cup cooked	14	3	11
barley, pearled*	1 cup cooked	6	2	4

Note: The analysis of dietary fiber is still in flux. At this time there is no satisfactory analytical method for identifying, characterizing, and quantifying the many components of fiber that exist in different foods. Thus, all information must be considered provisional.

Food Item	Amount	Total fiber (grams)	Soluble (grams)	Insoluble (grams)
bran muffin	2 ounces	4	1	3
buckwheat groats (kasha)	1 cup cooked	19	—	—
cornmeal, whole grain	1 cup cooked	2.5	1	1.5
flaxseed, ground	1/4 cup	7	3	4
matzoh, white*	1 cracker	1	<1	0.5
matzoh, whole wheat	1 cracker	3.5	1	2.5
millet	1 cup cooked	3	1.5	1.5
oat bran	1 cup cooked	6	3	3
oatmeal	1 cup cooked	4	2.5	1.5
quinoa	1 cup cooked	5	—	—
rice, brown	1 cup cooked	3.5	<1	3
rice, white*	1 cup cooked	<1	—	—
rye bread	2 slices	3.5	1.5	2
rye cereal	1 cup cooked	4.5	2	2.5
rye crackers (Wasa)	2 pieces	1.5	<1	1
shredded wheat	1 cup	5	—	—
spaghetti, corn	1 cup	5.5	—	—
spaghetti, regular*	1 cup	4	2	2
spaghetti, spinach*	1 cup	5	1	4
spaghetti, whole wheat	1 cup	6	<1	5.5
tortilla, corn	1	1.5	<1	1
tortilla, whole wheat	1	2	0.5	1.5
wheat berries	1 cup cooked	3.5	0.5	3
wheat bran	1 tablespoon	1.5	<1	1.5
wheat, cracked (bulgur)	1 cup cooked	8	1	7
Wheatena	1 cup	6.5	—	—
wheat germ	1/4 cup	4	<1	3.5
white bread*	2 slices	1	0.5	0.5
whole wheat bread	2 slices	4	1	3

*Not a recommended food. Included only for comparison.

Food Item	Amount	Total fiber (grams)	Soluble (grams)	Insoluble (grams)
Vegetables				
acorn squash, baked	1 cup	9	1	8
alfalfa sprouts	1 cup	1	—	—
artichoke	1 globe	7	1	6
asparagus	1 cup	3	1	2
avocado	1/2 (3 ounces)	4	2	2
beet greens, cooked	1 cup	4	0.5	3.5
beets	1 cup	3	1	2
broccoli	1 cup	4.5	2	2.5
brussels sprouts	1 cup	6	3	3
cabbage, raw	1 cup	2	1	1
cabbage, cooked	1 cup	3.5	1.5	2
carrots, raw	1 medium	2	1	1
carrots, cooked	1 cup	5	2.5	2.5
cauliflower	1 cup	3	1	2
celery	2 large stalks	1	—	—
chard, cooked	1 cup	3.5	—	—
collard greens, cooked	1 cup	5	2	3
corn	1 cup	4.5	<1	4.5
corn on the cob	1 medium ear	2	<1	2
fennel	1 cup	3	—	—
green beans	1 cup	4	1.5	2.5
green peas	1 cup	9	1	8
jicama	1 cup	6	—	—
kale, cooked	1 cup	1.5	<1	<1
lettuce	1 cup	1	—	—
mustard greens, cooked	1 cup	3	1.5	1.5
nopales (cactus)	1 cup	5	—	—
parsnips	1 cup	6	3	3

Food Item	Amount	Total fiber (grams)	Soluble (grams)	Insoluble (grams)
potato, baked	1 medium (4 ounces)	3	1	2
potato, boiled	1 cup	3	<1	2
rutabaga	1 cup	3	1	2
snow peas	1 cup	4	1	3
spinach, raw	1 cup	1	<1	<1
spinach, cooked	1 cup	4	1	3
summer squash	1 cup	2.5	1	1.5
sweet potato	1 medium (4 ounces)	3	1.5	1.5
tomato	1 medium (4 ounces)	1.5	<1	1
turnip	1 cup	3	1	2
Fruit				
apple	1 medium (5 ounces)	4	1.5	2.5
apple rings, dried	10	5.5	1	4.5
apricots, dried	6 halves	2	1	1
banana	1 (4 ounces)	3	1	2
berries blueberries raspberries strawberries	 1/2 cup 1/2 cup 1/2 cup	 2 4 2	 0.5 1 <1	 1.5 3 1
cherries	20	3	1.5	1.5
dates, dried	5	3	1	2
figs, fresh	2	3	<1	2.5
figs, dried	2	3.5	1.5	2
grapefruit	1/2	1.5	1	<1
grapes	20	1	<1	<1
kiwi	1 medium (2.5 ounces)	2.5	1	1.5
mango	1/2 cup	1.5	1	<1

Food Item	Amount	Total fiber (grams)	Soluble (grams)	Insoluble (grams)
nectarine	1 (5 ounces)	2	<1	1
orange	1 (4.5 ounces)	3	2	1
papaya	1 cup	2.5	—	—
peach	1 (3 ounces)	2	1	1
pear	1 (5 ounces)	3	<1	2.5
pineapple	1/2 cup	1	—	<1
plantain, cooked	1/2 cup	2	<1	1
plum	1 (2.5 ounces)	1	0.5	0.5
prunes, dried	2	1	0.5	0.5
raisins	1/2 cup	3	1	2
tangelo	1 (3 ounces)	2	1.5	<1
tangerine	1 (3 ounces)	2	1	0.5
Nuts				
almonds	1/2 cup	8	1	7
almond butter	1/4 cup	2	<1	2
Brazil nuts	1/2 cup	4	—	—
cashews	1/2 cup	2	1	1
chestnuts, roasted	1/4 pound	6	0.5	5
filberts (hazelnuts)	1/2 cup	3.5	1	2
peanut butter	1/4 cup	4	1	3
peanuts	1/2 cup	6	2	4
pecans	1/2 cup	4	1	3
pine nuts	1/2 cup	3	0.5	2.5
pistachios	1/2 cup	7	<1	7
pumpkin seeds	1/2 cup	2.5	<1	2
sesame seeds	1/4 cup	4	1	3
sunflower seeds	1/2 cup	7	2	5
tahini (sesame butter)	1/4 cup	5.5	1	4.5
walnuts	1/2 cup	2	0.5	1.5

CHAPTER 2

Walking the Dietary Fat Tightrope

❦

Although many people have come to view fats as an enemy, in truth we couldn't live without them. Fats are integral to all cell systems. They regulate cell membrane flexibility and are essential for cell growth and the healing of damaged tissue. Fats also provide the raw material for the manufacture of substances that regulate the immune system, response to inflammation, adrenal and sex gland activity, blood platelet stickiness, visual acuity, brain development, and neurological performance, among other things. The vitamins A, D, E, and K, and the phytochemicals known as carotenoids depend on fat to escort them into the bloodstream.

Widely publicized advice to reduce fat intake in order to prevent or overcome heart disease and cancer has left many people anxious, confused, and discouraged. In trying to follow low-fat diets, they often turn to contrived low-fat foods of limited nutritional value; then they reward themselves with foods containing precisely the wrong kind of fat to fulfill their meager fat allowance. Some people also set unrealistically low fat goals.

For optimal health, it's important to have a grasp of the nature of fats in order to distinguish the specific ways they act in the body. It's also important to recognize that genetic diversity plays a role in how people respond to eating fat. As in most areas of nutrition, the benefits—or problems—that occur in one individual aren't always seen in another. Some diet-related examples: (1) When the fat content of the diet of people with high measures of blood cholesterol and triglycerides is altered, they frequently react differently from normal subjects. (2) Where fat is concerned, it seems that no one fatty acid is favorable for all; nor does any one fatty acid appear to be universally detrimental.

In the standard North American diet of the late 1990s, fats account for 34 to 37 percent of average daily calorie intake. This is encouraging, as it is less than the 40 percent figure in the late 1970s. However, most health professionals involved with disease prevention believe this figure is still too high and view it as a contributing factor to obesity, heart disease, and cancer. A 30 percent ceiling is recommended by the American Heart Association (AHA) and the U.S. Department of Agriculture (USDA).

The reliability of the recommended fat allowances is open to question, starting with the standard 30 percent figure. Many popular regimens directed at reducing heart disease are based on a 10 to 20 percent fat ceiling. The World Health Organization recommends that at least 15 percent of calories come from fat. On the other hand, fat consumption in some countries with a much lower incidence of obesity, heart disease, and cancer is considerably higher than these recommendations. (In Greece, for example, estimated average daily fat intake is 40 percent of calories.)

Our extensive review of the research on fat reveals that the percent of calories from fat or total fat intake may be less important than the balance of fats in our diet. That is, where fats come from is a key factor in determining overall health and how we cope with many common ailments.

In order to maintain a sound diet with adequate calories and nutrients, we need to know what fats to limit and how to go about effectively replacing them. What must be resolved is (1) Which fats do the most damage and at what quantity do they become dangerous? (2) Is it best to replace avoided fats with other types of fats, and if so which ones? Or, (3) Are carbohydrates or protein better alternatives to fats? These concerns are addressed in this chapter.

What Are Fats?

The word "fat" itself can be somewhat confusing, since fat is found both within the body and in the foods we eat. Internally, fat is deposited in cells. Collectively these cells are known as adipose (or fatty) tissue. Fats are also found in the bloodstream; these circulating fats are called (serum or blood) triglycerides.

In describing dietary fats, the terms "fat" and "oil" are used to characterize different physical states of the same kind of substance. A fat that is liquid at room temperature is called an oil, whereas one that is a solid or semisolid is referred to as a fat.

Types of Fat

Fats are composed of smaller components known as fatty acids. The technical terms saturated, monounsaturated, and polyunsaturated relate to the number of hydrogen atoms they contain.

- In a saturated fatty acid, all of the possible sites for hydrogen are filled.
- In a monounsaturated fatty acid there is room for one more hydrogen atom.
- A polyunsaturated fatty acid has room for more than one hydrogen atom to be added.

Use of the words "saturated," "monounsaturated," and "polyunsaturated" gives the impression that individual foods are composed of just one type of fatty acid. Actually, the fats contained in food are a complex mixture of fatty acids. Therefore, when a food is referred to as saturated, monounsaturated, or polyunsaturated, this description simply pertains to the type of fatty acid that makes up most of its fatty portion.

The nutrition panels on food labels list total fat content and further break this down into saturated, polyunsaturated, and monounsaturated fats. Be aware that this information, as you are about to find out, is of limited use since individual fatty acids within each of these categories (which aren't specified on food labels) have quite different effects.

Saturated Fatty Acids (SFAs)

Saturated fats (SFAs) are most commonly associated with animal products. Among the family of saturated fatty acids there are four of note: lauric, myristic, palmitic, and stearic acids.

Lauric, myristic, and palmitic acids are all thought to adversely affect blood cholesterol levels. Many studies, but not all, declare stearic acid neutral in relation to blood cholesterol. However, all of these saturated fatty acids promote blood platelet stickiness, which can compromise one of the chambers of the heart or lead to obstructions in blood vessels (see Fat and Heart Disease, on page 323).

Monounsaturated Fatty Acids (MFAs)

Olive oil usually comes to mind when people mention monounsaturated fats (MFAs). The most commonly consumed MFA is oleic acid. Canola oil, avocados, and almonds are other prominent sources.

Polyunsaturated Fatty Acids (PUFAs)

People generally think of vegetable oils as a source of polyunsaturated fatty acids. PUFAs are divided into two categories, depending on their structure. One group is the omega-3 fatty acids and includes alpha linolenic acid and eicosapentaenoic acid; the other is the omega-6 fatty acids, to which linoleic acid belongs.

While the body uses many different fatty acids to perform various tasks, only two must be supplied by the diet. These "essential fatty acids" are linoleic acid (LA) and either eicosapentaenoic acid (EPA) or its precursor alpha linolenic acid (LNA). If the diet includes the proper amounts of these fatty acids, along with other conutrients that facilitate their use, the body itself can manufacture all the other fatty acids it needs.*

*Infants appear to have an additional need for the fatty acid called docosahexaenoic acid (DHA). DHA is essential for brain and eye development; during the last trimester of pregnancy—the period of most rapid brain development in the fetus—DHA is transmitted via the mother's blood supply. After birth, breast-fed infants continue to receive DHA from mother's milk. The fact that infant formulas don't contain this important fatty acid is a matter of concern.

Trans Fatty Acids

The technology used to transform vegetable oils into spreads or more stable oils for use by the food industry is called hydrogenation. This is how margarine and vegetable shortening are created.

During hydrogenation, the configuration of polyunsaturated fats changes; some previously unsaturated positions become saturated and some of the remaining unsaturated bonds move to new positions. These new fats, which are rare in nature and foreign to the human digestive system, are called trans fatty acids. From 7 to 24 percent of the fat in margarines and about 15 percent of the fat in vegetable shortenings is in this form. The partially hydrogenated fats and oils used extensively by the fast food industry contain approximately 30 percent trans fatty acids.

Due to the structural changes caused by hydrogenation, these synthetic fatty acids compete with important natural fatty acids, interfering with critical biological activities.

Enough vs. Too Much

Mainstream Guidelines on Fat

The guidelines from the USDA and the AHA both advocate obtaining no more than 30 percent of total calories from fat. Of this, they recommend limiting saturated fatty acids to no more than 10 percent of calories, or one-third of total fat. Unfortunately, they offer no details as to which particular saturated fats should be emphasized or deemphasized, even though the AHA acknowledges that different saturated fatty acids have varying effects on blood cholesterol. In addition, this organization notes that "wide guidelines do not address the specific needs of all individuals," and furthermore advises that people at risk due to elevated LDL cholesterol that responds to diet can benefit by restricting saturated fats to 7 percent or less of total calories.

The AHA recommends that monounsaturated fatty acids account for up to 15 percent of total daily calorie intake.

According to the AHA, polyunsaturated fatty acids should also comprise up to 10 percent of total daily calorie intake. Again, they give no instructions as to how this should be apportioned in terms of the omega-3 (LNA/EPA) and omega-6 (LA) factions. Nor do they specify a lower limit. This is quite remarkable from such a highly respected source, for a diet lacking these fatty acids cannot maintain health, and the balance between them is of utmost importance. This lack of direction could account for a variety of health problems.

The issue of how much trans fatty acids might be appropriate is rarely confronted. The fact is, despite evidence that they have a negative impact on blood cholesterol levels and cause narrowing of the arteries and possibly insulin resistance, trans fatty acids have been allowed to remain in our food supply without full evaluation of the consequences. On U.S. food labels, trans fatty acids are lumped in with polyunsaturated fats, but inside the body they behave more like saturated fats. In many other countries trans fatty acids are listed separately to avoid this confusion.

Designing New Guidelines

The amount of (omega-6) LA required to avoid symptoms associated with fatty acid deficiency is approximately 1.5 percent of calories, or from 2 to 4 grams per day. It appears that the essential role of LA is fully satisfied at 2 percent of calories.

There are no sanctioned guidelines in the United States, but Health and Welfare Canada recommends consuming LA in the amount of about 3 percent of total daily calories (or 7 to 9 grams for most age groups). At intakes considerably above this, the effect of LA on cardiovascular health, lung and kidney function, and immune and inflammatory response is unclear, but indications are it can undermine health. It's important to note that estimated daily per capita LA intake in the United States (1984) was reported as 16 to 20 grams for men and about 12 grams for women—substantially more than the Canadian government counsels. Just how much LA the body can comfortably handle before it becomes a problem depends to a great extent on how much (omega-3) LNA or EPA there is to counterbalance it.

Research as to the daily minimum requirement for LNA is limited, since recognition of the importance of omega-3 fatty acids is relatively recent. Health and Welfare Canada suggests that LNA should represent 0.5 percent of daily adult calorie intake, or a 6:1 ratio of LA:LNA. In the Japanese diet, which is often touted for its low incidence of heart disease and certain cancers, the LA:LNA ratio is 4:1.

While we still don't know for certain, emerging research indicates a LA:LNA ratio of 3:1 may be preferable in order to facilitate uptake of LNA and its transformation into EPA and docosahexaenoic acid (DHA), a fatty acid believed to be essential to infants, but possibly not adults. If this is the case, at an LA intake of 12 grams, 4 grams of LNA would provide a reasonable balance. Similarly, at an LA intake of 16 to 20 grams, a reasonable intake of LNA would be 5 to 7 grams. A substantially different proportion causes the two fatty acids to compete for the same enzyme that is needed to initiate their transformation into more usable metabolites.*

Per capita food availability studies estimate that the U.S. food supply (1990) offers 1.7 to 2.2 grams LNA daily. The amount of LNA available in the Canadian diet is judged to be somewhat higher at 2.5 to 3 grams per day. In the United States this translates to an LA:LNA ratio of about 10:1, which is much too low!

*Consuming 3 to 4 grams of LNA is believed to be equivalent to directly consuming 0.3 grams of EPA, based on estimates of typical conversion rates by the body; however, in diets with antagonistic amounts of LA relative to LNA, this LNA metabolism is crippled.

Are all these numbers necessary?

"I know that all these numbers and ratios are apt to make people's eyes glaze over. Unfortunately, balancing unsaturated fat intake is a complicated subject, and I suspect this is why health agencies have chosen to ignore the importance of individual fatty acids. I think the most relaxed approach to maintaining a suitable balance is to eat a wide variety of fat-providing wholefoods of vegetable origin. This means choosing different types of nuts and seeds, full-fat soy foods, wheat germ, avocados, and olives. To get more of the hard-to-obtain omega-3 LNA, flaxseeds can be ground and sprinkled on grains, added to spreads, or used in baking. ("In Nikki's Kitchen" will show you how.) It's best to minimize concentrated fats such as butter and most vegetable oils, or when needed give preference to virgin olive oil and cold-pressed canola oil. To boost LNA, flaxseed oil is useful, but it can't be used in cooking. Similarly, hemp oil—which is perfectly balanced—is only suitable for cold applications."

The Golden Combination

As we maintained earlier, the percent of calories from fat and total fat intake appear to be less important than achieving the proper balance. Fats can be safely consumed in a range as wide as 10 to 40 percent of total daily calories, depending on your health and the foods this fat comes from. Despite the specific nature of the following recommendations, don't become fixated on numbers. Instead, use them to devise an overall strategy for yourself when selecting fat-containing foods to achieve the most advantageous balance.

1. Once you have decided where you want to be within the 10 to 40 percent of calorie range based on the preceding information, fatty acids should be apportioned as follows:

Saturated = from 0 to 30 percent of fat intake

Monounsaturated = 50 to 80 percent of fat intake

Polyunsaturated = 20 to 30 percent of fat intake, with from three to six times more omega-6 (LA) than omega-3 (LNA)

For food sources of these fatty acids, see the table Foods and Their Fatty Acids (page 314).

2. How this translates into grams of fat (which is the way this nutrient is represented on food labels and in food reference tables) is shown in Calculating a Reasonable Fat Allowance, below. Although the calculations may seem complicated at first (they're not), you'll probably only need to do this once to set your fat goals.

3. Where diets are very low in calories and/or total fat, the proportion of polyunsaturated fat may need to be adjusted upward in order to satisfy the

To compute your total daily fat goal (in grams):

Your calorie intake × Desired % calories from fat ÷ 9* = Daily goal fat

Once you have this number:

Daily fat goal × .3 = (Maximum) daily saturated fat goal
Daily fat goal × .5–.8 = Daily monounsaturated fat goal
Daily fat goal × .1–.3 = Daily polyunsaturated fat goal
Daily polyunsaturated fat goal × .75–.86 = Daily omega-6 (LA) goal
Daily polyunsaturated fat goal × .25–.14 = Daily omega-3 (LNA) goal

Example: at 1800 calories with goals of total fat—25% calories; saturated fat—20% total fat; monounsaturated fat—55% total fat; polyunsaturated fat—25% total fat

Daily fat goal: 1800 × .25 (450) ÷ 9 = 50 grams
Daily saturated fat goal: 50 × .20 = 10 grams
Daily monounsaturated fat goal: 50 × .55 = 27.5 grams
Daily polyunsaturated fat goal: 50 × .25 = 12.5 grams
Daily omega-6 (LA) goal: 12.5 × .75 = 9 grams (3:1 ratio) to 12.5 × .86 = 11 grams (6:1 ratio)
Daily omega-3 (LNA) goal: 12.5 × .25 = 3 grams (3:1 ratio) to 12.5 × .14 = 2 grams (6:1 ratio)

*Fat, no matter what the source, furnishes 9 calories per gram.

body's requirement for the essential fatty acids—at least 2.5 to 3 grams LA and approximately 1 gram LNA. Foods should be chosen with this in mind.

4. Where diets are high in calories and/or total fat, monounsaturates should be emphasized to avoid overconsuming either saturated or polyunsaturated fatty acids. Again, the table Foods and Their Fatty Acids will help you decide which foods deserve more attention than others.

Right Fat Foods

"The microbe is nothing: the terrain is everything."

—LOUIS PASTEUR

In trying to reduce nutrition to simple lessons, the package in which individual nutrients are delivered is often ignored. While Pasteur's comment parallels our thoughts about the wholeness of food in general, when it comes to dietary fats this aphorism is particularly relevant. The framework in which they're delivered (that is "the terrain") plays a critical role in the competence of individual fatty acids (akin to Pasteur's "microbes"). Therefore, when deciding which fats to eat, the food that they're contained in must be considered.

In nature, all fats are part of a food. Once these fats are extracted from the source and isolated in a concentrated form (oils, butter, lard), at least three things happen: (1) they're subject to harmful oxidation, (2) the ratio of key constituents becomes unbalanced, (3) the likelihood of overconsumption increases.

Our hunter-gatherer forebears consumed their fat indirectly; that is, contained within animal flesh or seeds. As animals became domesticated and agriculture developed, this broadened to include eggs, dairy, and cultivated nuts and grains. Later, the rendering of fat from meat, the pressing of oil from seeds or fruit (olives), and the separating of fat from milk for butter increased the quantity and concentration of fats, as well as the number of choices. As technology and the industrial revolution took over the food-processing industry, new techniques developed for producing concentrated fats with a long shelf life and greater commercial versatility. All this modernization dramatically altered the form and context of human fat consumption.

There is little question among those who study nutrition that consuming concentrated fats in quantity isn't what nature originally intended. Thus it isn't surprising that fat has become a problematic component of our diets.

Today, the major fats in our diet come from extracted fats, as well as animal flesh and dairy foods. Nuts and seeds, soybeans, wheat germ, and certain fatty fruits like avocados and olives are additional sources, although in the standard U.S. diet they aren't as significant. Ironically, it is this latter group that merits attention, for these are the most healthful fat providers. We know this will be hard for many people to accept given the negative publicity regarding fat over the last few years. As soon as Nikki says "nuts" or "avocado" to a client, his or her immediate horrified response is "but they have fat!" It's time to redirect attention from "low fat" to the "right fat."

Nuts and Seeds

Because most people think of nuts as "fatty" and "fattening," Nikki's clients are surprised when nuts are included in her weight-loss plans, and even more so when they're touted as "heart healthy."

Despite the fact that from 73 to 90 percent of their calories come from fat, a look at the fatty acid makeup of nuts and seeds shows how compatible they are with good health. We think it's very important to pay attention to studies like these:

• Diet trials in which 30 percent of calories were derived from fat showed that eating 3 ounces of walnuts daily (providing about 20 percent of the fat calories) resulted in more favorable serum lipids compared with a diet that was nut free. This isn't unexpected considering the favorable distribution of fatty acids in walnuts. However, an additional interesting observation is that some of the improvement may have been due to other components in the walnuts, specifically the low ratio of the amino acids lysine to arginine (see Fat and Heart Disease, on page 323).

• Similar results have been seen using almonds, which are high in mono-unsaturated oleic acid. This was seen even when they added 23 grams of fat to the daily diet, increasing overall fat intake from 28 percent of calories to 37 percent.

Unlike concentrated oils, the fatty acids in nuts and seeds are accompanied by protein, vitamins, minerals, and fiber. Almonds and Brazil nuts are particularly high in calcium, while pistachios, sunflower seeds, and sesame seeds provide notable amounts, as well. Most nuts and seeds are rich in potassium and iron. As you will see later on, nuts and seeds also make a very important contribution in terms of vitamin E (see Other Nutritional Factors Related to Fats, on page 338).

Nuts and seeds are a significant source of selenium, copper, magnesium, and zinc. The essential role of these minerals is discussed in Chapter 3. In fact, Brazil nuts are the most reliable food when it comes to selenium; a single nut furnishes 140 mg, which is twice the U.S. RDA for this mineral and about what you find in a substantial selenium supplement.

Caution: If nuts are eaten on top of an already ample diet, they can increase calorie consumption enough to cause weight gain. Furthermore, if oil-roasted nuts and seeds are chosen, potential health benefits are likely to be offset by the damaging mode of preparation.

Flaxseed

Another fat-bearing food that gains prominence in *The Healthiest Diet in the World* is flaxseed. Flaxseeds are the tiny brown seeds of a graceful annual plant with delicate blue flowers. While an unfamiliar ingredient in most North American kitchens, its dietary use has been traced back thousands of years. Hippocrates wrote about the use of flaxseeds medicinally, and during the reign of Charlemagne in eighth-century France, it is said he considered flax so important for the health of his subjects that he passed regulations requiring its consumption.

Flax was first introduced into North America in 1617 as a fiber crop. Today, Canada is one of the world's leading producers, and flaxseeds are currently used by many commercial bakers in Canada and Europe. Their nutty flavor and unique nutritional composition are two big selling points.

Flaxseed is one of the few foods where (omega-3) LNA predominates, with a ratio of LA:LNA of 1:3.5. Because most commonly eaten foods provide only small amounts of LNA, flaxseed is extremely useful in shifting the balance of polyunsaturated fatty acids in a more favorable direction. Flaxseeds also contain soluble fibers that help lower blood cholesterol, and lignan precursors that are broken down in the digestive tract to form hormonelike substances that show antitumor activity. These topics are discussed in Chapter 1. Flaxseed is also known for its laxative effect.

While the tiny brown seeds provide the safest packaging for the easily spoiled oil within, the seed coating is resistant to the digestive process. Therefore, consuming the intact seed may not be of much use. To obtain the benefits, the seeds should be ground (see page 239) or in oil form (see below).

Avocado

Although thought of as a vegetable, avocados are a fruit native to Mexico and Central America, where they were considered an aphrodisiac.

Unlike other fruit, rather than being rich in sugars, avocados are high in fat. In Florida avocados, fat accounts for about 70 percent of the calories; about 90 percent of the calories in California varieties come from fat. This fat is predominantly monounsaturated oleic acid. Avocados also provide notable amounts of soluble and insoluble fibers, vitamins A, E, K, and C, several B vitamins (thiamin, riboflavin, niacin, B_6, biotin, folate, pantothenic acid), potassium, magnesium, iron, and copper.

Some influential health advocates have prejudiced people against avocados because of their high fat content. This is ironic, as the fat is actually one of the things that makes them so attractive from both a nutritional and culinary perspective. Noteworthy here is an experimental trial diet in which women eating from 1 to 1½ avocados daily lowered total cholesterol, LDL cholesterol, and the lipoprotein apo B significantly, despite an overall daily fat intake of about 37 percent of calories. When switched to a calorically comparable diet high in carbohydrate but with just 20 percent of calories from fat (and no avocado), the women demonstrated a smaller, less significant drop in total cholesterol; moreover, only protective HDLs were diminished. As a result, the total cholesterol:HDL ratio actually benefited when avocado was provided and suffered on the low-fat, high-carbohydrate regimen. (For more on the significance of this, see Fat and Heart Disease, on page 323.)

Olives

Like olive oil, olives are high in monounsaturated oleic acid. They don't offer significant amounts of other nutrients and are quite high in sodium. (A snack of just 4 or 5 olives can add 200 to 300 mg, or about one-tenth of the preferred daily sodium intake.)

Fish

Fish is considered by many to be the favored animal source of fats, mostly because fish are unique in their abundance of two of the fatty acids of the omega-3 type, EPA and DHA. Sadly, fish today may furnish a lot more than these desirable fatty acids: pesticides and heavy metals. This is a problem acknowledged by the U.S. Environmental Protection Agency. Since 1993, the EPA has been issuing state-by-state recommendations to avoid or limit certain fish from specific water bodies. These include warnings for the general population, as well as sensitive subgroups such as pregnant women, children, and people with compromised immune systems. Each year the number of advisories increase; between 1994 and 1995 they went up by 14 percent, and from 1993 to 1995 there was a 36 percent increase. This isn't necessarily due to rising fish contamination, but to some extent reflects a step-up in assessments. What this implies is that for years fish have been taken from numerous polluted sources; they just weren't identified. As of January 1996, there were advisories for water bodies in forty-seven states and the District of Columbia.

Some people look to farm-raised fish bred in controlled environments to reduce exposure to contaminants, but this may not be as good a solution as it first appears. Farm-raised fish can have as little as one-fourth to one-half the LNA content of free-swimming counterparts; EPA and DHA are less affected. The significance of these findings isn't known.

Fish eaters who want more information on these warnings can contact the U.S. Environmental Protection Agency (see "Resources").

Edible Oils

People are often confused about which fats are most suitable for cooking, salads, spreads, and other food uses. Since concentrated fats are all processed to some degree, they're never as desirable as fats within foods.

Salad dressing is among the top five sources of fat in the diet. Not surprisingly, people feel they're eating healthfully when they choose salads. But to make the salad more enjoyable, they pour on the dressing. Unfortunately, most people don't take time to make their own dressing, and the fat in most bottled dressings isn't generally among the best choices. Nikki's clients often report that they use commercial "low-fat" and "fat-free" dressings; while they may not add fat, most are high in sodium, and one of the principal ingredients is sugar in some form. In fact, a standard 2-tablespoon serving generally contains from 1 to 2½ teaspoons of sugar (4 to 10 grams). To make salads suitably enticing, our recipes provide you with delicious fat-free and low-fat/healthy-fat dressings (see pages 188 to 193).

Despite all the no-fat and low-fat approaches provided in our recipes, there are times when a little oil is useful or desirable. Sometimes oils are even necessary to improve the ratio of fatty acids in the diet. For such instances, here is a brief rundown of preferred choices. The fatty acids composition of a variety of oils is shown in the table Foods and Their Fatty Acids, on page 314.

★ COOKING WITHOUT ADDING FAT ★

In developing the recipes for "In Nikki's Kitchen," we were delighted by how easy it was to eliminate fats as a cooking medium. In their place we use such flavoring agents as orange juice, apple juice, bean cooking liquid, tomato products, wine, vinegars, soy sauce, as well as stewing vegetables in their own juices. Although some people swear by cooking sprays and nonstick pans, we haven't found either necessary. All you need are some pots with tight-fitting lids. Where sticking might be a problem, you can wipe the surface of a pan with a paper towel dampened with oil.

Olive Oil

Customarily, olive oil is the least processed of the commonly available oils. But to receive all the incidental constituents that make olive oil acceptable, only extra virgin or virgin olive oil qualifies. To make virgin olive oil, olives are pressed without the use of water, heat, or solvents. The oil is then filtered and judged for taste, color, and aroma, as well as residual acidity. Oils that don't measure up are refined chemically, resulting in olive oil that is colorless, odorless, and nutritionally inferior. To give these oils culinary appeal, a small amount of virgin olive oil is reintroduced. Olive oils described as "light" have no less fat in them. They're simply refined olive oil with little or no virgin oil added back.

Olive oil can be used in salads and spreads, as well as for cooking. It doesn't stand up well to high temperatures and therefore shouldn't be used for high-heat sautéing or frying (which isn't a cooking technique we endorse even with more suitable oils).

Canola Oil

The name of most oils indicates their origin. Thus, when it comes to canola oil, people are understandably puzzled. In fact, this oil comes from rapeseed, a source of oil once deemed unsafe due to unhealthy amounts of erucic acid in this plant.

This health problem was conquered when a new strain of rapeseed was developed in Canada. To circumvent the stigma attached to high-erucic rapeseed oil, the new low-erucic rapeseed oil was named after the country that introduced it: hence, Canada oil, which became canola oil.

We are usually wary of a food that hasn't been part of the human food supply for very long. But because of its relatively healthful balance of fatty acids (and lack of negative reports), canola oil appears to be a safe choice. We strongly urge you to seek out cold-pressed varieties, as the high temperatures used in other extraction methods may be damaging.

Canola contains respectable amounts of phytosterols (discussed in Fat and Heart Disease, on page 323), although refining reduces them by half. Among its strong points is a high temperature tolerance, making it a good choice for sautéing (and frying). Since it's tasteless as well, canola oil is a useful fat for baked goods.

Flaxseed Oil

If you wish to consume LNA (omega-3) in a concentrated form, flaxseed oil can be used. Although flaxseed oil doesn't contain the beneficial lignan or fibers found in the seeds, it does furnish a notable amount of valuable phytosterols.

Flaxseed oil is available in natural food outlets. Because it's vulnerable to oxidation, flaxseed oil must be purchased as fresh as possible from a supplier that either freezes or refrigerates it. It should be packaged in a nontransparent container, stored in the refrigerator, and, once opened, consumed within two months.

Flaxseed oil can be used in salad dressings, spreads, and other uncooked applications. It can be added to hot dishes after cooking (for example, to enhance pasta dishes, grains, or cooked vegetables), but it shouldn't be used as a cooking medium or subjected to direct heat since the fatty acids don't withstand high temperatures.

Hemp Oil

Hemp is derived from the plant known as *Cannabis sativa*, otherwise known as marijuana. In addition to being the source of a mind-altering drug, the hemp plant furnishes edible seeds, oil, and fiber for cloth. Despite this incredible versatility, products from *Cannabis sativa* are practically unknown in contemporary North America.

Although during World War II hemp was promoted as a crop that could help save the economy, cultivation of *Cannabis sativa* is currently prohibited in the United States. Its classification as a psychoactive drug doesn't justify this ban, since strains grown for commercial use—and oil, in particular—are low in the sticky resin that has earned this plant its infamous reputation. Furthermore, cleaning and washing the seeds prior to oil pressing eliminates any potentially active tetrahydrocannabinol (THC). All hemp seeds imported to the United States are sterilized (as required by law); fresh "live" seeds will remain unavailable until growing laws are revised.

Fat accounts for about 35 percent of the hemp seed. Of the remainder, 25 percent is protein. The flavorful, green-hued oil contains LA and LNA in what is considered to be an ideal balance (1:3), and it is one of the few edible oils containing gamma linolenic acid (GLA), an important fatty acid that most healthy people can manufacture from LA.

Hemp oil is easily oxidized. To preserve its healthfulness it requires cold storage in a nontransparent container. Once opened, it is best consumed within three months. If you can't find hemp oil in a natural food store, see "Resources."

Sesame Oil

Since ancient times, sesame has been an important oil seed not only because of its high fat content, but also because of its extraordinary resistance to oxidative deterioration (spoiling) and its reputed medicinal qualities. Traditional Chinese medicine books claim that sesame increases energy and prevents aging.

Despite a relatively high omega-3 content, the oil from roasted sesame seeds is extremely stable, and even refined oil from unroasted sesame seeds resists oxidation much better than soy, rapeseed, safflower, or corn oils. In comparison tests, roasted sesame oil remained sound at 50 days (when testing ended); refined unroasted sesame oil began to show signs of oxidation at 35 days, while the other oils began to oxidize after 5 to 20 days.

Sesame seeds contain some unusual lignan components, including sesamin and sesamolin, and because of them the extracted oil exhibits unique chemical and physiological properties. The phenolic compounds sesamol and sesaminol, among others, that are produced from these lignans, are credited with giving sesame its strong antioxidant power. This affects not just the integrity of the fat itself, but also its capacity to act inside the body as a protective factor against oxygen-generated aging, mutation, cancer, and other diseases.

These compounds have been shown to act synergistically with the vitamin E present in the oil. What is especially interesting about this is that the form of vitamin E in sesame is gamma-tocopherol. It was always assumed that only the vitamin E compound alpha-tocopherol is biologically active. This is a nutritional misconception that is finally receiving some attention. (For more on this see Other Nutritional Factors Related to Fats, on page 338, and Chapter 3, "Preventing System Breakdowns." Sesamin has also been touted as a cholesterol regulator in studies on rats.

Another quality of sesame oil is its extremely high phytosterol content. As discussed later in this chapter in Fat and Heart Disease, phytosterols may have a significant impact on reducing blood cholesterol. Even refined sesame oil, in which less than a third of the phytosterols remain, is higher than most other oils.

Roasted sesame oil has an exquisite flavor. Just a small amount contributes enormously to the taste of whatever food it's added to. Because of its heat tolerance, it can be used in all cooking applications. You can find sesame oil in natural food stores, some supermarkets, Asian food outlets, and gourmet shops.

FOODS AND THEIR FATTY ACIDS

I. Percent of Various Fatty Acids in Concentrated Fats

Fat	% Saturated	% Mono-unsaturated	% Poly-unsaturated	% Trans
Vegetable Oils*				
canola	7	59	30	<1
coconut	87	6	2	—
corn	14	25	60	—
flaxseed	10	17	69	—
hemp	21	30	41	—
olive	14	74	10	1
palm	50	39	9	—

*100 percent of product is fat.

Fat	% Saturated	% Mono-unsaturated	% Poly-unsaturated	% Trans
peanut	19	46	33	—
safflower	9	12	75	—
safflower, high oleic	6	75	14	—
sesame	14	40	42	—
soybean	14	23	58	—
sunflower	12	19	66	—
sunflower, high oleic	9	84	4	<1
walnut	9	23	63	—
wheat germ	19	16	62	—
Fish Oils*†				
cod liver	23	47	23	—
menhaden	30	27	34	—
salmon	20	29	40	—
Other Concentrated Fats†‡				
beef fat	71	32	36	3
butter	51	24	3	—
cocoa butter	60	33	3	—
lard	40	42	14	1
margarine, stick	17	39	21	23
margarine, tub	8	21	18	6

†These foods not recommended but included for comparison.
‡Figure represents percent of fatty acids in total product, not as percent of total fat. Butter is composed of only 81 percent fat; stick margarine (Blue Bonnet), 80 percent fat; tub margarine (Blue Bonnet), 49 percent fat; figures for beef fat, lard, and cocoa butter are based on a product that is 100 percent fat.

II. Percent Breakdown of Saturated Fatty Acids in Concentrated Fats

Fat	% Lauric	% Myristic	% Palmitic	% Stearic
Vegetable Oils*				
canola	—	—	4	2
coconut	45	17	8	3
corn	—	—	11	2

Fat	% Lauric	% Myristic	% Palmitic	% Stearic
flaxseed	—	—	6	3
hemp	—	—	19	2
olive	—	—	11	2
palm	<1	1	44	4
peanut	<1	<1	10	2
safflower	—	<1	6	2
safflower, high oleic	—	—	5	1
sesame	—	—	9	5
soybean	<1	<1	10	4
sunflower	—	—	6	5
sunflower, high oleic	—	—	4	4
walnut	—	—	7	2
wheat germ	—	<1	17	1
Fish Oils†				
cod liver	—	4	11	3
menhaden	—	8	15	4
salmon	—	3	10	4
Other Concentrated Fats†‡				
beef fat	<1	2	18	8
butter§	2	8	21	10
cocoa butter	—	<1	25	33
lard	<1	1	23	15
margarine, stick	—	<1	10	7
margarine, tub	—	—	5	3

§7 percent of product is short-chain fatty acids not represented in table.

III. Percent Breakdown of Polyunsaturated Fatty Acids in Concentrated Fats

Fat	% Linoleic (LA)	% Linolenic (LNA)	Ratio omega-6: omega-3
Vegetable Oils*			
canola	20	9	2:1

Fat	% Linoleic (LA)	% Linolenic (LNA)	Ratio omega-6: omega-3
coconut	2	0	—
corn	58	2	29:1
flaxseed	13	55	1:4
hemp	30	11	3:1
olive	9	<1	15:1
palm	9	<1	31:1
peanut	32	1	32:1
safflower	74	<1	—
safflower, high oleic	14	0	—
sesame	41	<1	—
soybean	51	7	7.5:1
sunflower	66	0	—
sunflower, high oleic	4	<1	19:1
walnut	53	10	5:1
wheat germ	55	7	8:1
Fish Oils‖			
cod liver	1	1	1:10
menhaden	2	1.5	1:7
salmon	1.5	1	1:15
Other Concentrated Fats†‡			
beef fat	3	<1	5:1
butter	2	1	1.5:1
cocoa butter	3	<1	28:1
lard	13	1	21:1
margarine, stick	19	1.5	13:1
margarine, tub	16	1	16:1

‖The principal polyunsaturated omega-3 fatty acids in fish oils are EPA and DHA; values for cod liver oil are 7 percent and 11 percent, respectively; for menhaden oil, 13 percent and 8.5 percent, respectively; for salmon oil, 13 percent and 18 percent, respectively. These oils also contain additional omega-6 fatty acids not listed here. The omega-6:omega-3 ratio reflects these other fats.

IV. Grams of Fat in Common Measures of Golden Pantry Selections

Food	Amount	Total Fat (grams)	Saturated (grams)	Mono-unsaturated (grams)	Omega-6 (grams)	Omega-3 (grams)
almonds	1/4 cup	18.5	2	12	4	<1
almond butter	2 Tbs	19	2	12	4	<1
avocado, CA	1/2 cup mashed	20	3	13	2	<1
avocado, FL	1/2 cup mashed	10	2	5.5	1.5	<1
Brazil nuts	1/4 cup	23	6	8	8.5	—
cashews	1/4 cup	16	3	9	2.5	—
egg	1 large	5	1.5	2	<1	—
flaxseed	2 Tbs ground	6.5	<1	1	<1	2.5
hazelnuts/ filberts	1/4 cup	18	1	14	1.5	—
olives	10	5	<1	4	<1	—
peanut butter	2 Tbs	16	2	8	5	—
peanuts	1/4 cup	18	2.5	9	6	—
pecans	1/4 cup	18	1.5	11	4	<1
pine nuts	1/4 cup	17	2.5	6.5	7	<1
pistachios	1/4 cup	15.5	2	10.5	2	—
pumpkin seeds	1/4 cup	16	3	5	7	—
soybeans	1 cup cooked	15	2	3	8	1
soybeans, roasted	1/4 cup	10	1.5	2.5	5	<1
soy flour, full fat	1/4 cup	4.5	<1	1	2	<1
sunflower seeds	1/4 cup	16	2	3	10.5	—
tahini	2 Tbs	17	2	6	7	—
tempeh	4 oz	6	1	1.5	3	<1

Food	Amount	Total Fat (grams)	Saturated (grams)	Mono-unsaturated (grams)	Omega-6 (grams)	Omega-3 (grams)
tofu, firm	4 oz	5	<1	1	1.5	1
vegetable oils#	1 Tbs	14				
walnuts	1/4 cup	15.5	1.5	3.5	8	2
wheat germ	1/4 cup	3	<1	<1	1.5	<1
yogurt, whole milk	1 cup	8	5	2	<1	—

#For the fatty acid composition of various vegetable oils, refer back to sections I, II, and III.

How the Body Uses Fat

Most people think of fat as a "problem." In reality, fat is responsible for so many functions in the body, it should be embraced. A good way to begin is by reading the following somewhat technical description of how fat keeps you alive and well. Even if you don't understand all of it, this section is sure to give you respect for fat's importance.

When food fats enter the digestive system they're broken apart by digestive enzymes and absorbed into the bloodstream.* Once taken into the cells, fatty acids can become a source of immediate energy or they can remain stored as adipose tissue. Fat actually furnishes 2.25 times more energy than equal amounts of either carbohydrate or protein, and unlike these two nutrients it can be stored in the body indefinitely. In addition, some fatty acids aren't oxidized for energy or stored; they are selectively converted into materials that can impact many cell functions.

Dietary fats can affect us in both complementary and competing ways. One thing they are used for is to manufacture compounds called eicosanoids, "chemical messengers" crucial to cell behavior and cell-to-cell interactions. Eicosanoids are synthesized in varying amounts by all cells of the immune system and are manifested in a number of different substances, including prostaglandins and leukotrienes. Among other things, eicosanoids regulate insulin secretion, muscle contractions, the immune system, the body's response to inflammation, and early

*Some fatty acids are released more readily than others. For example, short-chain fatty acids (with only four to ten carbons) are quickly absorbed and easily turned into usable energy. The particles of longer-chain fatty acids (lauric, myristic, palmitic, and stearic) must undergo reassembly in the liver before they can be used. There they are transformed into very-low-density lipoprotein (VLDL) particles, which ultimately form cholesterol-rich low-density lipoproteins (LDL). These LDLs are potentially harmful to the arteries, but receptors in the liver can remove them and prevent this from happening. Whether this happens or not depends to some degree on diet. When saturated fatty acids are too concentrated they impair LDL removal, whereas unsaturated fatty acids facilitate this activity.

brain and retina development. They operate via a complex system of balances, with the actions of some directly opposing the actions of others. Either a deficiency or an imbalance of eicosanoids can result in a number of pathological states, including arthritis, asthma, angina, thrombosis, impaired immune response, allergic reactions, and various chronic conditions caused by people's response to inflammatory stimulants.

An area of major importance is the effect fatty acids have on cell permeability and the fluidity of cell membranes. This, in turn, influences hormone receptors, enzymes, and nutrient flow within and between cells. The sensitivity of cells to both insulin and cholesterol is accordingly mediated by dietary fats.

Ordinarily, the presence of fat in the bloodstream moderates the output of cholesterol by the liver. If the supply of essential polyunsaturated fatty acids (PUFAs) is too low, the liver increases cholesterol production in order to keep cell membranes pliable. When intake of PUFAs is adequate, cholesterol production is suppressed. In addition, eating large amounts of saturated fat stimulates the body to make more cholesterol, while consumption of trans fatty acids, found in margarine and many processed foods, impairs its clearance.

If fat is replaced with additional calories from sugars and starches, the body converts these nutrients into fat and then uses this to make more cholesterol. This is how a diet low in essential fatty acids and high in carbohydrates can actually provoke elevated cholesterol and triglyceride levels rather than improving them.

The table Fat Facts at a Glance (page 321) lists the common dietary fatty acids and some of their prominent functions and effects. It also enumerates many of the conditions brought about by the three most widely studied prostaglandins (PG_1, PG_2, PG_3).

A number of different elements from a variety of foods assist fat metabolism and facilitate the conversion of fat into regulatory substances and energy. These are discussed in Chapter 3.

As noted earlier, fats serve as indispensable carriers for vitamins A, D, E, K, and the phytochemicals known as carotenoids. This is a very important function. For instance, in experiments measuring the absorption of carotenoids, when either carrots or tomatoes were cooked with modest amounts of olive or corn oils, blood levels of the specific carotenoids being measured increased strikingly compared with carrots or tomatoes consumed in a fat-free setting. Due to the growing body of information pertaining to the health-protective potential of carotenoids, as well as vitamins A, D, E, and K, completely avoiding fat at mealtimes could be an unsound strategy.

Also keep in mind that many flavors are fat soluble, and therefore adding a little fat can render food more tasty. Moreover, fat can make a meal more satisfying, because its presence in the stomach delays gastric emptying.

FAT FACTS AT A GLANCE

For food sources, see the table Foods and Their Fatty Acids, on page 314.

Fatty Acids	Function/Effects
Saturated	associated with increased macular degeneration and coronary disease; possible connection to increased cancers
short-chain saturated fatty acids (4 to 10 carbon)	the most easily digested saturated fats
lauric, myristic, and palmitic acids	raise blood cholesterol and triglyceride levels; atherogenic; increase blood platelet stickiness; may promote tumor growth
stearic acid	most but not all research shows no effect on blood cholesterol and triglycerides; increases blood platelet stickiness
Monounsaturated	no adverse health effects known at this time
oleic acid	neutral or lowering effect on blood triglycerides and cholesterol; lowers LDL but not protective HDL cholesterol
Polyunsaturated	several health-protective roles if individual fatty acids are properly balanced; improper ratios may lead to tumor cell growth, inflammatory disorders, impaired mental function, decreased immune performance, and more
linoleic acid (LA) omega-6	an essential fatty acid required for health; promotes clearance of triglycerides from blood following meals; enhances muscle recovery; high levels associated with behavior problems and decline in cognitive function; may promote tumor growth if not balanced with omega-3 fatty acids; increases PG_1 levels* (converted by body into arachidonic acid)
arachidonic acid (AA) omega-6	increases PG_1 levels*

*PG_1 prostaglandins decrease platelet stickiness; help kidneys remove sodium and fluids; improve circulation; decrease blood pressure; improve angina; reduce inflammation; improve insulin function; regulate calcium metabolism and improve nerve function; increase T cells and immune performance; inhibit PG_2 prostaglandins.

Fatty Acids	Function/Effects
alpha linolenic acid (LNA) omega-3	an essential fatty acid required for health; decreases levels of total and LDL cholesterols; promotes clearance of triglycerides from blood following meals; increases cell membrane fluidity; enhances muscle recovery; inhibits tumor growth; may protect against osteoporosis by inhibiting tumor necrosis factor; adequate levels associated with improved cognitive function and mental outlook; excess amounts can suppress immune function; decreases production of PG_2[†]; increases production of PG_3[‡]
eicosapentaenoic acid (EPA) omega-3	healthy people convert LNA into EPA; prevents sticky blood platelets; lowers blood triglycerides; lowers blood pressure; enhances adrenal and sex gland activity; decreases synthesis of arachidonic acid and production of PG_2[†]; increases production of PG_3[‡]
Docosahexaenoic acid (DHA) omega-3	healthy people convert LNA to DHA, but possibly essential for newborns; functions similar to EPA; enhances brain cell development and vision
Trans fatty acids	fats rarely exist in the trans form in nature, but are created during hydrogenation; raise blood cholesterol levels by interfering with body's cholesterol-clearing capability; cause narrowing of the arteries; contribute to blood platelet stickiness; may be a factor in insulin resistance; associated with elevated risk for breast cancer

[†]PG_2 prostaglandins increase platelet stickiness; increase blood pressure; increase inflammation. Note PG_2 is inhibited by PG_1.
[‡]PG_3 prostaglandins regulate blood pressure; reduce platelet stickiness; enhance kidney, immune, and arterial functions; reduce inflammation; regulate calcium and energy metabolism.

Fat and Body Weight

Sometimes there appear to be as many weight-loss strategies as there are people seeking to lose weight. One of the popular themes echoed both by Nikki's clients and even some health professionals is that as long as people restrict fat they can eat as much as they want and not gain weight. In Chapter 1, we exposed the fallacy of this viewpoint by presenting the deleterious effects of high carbohydrate intake on fat storage. But there is another reason to challenge this claim.

One way the body appears to protect itself from weight gain due to increased fat consumption is by speeding up the rate of energy metabolism. This was demonstrated in two 10-day studies of identical male twins conducted at Tufts University. When the men were fed diets with comparable amounts of calories, those consuming 40 percent of calories from fat used up 55 calories more per day than those fed 20 percent calories from fat. (In the course of the study there were no meaningful changes in body weight, but this isn't surprising; ten days account for only 550 calories, while the loss of a pound of fat correlates to 3,500 calories.) What this study showed was that diets higher in fat can increase the amount of energy the body expends.

If the Tufts researchers are right—and indeed this outcome has been corroborated elsewhere—replacing fat calories with carbohydrate calories may actually impede weight loss, not assist it.

What Happens When Fat Consumption Is Out of Balance

Substituting one source of fat for another, for example replacing saturated fats with polyunsaturated fats, can be helpful for some conditions (such as reducing blood lipids) but can compromise others (such as immune response). We have already mentioned that replacing fats with carbohydrates can also have unwanted consequences. This is precisely why *The Healthiest Diet in the World* is about total diets, not just individual foods or nutrients, and why food selection must pertain to the individual, not the general population.

In the next few sections we discuss the influence various fatty acids can have on your health. Rather than continually repeating the foods in which the specific fatty acids referred to are found, we ask that you look back at the table Foods and Their Fatty Acids, on page 314, to obtain this information. You should also explore the table Fat Facts at a Glance, on pages 321–22, which summarizes the effects of different fatty acids.

Fat and Heart Disease

In most instances, coronary heart disease (CHD) is caused by obstruction of vessels leading to the heart due to arteriosclerosis (thickening of arterial walls accompanied by a loss of elasticity) or thrombosis (coagulation or clumping of blood in some part of the circulatory system). These events may occur singly or in combination. What causes either of these conditions isn't clear, although there are numerous theories and a lot of clues.

For many years the standard approach to risk reduction and treatment has been restricting total fat consumption and replacing saturated fats with polyunsaturated fats in order to reduce blood cholesterol levels. Although this is still the usual protocol, the precise relationship between cholesterol and CHD is baffling.

One thing that is obvious is that this narrow focus on cholesterol is limiting

Triglycerides: Triglycerides is another word used for fat—both the kind of fat found in food and the form in which fat occurs in the body. This technical term comes from the chemical structure of a fat molecule, which consists of three fatty acids (hence "tri") held together by a molecule of glycerol.

During digestion, dietary fats are broken down into individual fatty acids and later reassembled into new triglycerides. Most of the triglycerides within the body are stored in fat tissues. Small amounts of triglycerides are always circulating in the bloodstream, and there generally is an increase in their amount soon after eating. When calories from carbohydrates are unavailable, the liver is responsible for releasing triglycerides into the bloodstream.

The triglycerides in the bloodstream that come directly from dietary fats may affect the body differently than triglycerides generated by the liver. The reason for this is the dissimilar forms in which they are transported in the blood (see Individualistic Lipoproteins, on page 328).

Lipoproteins (HDL, LDL, VLDL): The term "lipoproteins" refers to the form in which the body transports fats from place to place. Rather than carrying fats to the tissues as triglycerides or individual fatty acids, the body encapsulates them in protein-covered particles called lipoproteins (lipid—for fat—plus protein). To keep these lipoproteins stable, they also contain cholesterol. The purpose of the cholesterol is to keep the particles from breaking apart.

Lipoproteins route fats from the blood to their final destination in various body tissues. These delivery proteins are sometimes called apo A lipoproteins (from the derivation away) or chylomicrons. They are relatively large in size. After delivering the lipid to its destination, the remaining fraction (called high-density lipoproteins or HDLs) is rapidly cleared from the blood. As a result, these lipoproteins seem to have minimal impact in the arteries. In fact, the ability to generate HDLs, which is reflected in blood analysis by a high level of HDL cholesterol, is an indication that the body is capable of handling fat in a satisfactory way.

Triglycerides that originate in the liver are packaged somewhat differently. These lipoproteins, called very-low-density lipoproteins (or VLDLs), contain a substance referred to as apo B and are much smaller in size. When they reach fat tissues, they too deposit their triglyceride portion. However, the "packaging" material they leave behind continues to circulate in the blood in a form known as low-density lipoproteins (LDLs), until the liver removes them. When these LDLs remain too long in the bloodstream they begin to deposit their cholesterol particles on the inside of artery walls. This is sometimes called arterial plaque and over time it can cause the arteries to close up, a condition known as atherosclerosis. This narrowing of the arteries can lead to heart attacks and strokes.

the use of other ways of handling this health problem. The fact is, current advice regarding fat is poorly conceived, as not all fats are detrimental and often the foods that replace them present a new set of problems. Moreover, dietary intervention can change risk through mechanisms that don't involve serum cholesterol at all.

As discussed in Chapter 1, increasing carbohydrates to compensate for eating less fat frequently elevates blood triglycerides and lowers the protective HDL cholesterol. Furthermore, it has been demonstrated that the fats made by the body during a low-fat, high-carbohydrate regimen mimic the fatty acid pattern associated with heart disease.*

Even those who believe in the conventional modified-fat model recognize that it needs to be improved upon so that the HDL cholesterol doesn't suffer and cancer risk doesn't increase, as can happen when people alter fat intake incorrectly.

The Rich-Diet Heart Theory

The frequent association between a "rich" diet and cardiovascular disease was the basis of the original diet-heart connection. This rich diet is described as a habitually high caloric intake compared to energy expenditure, coupled with generous amounts of saturated fat (and cholesterol) coming from meat, eggs, and dairy. The rich diet is high in total fat, concentrated sugars, salt, and alcohol. During the last few decades this way of eating has become more widespread and patterns of heart disease seem to coincide.

The pioneer study of the relationship between dietary fats and heart disease was initiated in 1958 by Ancel Keys. This Seven Countries Study, using cross-cultural data, followed more than 12,400 men aged forty through fifty-nine over a twenty-five-year period. After only five years investigators had already found evidence for an association between saturated animal fats and serum cholesterol, and between serum cholesterol and the incidence of CHD. Since this initial data implicating animal fat, there have been many corroborative studies pointing to as much as a 60 percent higher frequency of CHD in individuals whose diets are highest in saturated fats compared to people at the lowest end. However, the basis for this theory—that elevated blood cholesterol is a *cause* of heart disease—has been widely contested. Despite the almost universal application of cholesterol-lowering therapies, numerous clinical trials fail to show that cholesterol-reducing dietary treatments or drugs improve outcome.

Toward a New Diet-Heart Theory

Scientific advances since these early studies have improved our knowledge of the various cholesterol components and precursors. There has also been a shift in what is believed to cause CHD. In time this will alter the medical assessment of risk and bring about the refining of dietary recommendations. But until clinicians are willing to consider a new diet-heart hypothesis, progress in preventing and treating CHD will remain impaired.

*In subjects fed a liquid diet containing 75 percent carbohydrate and 10 percent fat for 25 days, circulating palmitic acid increased, while linoleate triglyceride content decreased. Subjects in the same study who drank a calorically equal formula consisting of 40 percent fat and 45 percent carbohydrates showed a completely different fatty acid pattern, reflecting the composition of the diet. The researchers found the negative change in the blood triglyceride pattern on the low-fat, high-carbohydrate diet quite disconcerting.

The Oxidized-Fat Theory. The events that initiate CHD are still unresolved, although there is a great deal of conjecture and theory. One plausible hypothesis that is gaining followers is that narrowing of the arteries (atherogenesis) begins as a response by vascular tissues to injury. Initially, fat-laden cells concentrate at the injury site, forming arterial plaque; later these cells are replaced with more rigid connective tissue. A heart attack or unstable angina may be the result of this plaque becoming destabilized and rupturing.

The precise role of cholesterol in this process is uncertain. Cholesterol particles attached to low-density lipoprotein (LDL) and very-low-density lipoprotein (VLDL) are connected with higher risk of coronary disease. A substantial body of evidence suggests that some LDL particles become altered—for example, by oxidation—and this makes them particularly atherogenic. When the altered LDL particles are taken into arterial cells they cause them to become laden with cholesterol and lose flexibility. They remain in the arterial wall as the "foam cell" component of plaque that is responsible for forming the infamous fatty streaks that are characteristic of arteriosclerosis.

The presence of more cholesterol in the bloodstream increases the odds that LDL particles will become oxidized. But the implication of this theory is that cholesterol itself isn't the culprit: The oxidation damage to part of the cholesterol molecule is at fault. If this can be prevented, the course of the disease can be inhibited.

The way in which high-density lipoprotein (HDL) is deemed to be protective is related to the capacity of HDL to pick up cholesterol from the artery wall and convey it elsewhere. In addition to possibly removing the potentially damaging LDL, HDL particles might even prevent LDL oxidation from taking place.

Three saturated fats are judged the most likely promoters of CHD due to their role in raising serum cholesterol. They are lauric, myristic, and palmitic acids, found in the highest concentrations in animal fat (and thus meat, eggs, and dairy foods), cocoa butter, coconut, and palm oils. These fats stimulate the liver to produce VLDL and LDL and disable the body's system for clearing LDL cholesterol from the bloodstream. There are no known benefits from consuming these fats. Short-chain saturated fatty acids, as well as stearic acid (found in greatest concentrations in butter, lard, beef, pork, lamb, and cheese), don't seem to raise blood cholesterol. But as you will soon see, this doesn't give them a clean bill of (heart) health.

Polyunsaturated fatty acids (PUFAs) lower blood cholesterol levels. Unfortunately, the omega-6 PUFAs (most concentrated in corn, safflower, sunflower, and soybean oils) lower not only damaging LDL and VLDL, but also beneficial HDL. Consequently, the total cholesterol to HDL ratio isn't enhanced. This doesn't seem to be the case with omega-3 fatty acids. Research trials in which 50 grams (2/3 cup) of ground flaxseed were added to the daily diet of healthy females for four weeks brought about decreased total cholesterol and an improved HDL ratio. Since similar results were obtained using flaxseed oil, the effects were attributed to LNA, flaxseed's principal fatty acid.

An additional drawback to PUFAs in general is that they're easily oxidized. Therefore, care must be taken to prevent this. Handling foods containing PUFAs properly before they're eaten is the one line of defense against external oxidation. Moreover, providing the body with an ample supply of antioxidants is the best way to defend against internal oxidation (see Chapters 3 and 4).

Researchers frequently cite the low incidence of heart disease in Mediterranean countries, despite relatively high fat intakes. They attribute this to the cardioprotective effects of oleic acid, the monounsaturated fat that is dominant in olive oil. The effect of oleic acid on cholesterol is at the least neutral; there is some evidence that it might even raise the preferred HDL cholesterol and lower the undesirable LDLs when used to replace saturated fatty acids. Compared to oils high in PUFAs—such as soybean, corn, safflower, and sunflower—olive oil, with its high oleic content, doesn't depress HDL cholesterol. But this may be a unique characteristic of olive oil, since canola oil, which is also high in oleic acid, has a depressive effect on HDLs similar to more highly polyunsaturated oils.

Some of the differences between test results comparing diets rich in monounsaturated fatty acids may be due to plant sterols and other miscellaneous constituents. Plant sterols (sometimes called phytosterols) are structurally similar to cholesterol, but differ slightly in their construction. Some of these plant sterols have been reported to compete with cholesterol for absorption. Sitosterol, for example, has been identified as a cholesterol-lowering compound that may be preferable to drug therapy. (Other principal sterols in edible fats and oils include campesterol and stigmasterol.) Consequently, despite comparable fatty acid distribution, it may make a difference whether the source is olive oil, canola oil, specially bred high-oleic varieties of sunflower and safflower oils, avocados, or almonds. All of these foods, however, are advantageous to some degree.

If oxidized LDL is indeed a major culprit in CHD (and a growing body of data suggests it is), another factor in favor of eating monounsaturates is that, unlike polyunsaturated fatty acids, they're resistant to oxidation. The specific fatty acids found in blood triglycerides and fat-containing tissues reflect dietary intake. Thus, the fat you eat can enhance or inhibit LDL susceptibility to oxidation. In fact, LDL particles that are high in oleic acid can slow progression of atherosclerosis not only by their own resistance to oxidation, but also by using up fewer antioxidants, leaving them free to protect more reactive LDL particles.

This issue of fat oxidation is extremely important on another level as well. If the oxidized-fat theory is valid, then consuming fats that are already oxidized or ones that are highly susceptible to oxidation can promote CHD. The more fragmented (processed) a food is, the more susceptible it is to oxidation. For example, spray-dried powdered eggs that have been measured for oxidized particles show high quantities compared to fresh eggs. Ground meat and poultry are more prone to oxidation than whole cuts. Improperly fried foods and poorly stored solid fats and oils are other potential avenues for consuming preoxidized fats.

Individualistic Lipoproteins. It has been theorized that the size of LDL particles may be key. That is, large particles, which are rapidly absorbed by the liver and degraded, show no atherogenic potential; small VLDLs and other lipid remnants aren't used as efficiently; they are likely to be converted to LDLs and remain for a longer time in the bloodstream.

Because lipoproteins aren't all alike, controlling HDL, LDL, and VLDL lipoproteins isn't as straightforward or as productive as the simplistic advice to "reduce total fat and saturated fat" makes it seem. There are many different lipoprotein particles and these undergo multiple enzyme-triggered reactions and interactions within the body. Differences not only in size, explained above, but also in composition make them more or less atherogenic. For example, the lipoprotein known as apo B that is incorporated into VLDL and goes on to become the main component of LDL is the fraction most likely to induce atherogenesis. Omega-3 fatty acids depress VLDL by reducing the rate of apo B synthesis.

Troublesome Triglycerides. The relationship between circulating fatty acids (triglycerides) and CHD is even more ambiguous than the cholesterol-heart relationship. The frequent inverse association between triglycerides and HDL points to a connection. A number of studies suggest that in addition to fasting levels of triglycerides, triglyceride levels that rise above normal after eating and remain in the blood following a fatty meal are predictive factors of CHD. Both omega-3 and omega-6 fatty acids appear to facilitate triglyceride clearance following consumption of fatty meals.

Sticky Blood. When it comes to dietary intervention, blood cholesterol and triglycerides have received most of the attention. However, there is another determinant with at least equal weight that can be manipulated by diet. It is the stickiness of blood platelets, or what is technically called aggregation. Sticky platelets are more apt to clump together and block arterial blood flow, precipitating a stroke or heart attack.

Dietary fats have a notable influence on blood platelet aggregation and there is also data connecting high triglyceride levels with increased measurements of several blood-coagulating factors. Unlike other dietary changes that can take years before results are apparent, in this realm even short-term measures are instrumental. Saturated fatty acids (including stearic acid, which was exonerated as a cholesterol-raising fat) increase platelet stickiness. Conversely, polyunsaturated fatty acids—and to a greater degree the omega-3s—improve blood viscosity and inhibit production of platelet-aggregating prostaglandins, reducing the likelihood of clumping.

Other Heart-Fat Considerations. In addition to helping to keep blood platelets from clumping and decreasing total cholesterol without suppressing HDLs, omega-3 fatty acids decrease vasoconstriction. This ability to counter nerve-stimulated constriction of blood vessels suggests another way in which these fatty acids might reduce heart attacks.

As a result of increased public promotion, consumption of polyunsaturated fatty acids in the United States has risen to about 7 percent of calories. This is an amount conspicuously higher than in either the recent or distant past. (In the 1930s polyunsaturated fat accounted for only 4 percent of daily calorie intake.) As noted later in other sections on fats and health, the long-term effect of this increase may have some unwelcome consequences.

Trans fatty acids have also been implicated in heart disease. In his presentation at the First International Conference on Fats and Oil Consumption in Health and Disease, Dr. Walter Willet, Harvard Medical School researcher and chairman of the department of nutrition at Harvard School of Public Health, stated that when the effects of trans fatty acids on HDL and LDL are correlated with CHD risk, "it can be conservatively estimated that approximately 30,000 deaths per year in the U.S. are attributable to trans fatty acids from partially hydrogenated vegetable oil." In addition to findings that they raise total cholesterol and depress HDL, trans fatty acids elevate concentrations of a compound called lipoprotein(a) or LP(a), which increases blood clotting. Elevated levels of LP(a) are associated with heart attacks and angina in both men and women.

Looking Beyond Fat. A new direction in the diet-heart theory is the possible protection afforded by antioxidant vitamins, minerals, and other plant constituents, including phytosterols and tocotrienols. This connection receives more of our attention in Chapter 3. We want to repeat here that phytosterols and tocotrienols are amply supplied by many of the healthy fat foods, especially nuts, seeds, soybeans, and avocados, as well as wheat germ.

Another interesting hypothesis in the diet-heart drama is the helpful role played by the amino acid arginine. A factor in the blood called endothelium-derived relaxing factor (EDRF) has been identified as a powerful vasodilator (it relaxes blood arteries), as well as an inhibitor of blood platelet aggregation. EDRF is actually nitric oxide. People with CHD, as well as people with high cholesterol levels, have reduced concentrations of EDRF in their arteries. Arginine is a precursor of nitric oxide. It is easily obtained by eating sunflower and pumpkin seeds, sesame tahini, walnuts, almonds, butternuts, Brazil nuts, pine nuts, and pistachios. Nuts and seeds are also high in magnesium, a mineral that has cardio-protective activity during acute heart attacks.

Diet-Heart Summary

When you factor in all this research, the standard recommendation to limit saturated fat intake to less than 10 percent of calories in order to lower cholesterol is only relevant regarding certain saturated fatty acids. However, it's probably good advice nonetheless due to the negative impact of saturated fats in general on platelet aggregation.

Replacing saturated fats with up to 10 percent calories from polyunsaturated fatty acids could have a palliative effect. However, if the balance between omega-6 and omega-3 fatty acids isn't taken into account, the outcome in terms of CHD may be only slightly better; moreover, as you will see in later sections, ignoring this ratio could seriously damage other health outcomes.

Instructions to dramatically reduce total fat intake seem overly severe, unless obesity is a contributing factor. Since there's no indication that monounsaturated fats worsen CHD (or other disease processes), fats high in monounsaturated oleic acid could provide an excellent way to offset the shift away from animal fats.

Fat and the Immune System

The body manufactures a variety of substances in order to fight infection and deactivate the toxins we are exposed to during the course of everyday life. Polyunsaturated fatty acids play a major role in both enhancing and suppressing this activity.

Linoleic acid (which must come from the diet) and arachidonic acid (which can come from food or be made in the body from linoleic acid) are integral to immune system function. When diets are deficient in linoleic acid (LA), the body can't manufacture the antigen interleukin-1, which activates infection-fighting T cells and B cells. As a result, immune response is compromised. But equally important, chronic overproduction of PG_2 prostaglandins formed from LA and arachidonic acid (AA) depresses the immune system as well. Furthermore, high concentrations of PG_2 promote tumor growth. As a result, diets that favor foods containing AA (found in animal fat) or LA (which is particularly prominent in safflower, sunflower, and corn oils) can be immunosuppressive.

What this means is that while modest amounts of (omega-6) LA are required for the immune system to operate, overstimulation due to immoderate ingestion of foods rich in this fatty acid can overwhelm the body's ability to fight invaders. This is a matter of concern for people who are trying to heed dietary advice that encourages a shift in fat away from animal sources.

One way the negative impact of these fatty acids can be offset is to increase intake of the competing polyunsaturated fatty acids that make up the omega-3 series. Once again, the predominant fatty acids in this group are alpha linolenic acid (LNA), eicosapentaenoic acid (EPA), and docosahexaenoic acid (DHA). In numerous experiments, diets high in omega-3 fats decrease AA levels and encourage production of antigens essential for the host defense system. Such diets could significantly improve inflammatory and immune diseases. Another thing that is clear from the research is that we need to consume omega-3 fatty acids on a regular basis, not just once in a while.

Fat and Cancer

Much research has been done to seek out a link between cancer and fat consumption. Although most guidelines for reducing cancer risk recommend lowering dietary fats, the evidence for this is inconsistent. The challenge is to discover whether total fat intake or just certain kinds of fat are culpable, which cells are at risk, and at what stage of cell growth this is really consequential. The answers to these questions are elusive, but as the body of research grows, more valuable information becomes available.

While evidence points to a strong association between fats and certain cancers, much of it is based on epidemiological studies in which dietary patterns are matched against medical incidents. These studies are complicated by multidietary and lifestyle factors; often certain foods appear to be causal or protective, but this doesn't necessarily define the role of any specific nutrient. Nonetheless, studies have displayed links between fat intake and cancers of the stomach, pancreas, colon, respiratory tract, prostate, breast, ovaries, and endometrium. Moreover, both saturated fats and polyunsaturated fats are implicated.

Until quite recently, no attempt was made in most cancer studies to differentiate between the various categories of polyunsaturated fatty acids. It's now recognized, however, that individual fatty acids have quite different effects. We spoke of eicosanoids extensively in the section How the Body Uses Fats. Tumor cells stimulate production of large amounts of the eicosanoids known as PG_2. PG_2 inhibits production of antigens that are necessary for cell differentiation, and this may be a clue to how tumors grow and spread. Another indication that PG_2 is somehow involved in cancer promotion is its ability to induce high levels of calcium in the bloodstream, a state often associated with lung, breast, pancreatic, and kidney cancers. In all these conditions natural killer cells and infection-fighting T cells are inhibited by this uncontrolled release of PG_2. Increased amounts of PG_2 have been associated with aggressive growth of both basal and squamous cell skin carcinomas as well.

Eicosanoids also control production of cytokines, regulatory compounds produced by cells of the immune system that influence the progression of many diseases. Two of these cytokines, interleukin (IL)-1 and tumor necrosis factor, decrease appetite and contribute to anorexia and cachexia, a type of wasting away seen in cancer patients.

Omega-6 fatty acids are the raw materials used by the body to manufacture PG_2 eicosanoids, IL-1, and tumor necrosis factor. This probably accounts for the frequent connection between diets high in polyunsaturated fats and several types of cancer. This doesn't mean foods that furnish omega-6 fatty acids should be avoided. Instead, it reinforces the need for a complementary intake of foods rich in omega-3 fatty acids, as they inhibit PG_2, IL-1, and tumor necrosis factor, and encourage synthesis of the countervailing prostaglandins PG_1 and PG_3.

Where animal fat is concerned, the real culprit remains unclear. In some studies of colon and prostate cancers the connection appears to be strongest with red meat in particular. Moreover, certain fats that are highest in dairy foods may be protective (see A Positive Role for Animal Fats? on page 334).

Monounsaturated fatty acids such as oleic acid don't appear to have any cancerous aftermath.

Prostate Cancer

The most comprehensive study of diet in relation to prostate cancer—the Health Professionals Follow-up Study of more than 51,000 U.S. men aged forty to seventy-five—has provided interesting (and puzzling) data. While red meat consumption was implicated, it hasn't been determined whether fat, the cooking process, or some other component in meat is the causative agent.

Contrary to many other cancer studies, the researchers here found a positive link between LNA and advanced prostate cancer. This was quite perplexing since most of the LNA in the subjects' diets came from vegetable oil, yet only animal fat appeared to be related to risk. The researchers concluded that there is some interactive factor pertaining to LNA that is present in animal sources (which are simultaneously high in saturated fatty acids and low in LA), but absent in oil (which is low in saturated fatty acids and high in LA and/or monounsaturated fatty acids). Oxidation byproducts of the LNA formed during the cooking of meat, for example, may be the carcinogenic culprits. Or, the connection may be to some other causative factor associated with LNA in meat but not LNA itself.

Although low-fat diets appear to inhibit growth of prostate cancer cells, scientists at Memorial Sloan-Kettering Cancer Control Center in New York admit they don't know what forms of fat might be responsible for tumor promotion. This discovery will prove important, since in other studies of prostate cancer inhibitors, the cancer-fighting component in tomatoes (lycopene) apparently wasn't well absorbed unless the tomatoes were cooked with some oil.

One interpretation of how fat contributes to prostate cancer is in relation to the effect of diet on male hormone metabolism. Studies assessing men's blood levels and urinary secretion of male hormones (testosterone) and female hormones (estrogen) show notable changes when dietary fat is manipulated. That is, men consuming diets high in overall fat with a greater emphasis on saturated fat (and simultaneously low in fiber) exhibit markers indicative of greater production of various forms of testosterone compared to low-fat (and high-fiber) diets. There is also a trend toward reduced production of estrogens; however, this is less consistent. The implication of these fluctuating hormone levels is uncertain, but since a number of studies show that testosterone excites prostate cancer cells while estrogen suppresses them, dietary fat and fiber may play a role in altering hormone-related enzyme activity in target cells in a manner that influences prostate cancer risk.

Breast Cancer

Regarding breast cancer, research results have been contradictory. There is a strong association with animal fat consumption in studies of populations, but in case-controlled studies they're only weakly linked, if at all. Many researchers in the United States believe fat intake is implicated in breast cancer; however, in other countries the majority of researchers do not. This lack of clarity is caused by the complexity of the cancer process. In 1990, after conducting a combined analysis of twelve studies of diet and breast cancer, an international team of researchers concluded that if all postmenopausal women in the United States were to limit saturated fat intake to 9 percent of total calories, the current rate of breast cancer in this population would be reduced by 10 percent. Antithetically, a 1996 review of seven studies from four countries found no evidence of an association between breast cancer and total dietary fat or any single category of fat. Based on these findings the reviewers stated that lowering fat in midlife is unlikely to have any notable effect on breast cancer incidence.

The aforementioned studies didn't rule out the possibility that controlling fat intake during childhood or adolescence might be of value. In fact, several studies suggest that dietary intervention possibly decreases breast cancer risk if undertaken early in life, but not once women reach the high-risk postmenopausal stage.

Other breast cancer surveys suggest that olive oil consumption correlates to a significantly reduced breast cancer risk, especially among postmenopausal women. Furthermore, at least five case-controlled studies implicate margarine (which is high in trans fatty acids) with an elevated risk for this disease. What hasn't been addressed in these human studies is whether individual fatty acids or their relative proportions could play a part.

Animal studies provide some direction, but whether the results are species-specific or applicable to humans isn't yet known. What they do indicate is that the formation of tumor-enhancing prostaglandins in breast cancer cells is essential for their growth, and that fats rich in LNA are able to prevent the progression of precancerous breast disease and help keep early, noninvasive breast cancer from becoming invasive. Researchers have shown that the cancer process can be interrupted by (1) reducing dietary intake of LA and (2) blocking the conversion of this omega-6 fatty acid by dietary supplementation with an omega-3 fatty acid. Once again, these studies illustrate how crucial the balance between (omega-6) LA and (omega-3) LNA is.

When breast cancer investigations are assessed from a different perspective, potential explanations sometimes appear. For example, when high-fat diets are consumed in the absence of carcinogens, tumors don't materialize. But in a cancer-promoting environment, fat seems to play a contributing role, suggesting it isn't a direct cause—or initiator—but a promoter.

Another notable piece of the puzzle illuminated by animal research is that the influence of fat is greater when coupled with a diet containing an excess of calories, leading to high body weight. Insulin, a known tumor-promoter, could be a key factor in this scenario.

Fat and Inflammatory Ailments

Hormonelike substances called prostaglandins are a subcategory of the eicosanoids. Excessive synthesis of PG_2 prostaglandins increases inflammation and may be a contributing factor in many perplexing conditions, including fibromyalgia, polymyalgia, arthritis, multiple sclerosis, lupus, ulcerative colitis or Crohn's disease, chronic fatigue, asthma, and psoriasis, among others. For example, studies clearly show an inhibition of T suppressor cells, permitting continued production of substances involved in rheumatoid diseases, and higher measures of PG_2 in the fluids of rheumatoid joints.

As explained above, the omega-6 polyunsaturated fatty acids, including LA and AA, are the precursors of PG_2, while the omega-3 fatty acids suppress PG_2

production. Research trials using flaxseed oil to treat rheumatoid arthritis reveal increased LNA and EPA in participants' white blood cells and a simultaneous decline in the production of proteins associated with this disease. When mice with induced lupus were treated experimentally with diets supplemented with ground flaxseed, they lived longer than control animals. Symptoms of patients suffering from inflammatory bowel disease and psoriasis have improved with omega-3 intervention. In fact, human studies consistently demonstrate a decrease in proinflammatory compounds when omega-3 fatty acids are increased.

It is important to emphasize that no nutrient stands alone in defending against illness. Overconsumption of LNA at the expense of LA can depress crucial T cell production, as well as some of the body's other important defense systems. It can also interfere with normal platelet aggregation, resulting in cerebral hemorrhage. Interestingly, all of these problems are more likely to occur when omega-3 enrichment comes from fish and supplements of fish oil, as opposed to plant sources.

Fat and Diabetes

Type II, non-insulin-dependent diabetes has been described as a disease that results from the interaction between nature and nurture. A genetic predisposition is essential, but the condition only flourishes in environments where rich food is plentiful.

The ideal composition of diets for diabetics is controversial. The need to restrict saturated fat intake is widely accepted. However, many diabetes researchers contend that monounsaturated oleic acid deserves a more prominent position in the diet of diabetics, rather than the low-fat, high-carbohydrate model that has received support in recent years. The virtues of low-fat, high-carbohydrate regimens are that they are filling without providing lots of calories, and with proper

335

Mentor

selection, as explained in Chapter 1, carbohydrate-rich foods can flatten blood glucose peaks following meals. Nonetheless, compared with diets high in monounsaturated fats, high-carbohydrate diets have the undesirable traits of prolonging periods of elevated plasma insulin and increasing plasma triglycerides.

Experimental diets using avocados, olive oil, and canola oil have showed improved blood sugar control without negative impact on coronary risk factors. Based on this success, it is presumed that specially bred high-oleic safflower and sunflower oils, as well as nuts and seeds that are rich in monounsaturates such as almonds, cashews, hazelnuts, peanuts, pistachios, pecans, and sesame and pumpkin seeds (see Foods and Their Fatty Acids, on page 314), can be safely included in diabetic diets, as long as caloric needs aren't exceeded.

There is also evidence for a protective role for omega-6 and omega-3 polyunsaturated fatty acids in modest, properly balanced amounts. As noted earlier, polyunsaturated fats improve cell membrane fluidity, making insulin receptor sites potentially more responsive. When insulin resistance is the underlying cause of hyperglycemia and hyperinsulinemia, the enhanced glucose uptake conferred by these fatty acids can improve these states.

Fat and Osteoporosis

Osteoporosis is a disease characterized by low bone mass, leading to bone fragility, resulting in fractures. Osteoporotic fractures can occur anywhere, but mainly affect the spine, leading to loss of height and chronic back pain, the wrist, and most clinically serious, the proximal femur (hip).

Osteoporosis affects more than 20 million people in the United States, and although more common in women, it isn't exclusively a female problem. It accounts for an annual toll of about 250,000 hip fractures and 1.5 million fractures in total.

There are two basic causes of low bone mass: insufficient bone matter deposited in the skeleton during the growth period, or loss later on in life at an excessive rate. The ultimate production of bone mass that can be achieved is largely under genetic control, but the capacity to reach genetic potential depends on outside factors. Because bone contains large amounts of calcium, calcium intake can increase bone mineral density throughout childhood. Individuals who have less than average bone mass when they become young adults may be at increased risk of osteoporosis in the future.

Rather than being a stable tissue, bone undergoes constant rebuilding (technically referred to as remodeling) throughout life. During this process there is continuous loss and replacement of many bone constituents (called turnover). Factors that provoke turnover at a particular site aren't clear, but a complete remodeling cycle takes at least five to six months.

Disruption of remodeling at any point leads to bone mass loss. For example, a decrease in sex hormones, especially estrogen, accelerates bone turnover, which is why postmenopausal women and older people in general are more susceptible.

But other intermediaries seem equally interactive, including the fat-induced eicosanoids that release PG_2, interleukins, and tumor necrosis factor. These three substances are potent stimulators of bone resorption, which leaves empty cavities in the skeletal mass. After menopause, production of interleukins in women increases, probably as a result of diminished steroid hormones. Defending against bone resorption—in other words slowing down the remodeling process—is an effective preventative step.

Treatment of both men and women with omega-3 supplements results in decreased production of PG_2, interleukins, and tumor necrosis factor. This implies a role for foods that can improve the LA:LNA ratio, including flaxseeds, hemp oil, canola oil, walnuts, wheat germ, and soy products.

Fat and Behavior

Epidemiological studies in various countries and in the United States hint at a connection between increased rates of depression and decreased omega-3 consumption. Researchers feel this is consistent with the frequency of depression in people who suffer from coronary artery disease, another ailment associated with insufficient omega-3 relative to other fatty acids. Other links with omega-3 deficiency are reflected in depressive symptoms in alcoholism, multiple sclerosis, chronic fatigue, and the like, as well as postpartum depression.

The nutritional connection is the body's use of omega-3 fats in conjunction with niacin and other B vitamins to form the PG_3 prostaglandins that regulate brain and neurological circuits throughout the body. In an evaluation of the role of dietary fats in cognitive function, a study of elderly Dutch men found a correlation between high intakes of linoleic (omega-6) fatty acids and cognitive impairment and decline. Conversely, omega-3 fatty acids appeared to preserve mental function in this population.

NIKKI'S DIALOGUE BOX

"If asked to give dietary advice to a parent whose child has been diagnosed with ADHD I would suggest the following regarding fat:

"Incorporate more nuts, seeds, soy foods, and wheat germ into the diet.

"Use olive or canola oils (and mayonnaise, salad dressing, and other foods made with these oils) rather than such oils as corn, safflower, or sunflower.

"Add a few tablespoons of ground flaxseeds or a tablespoon of flaxseed oil to the daily diet. Ground flaxseeds can be mixed into cereals, spreads, sprinkled on vegetables, incorporated into pancakes and baked goods; flaxseed oil can be used in salad dressings, spreads, or as a seasoning for vegetables, pasta, and grains (see 'In Nikki's Kitchen').

"Avoid foods that are high in fat and lack other essential nutrients—in other words, many contrived snack foods, sweets, processed meats, and the like."

The relationship between fatty acids and attention-deficit hyperactivity disorder (ADHD) is under investigation. ADHD is the term used to describe children who are inattentive, impulsive, and hyperactive. The cause is unknown and believed to be multifactorial. Several studies of children diagnosed with ADHD show an association with certain patterns of fatty acids that show up in blood analysis. Moreover, when their diets were compared with those of control subjects, intake of calories, protein, carbohydrate, vitamins, and minerals were all similar. What was different was fat consumption: ADHD children generally ate more overall fat and had a higher ratio of omega-6 to omega-3 fats.

Other Fat-Related Ailments

Age-related macular degeneration is a condition that affects the macula of the eye—the most sensitive part of the retina—and alters the visual field. There is no effective treatment for this disease, which is the leading cause of legal blindness in the United States. There is evidence that protection against macular degeneration is afforded by diets high in certain fruits and vegetables (see Chapter 4). Increased incidence of macular degeneration is also associated with diets high in saturated fats. Proposed mechanisms of causation are: (1) narrowing of the arteries, provoked by dietary saturated fats, reduces blood flow to the retina, or (2) a high saturated-fat intake causes lipids to collect in the retina and impede the supply of nutrients.

A large intake of polyunsaturated omega-6 fat is reported to increase gallstone formation. Remember, too, without adequate protection from antioxidants, cellular membranes rich in polyunsaturated fatty acids are subject to increased oxidation damage. This not only raises the risk of heart disease and certain cancers, but also stroke, emphysema, and cataracts.

Other Nutritional Factors Related to Fats

Cholesterol

Cholesterol is a fatlike substance manufactured by the body and also found in food in conjunction with fats. It occurs only in foods of animal origin. There is wide variation in the way people respond to dietary cholesterol. This is due partly to genetics and partly to factors such as exercise, body weight, age, menopausal status in women, overall health, and a host of dietary influences. Despite what many people believe, for the majority of us dietary intake of cholesterol has only a small effect on total blood cholesterol levels, and even less effect on the proportion of various lipoproteins (HDL, LDL, VLDL).

When cholesterol is consumed, a certain amount is absorbed directly by the intestines. Depending on other dietary factors (including the amount of fiber and resistant starch, as explained in Chapter 1), some of this cholesterol is excreted in the stool. In most individuals, the liver maintains proper balance by turning down cholesterol production in response to ingested cholesterol or converting some of it into bile acids.

Unlike cholesterol-raising saturated fats, which are implicated in a number of disease states, cholesterol isn't suspected of causing any other disorder. Although some health practitioners still advise people to limit intake of cholesterol, all agree that the danger of dietary cholesterol is far outweighed by the problems created by eating saturated fats.

Vitamin E

Vitamin E is an essential vitamin that is soluble in fat. Actually, there are eight naturally occurring compounds that have been identified in vitamin E. These have been divided into two groups: tocopherols and tocotrienols.

It has generally been thought that only one form of vitamin E, alpha-tocopherol, plays an active part in human nutrition. New data refute this and suggest a role for the other compounds within this family. Noted cancer researcher Bruce Ames and his colleagues have tested the activity of gamma-tocopherol and found it to be more protective against certain mutagenic compounds than alpha-tocopherol. They believe it may play a role in fighting cancer, heart disease, and other degenerative diseases. Of particular note is their thesis that the two forms of tocopherol may complement each other and the presence of both may be required for optimal benefit. Special mention is made of the contribution of nuts and seeds, as well as endorsement of the ratio of tocopherols found in food. In fact, the researchers state that alpha-tocopherol alone (as common in many vitamin supplements) may have the unfavorable effect of displacing gamma-tocopherol in blood and other tissues.

Vitamin E is essential for neurological function and maintaining the integrity of red blood cells. It's involved in immune performance, cardiovascular health, and cancer prevention. Despite a universal recommended daily intake of 8 to 10 mg of alpha-tocopherol for women and men, respectively, actual need is in direct proportion to the amount of polyunsaturated fatty acids in the diet. Analysis of data from the 1987–1988 National Health and Nutrition Examination Survey (NHANES) indicates a lower than desirable ratio of vitamin E to polyunsaturated fat in 23 percent of men and 15 percent of women.

Certain fatty foods are major suppliers of vitamin E, including nuts, seeds, olives, soybeans, avocados, and the oils extracted from these foods, as well as whole grains and wheat germ. Sunflower seeds are uncommonly high in alpha-tocopherol, and filberts furnish substantial amounts as well. Other tocopherols are amply supplied by Brazil nuts, peanuts, pecans, sesame seeds, and walnuts. There are still only preliminary measurements of tocopherols and tocotrienols within foods; therefore, other foods may prove significant in the future. In any event, animal products are poor sources.

Understandably, diets low in fat from plant sources are apt to be deficient in vitamin E. Where monounsaturated fatty acids predominate there is likely to be a good balance of intake to need. If polyunsaturated fats are emphasized, vitamin E requirements go up. When nuts and seeds are a part of the diet, adequate consumption of vitamin E can be accomplished; but if refined oils are the primary source of polyunsaturates, other vitamin E–rich foods (or supplements) should be added to the diet.

Vitamin K

Vitamin K is required for blood to clot and for activation of at least three proteins involved in bone formation. Vitamin K is also a cofactor in the synthesis of proteins found in blood, liver, kidney, lung, skin, spleen, placenta, reproductive organs, and vascular tissue, although the functions of most of these proteins have yet to be determined.

In order for vitamin K to be absorbed, fat must be provided at the same time. The data currently available on the vitamin K content of foods indicate that the richest sources are dark leafy green vegetables, followed by soybean, canola, and olive oils. Lesser amounts are found in almonds, pistachio nuts, walnuts, sunflower seeds, sesame seeds, safflower seeds, and their oils. Corn and peanut oils contain very little vitamin K and animal foods are poor sources.

Vitamin K remains stable during processing, but is rapidly destroyed by both daylight and fluorescent light. Accordingly, oils should be stored in nontransparent packaging to protect their natural vitamin K content.

Plant Sterols

Minor components in oils called sterols and terpenes presumably contribute to the capacity of some oils to reduce oxidative damage to the body, a factor involved in most degenerative diseases. In research done on both olive and sesame oils, some of their antioxidant capacity is attributed to these constituents. Plant sterols (phytosterols) have also been viewed as potential blocking agents to cholesterol absorption. As phytosterols become more widely recognized, we will undoubtedly learn more about their role in health protection.

The highest levels of phytosterols are found in rice bran oil, sesame seed oil, wheat germ oil, and corn oil. Refining reduces the phytosterol content of these oils by one- to two-thirds, but even then they're richer than most other oils. While all oils make some contribution, refining dramatically reduces phytosterol content and hydrogenation lowers it an additional 20 to 40 percent.

Other excellent food sources include wheat germ, sesame seeds, and sunflower seeds, with lesser but still significant contributions from other seeds and nuts, as well as soybeans and avocados.

Fat Substitutes

In 1990, to help Americans reduce dietary fat, Healthy People 2000, a government-sponsored project, called upon food manufacturers to double the availability of lower-fat food products by the year 2000. To meet the challenge, more than a thousand new lower-fat and fat-free products have been introduced annually since 1990.

A number of potential fat substitutes have been formulated in the United States, but the product that has been most widely embraced by food manufacturers is Olestra, an artificial fat conceived by Procter & Gamble. The allure of Olestra, formulated from sugars and vegetable oil, is that it passes through the body without being digested or absorbed. As a result, it doesn't add any fat or calories. The potential uses are vast: Olestra can be formulated for baked and fried foods, dairy products, cooking oils, margarine, spreads, and shortening.

Unfortunately, Olestra brings with it a new set of problems. Not only could it conceivably displace fats that might have health benefits, researchers say it binds and flushes away some key nutrients. Even the manufacturer agrees that fat-soluble vitamins A, D, E, and K are at risk. The fake fat can also sweep out numerous other health-enhancing food elements, such as the carotenoids found in many fruits and vegetables (see Chapter 4). While companies that use Olestra have made some attempt to fortify foods with supplemental vitamins, whether the body will be able to assimilate these added nutrients hasn't been established. Moreover, it's virtually impossible to add back the multitude of elements that are vulnerable, even if they were all known—in itself an impossible task.

By the manufacturer's own admission, consuming the equivalent of 15 to 20 Olestra-containing potato chips a day reduces blood concentration of various carotenoids in the range of about 60 percent. Using data generated by Procter & Gamble, Harvard School of Public Health epidemiologist Meir Stampfer has made some rather grim estimates of the potential impact of eating just three small Olestra-containing snacks with a meal over the course of a week. (In other words, a 1-ounce bag of potato chips with lunch or dinner three days out of the week.) According to Stampfer, on a yearly basis, the projected loss of carotenoids could mean:

- 390 to 800 additional cases of blindness due to macular degeneration in the United States every year (and 1,950 to 4,000 cases of partial visual deficit)
- 2,400 to 9,800 added cases of prostate cancer, leading to 1,500 more deaths
- 32,000 subsequent coronary-related deaths
- 1,500 to 7,500 cases of lung cancer, most of them fatal

Although Stampfer admits that these projections are speculative, in developing these figures he made a point of using conservative outcomes, not extreme-case scenarios.

Even if the fear of its health impact is exaggerated, Olestra can cause a range of gastrointestinal problems, including nausea, abdominal cramping, and diarrhea.

A panel of renowned scientists and health professionals who participated in the Olestra Project, sponsored by the Harvard School of Public Health, overwhelmingly agreed that questions regarding Olestra's potential to do harm far surpass any foreseeable health benefits. Nevertheless, the issue won't end regardless of whether or not the FDA permits Olestra to remain in the food supply and approves its use in more product formulations (and in all likelihood it will); nor does it depend on the public's ultimate decision to accept or reject Olestra on their own. "Fear of fat" will continue to lead to more and similarly problematic fat substitutes until we acknowledge the health benefits and risks of various fats. Once diets are constructed from whole, naturally occurring foods, the quest for fat substitutes will vanish.

The final irony in all this for those who believe fat substitutes will provide the sensory effect of fat without the calories is that the body isn't so easily deceived. Numerous studies demonstrate that when fat is restricted people make up for it instinctively by increasing calories from other sources—usually carbohydrates. This occurs even when the illusion of fat is present.

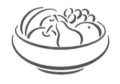

CHAPTER 3

Preventing System Breakdowns

A multitude of vitamins, minerals, amino acids, and diverse components found *within* foods are needed for the body to run effectively. Without them the body's entire metabolic system and line of defense would falter. The responsibilities of these nutrient helpers cannot be fulfilled with supplements, no matter how well chosen.

One of the principal jobs of the nutrient helpers is in the production of enzymes. Enzymes are the catalysts for all chemical reactions in the cell, thereby allowing life to continue. They participate in the transformation of food into energy, the building and rebuilding of tissues and cells, the body's defense against oxygen-induced damage, and more. An individual cell may contain literally hundreds of different enzymes, each one very specific in regard to the substances it acts upon and the reactions it triggers. The ultimate fate of numerous compounds in the body depends on which enzymes exert their action upon them.

Enzymes consist of two parts: a protein portion and a cofactor. The protein portion is supplied directly by dietary amino acids (from protein-providing foods) and indirectly by using these amino acids to build other needed proteins. While many amino acids can be synthesized within the body, certain ones must be obtained from outside sources. These are described as "essential amino acids." If the body runs short of any amino acid required to assemble a particular enzyme, production of that enzyme will cease and the specific function dependent on it will not proceed.

The cofactor portion of an enzyme is composed of particular minerals, a B-complex vitamin, or in some cases both of these nutrient helpers.

Nutrient helpers also serve as antioxidants. Body cells and tissues, along with various other internal constituents such as lipids and cholesterol, are susceptible to damage caused by contact with oxygen. Antioxidants shield vulnerable sites from oxidation. This protection is conferred by specialized enzymes, as well as certain vitamins, minerals, and plant chemicals that are found in food. Antioxidants work on many different fronts. Among other things, they can prevent damage to DNA, keep lipids from oxidizing, and inhibit malignant transformation of cells. They are associated with lower incidence of certain types of cancer and such degenerative conditions as coronary heart disease, macular degeneration, and cataracts.

Nutrient Helpers at Work

Glucose Metabolism Needs Nutrient Helpers

After carbohydrates are acted upon in the digestive system and pass into the bloodstream, the real work of transporting them into the cells and releasing their potential energy begins. The process starts with the hormone insulin, which was discussed in Chapter 1.

The mineral chromium is a crucial companion to insulin. It facilitates the binding of insulin to cell receptors, making the hormone more efficient. Chromium's presence in a substance known as glucose tolerance factor is presumably what enables it to normalize blood sugar that is either too high or too low.

When chromium is in short supply the body pumps out more insulin, which means inadequate chromium intake can provoke hyperinsulinemia. This ability to influence insulin levels also helps explain why, with sufficient chromium, levels of blood triglycerides, total cholesterol, and the preferred HDL cholesterol also improve.

Chromium is one of the most studied minerals. Although a 1995 study done at Dartmouth College using the supplement chromium picolinate caused quite a stir when hamster cells cultivated in a dish showed signs of genetic damage, there has never been an association between dietary chromium and any ill effects. Actually, people are more apt to have a deficiency of this nutrient, as it isn't widely available in the food supply and concentrated sugars stimulate urinary excretion. In fact, any situation that overstimulates insulin release puts a drain on chromium stores.

Zinc is another mineral involved in the synthesis, secretion, and utilization of insulin. In addition, it has a protective effect against damage to the beta-cells of the pancreas, where insulin is produced.

Several B vitamins play a part in glucose metabolism, primarily as structural components of enzymes involved in energy production. In this capacity, thiamin, pantothenic acid, biotin, and niacin are all required for the conversion of glucose into energy. Nicotinic acid (a form of niacin) is an ingredient, along with chromium, in glucose tolerance factor. This is only part of niacin's vital functions, for it participates in more than fifty unrelated biochemical reactions, including synthesis of fats and steroids, the metabolism of amino acids, and DNA repair.

Foods for Glucose Defense

In light of the above, people with high or low blood sugar or insulin levels should increase their intake of foods providing chromium. Because chromium isn't found in large amounts in any one food, and food analysis for this nutrient isn't adequately sensitive, it's important to eat a variety of potential contributors, which include whole grains, nuts, seeds, vegetables, and fruit.

People with blood sugar concerns, along with anyone looking to get the most energy out of what they eat, should also consume a variety of foods containing zinc and B vitamins. Some nutritional considerations concerning zinc are covered on page 359, along with specific providers. Eating a broad diet containing legumes, nuts, and whole grains is of special note to vegetarians, as zinc is found in association with protein foods and is most concentrated in red meat.

The B vitamins used to transform glucose into energy come from legumes, nuts, seeds, whole grains, egg yolks, avocado, mushrooms, and a few other vegetables (for details see page 357).

Fatty Acid Transformation Needs Nutrient Helpers

The fatty acids that circulate in the bloodstream are hooked together in a variety of configurations that determine how they act. In addition to performing specific functions, excess dietary fats may be converted to energy or stored as adipose tissue for future use.

Nicotinamide (a form of niacin) is an essential part of the coenzymes NAD and NADP, which are intermediaries in the release of energy from dietary and stored fats. These niacin-dependent coenzymes are also involved in the creation of long-chain fatty acids used in cell membranes, steroids and eicosanoids, and cholesterol regulation. (NAD and NADP are responsible for numerous reactions throughout the body and hundreds of enzymes require the niacin furnished by NAD and NADP.) The B vitamins biotin, thiamin, and pantothenic acid all play similar supporting roles.

The polyunsaturated fatty acids linoleic acid (LA) and alpha linolenic acid (LNA) are the precursors of the longer-chain fatty acids that the body synthesizes and uses to make the chemical messengers called eicosanoids (discussed in Chapter 2). Here, again, we encounter a number of middlemen along the way.

Magnesium, for example, plays a role in the production of PG_1, the prostaglandin that, among other things, influences fluid balance, regulates levels of circulating and tissue calcium, and participates in nerve impulses and muscle contractions. In this last capacity it is believed to impact significantly on heart disease and the symptoms associated with toxemia during pregnancy. A lack of magnesium has been suggested in premenstrual syndrome (PMS), where fluid retention, cramps, and food cravings are prevalent. (Magnesium's activities are quite extensive; it is used in more than three hundred different enzyme systems, where it joins in the body's handling of carbohydrates and proteins, among other applications.)

Zinc is another cofactor involved in the metabolism of fats and prostaglandin synthesis. In humans, there are distinct similarities between zinc deficiency and essential fatty acid deficiency symptoms. In experiments with rats, restricting zinc intake dramatically depresses prostaglandin production, especially in the cells of the digestive system where they play an important role in immune and inflammatory responses. Likewise, zinc-deprived rats exhibit impaired blood platelet coagulation. Evidence suggests that zinc is required for the transformation of linoleic acid to arachidonic acid, and ultimately the generation of PG_1 prostaglandins.

The desaturation of saturated fatty acids that is a normal part of fat metabolism is curtailed when copper is missing. Therefore, it isn't surprising to learn that copper deficiency results in elevated levels of serum triglycerides and cholesterol. In fact, a lack of copper appears to cause a rapid release of cholesterol from the liver into the bloodstream.

In Chapter 2, we noted that vitamin E requirement increases in proportion to polyunsaturated fat consumption. In this circumstance, vitamin E plays a helper role in prostaglandin production, enhancing the use of omega-3 fatty acids and thereby reducing levels of the prostaglandin PG_2, which is generated by competing omega-6 fatty acids. As a result, vitamin E assists in improving the body's inflammatory response and immune function.

Three sulfur-rich amino acids—methionine, cysteine, and cystine—modulate the conversion of arachidonic acid to eicosanoids. Thus, they too play a critical part in how fatty acids impact on immune function, cell division and multiplication, growth of normal and cancerous tissues, inflammatory response, the behavior of blood platelets, and more.

Foods That Get Fats to Do Their Job

Niacin, magnesium, zinc, copper, vitamin E, and the sulfur-containing amino acids methionine, cysteine, and cystine all have complementary roles to play in order for the fats you eat to fulfill their job. Foods in the legume family are particularly commendable, along with nuts, seeds, and certain vegetables, all enumerated in Dietary Sources of Nutrient Helpers, on page 356.

Liver Functions Need Nutrient Helpers

Substances that facilitate the handling of fat by the liver are called *lipotropic factors*. Lecithin was one of the earliest substances recognized to take part in this process. The active ingredient in lecithin—choline—is an indispensable dietary constituent, and one of its functions is to prevent lipids from accumulating in the liver. In order to be exported from the liver, triglycerides must be incorporated into very-low-density lipoprotein (VLDL). One of the essential components of VLDL is a compound that contains choline; if choline is unavailable, VLDL can't be manufactured and liver triglycerides build up, eventually resulting in liver dysfunction. Any condition that increases triglyceride synthesis by the liver, such as a high-carbohydrate diet, increases the need for choline.

In addition to its protective role in the liver, choline is used to make certain phospholipids that are essential components of all cell membranes. It is also critical to the production of neurotransmitters and other messenger molecules responsible for sending messages to the brain and central nervous system. In this capacity it affects mood, movement, cognition, and behavior. As we age, uptake of choline into the brain is curtailed, perhaps indicating an increased dietary need to offset this diminished capacity.

Another lipotropic factor that prevents infiltration of fat into the liver is the amino acid methionine. Methionine is an essential amino acid, meaning it must be supplied by food sources. A most important function of methionine is to provide a complex of molecules called methyl groups that the body needs to manufacture a variety of compounds, among them choline. The liver also uses methionine (along with the amino acid lysine) to create carnitine. Carnitine serves as a carrier for fatty acids into cells so they can be used to generate energy.

The body can use methionine to manufacture another amino acid, cysteine. Or cysteine can be consumed directly, thus sparing methionine for other functions. Cysteine improves the body's handling of fat by inhibiting production of fat by the liver, increasing fat breakdown and elimination by the intestinal tract, and mobilizing fats deposited in adipose tissues and facilitating their excretion. These activities help curb blood triglyceride and cholesterol levels.

Foods That Help the Liver Do Its Job

Choline and the amino acids methionine and cysteine (alternately referred to as the sulfur-containing amino acids) help control the flow of nutrients that interact with the liver—one of the most vital organs in the body. Egg yolks, soybeans, and a variety of nuts and seeds are among the most reliable sources (see pages 358 and 360 for more).

Countering Oxygen Damage

In the natural course of life, our bodies, like many other things, are continuously challenged by exposure to oxygen. Although they don't rust, cells and tissues, along with various other internal constituents such as lipids and cholesterol, are similarly vulnerable to damage initiated by contact with oxygen. To counter this, we have the capability to mount a defense that employs a variety of strategies. But if at any time the pro-oxidant forces outweigh the antioxidant shield, target sites can become victims of attack.

Oxidative damage may be a causative mechanism in the degenerative diseases of aging, including cataracts, brain dysfunction, heart disease, and the initiation and promotion of cancer. It is the high lipid content of immune cells that puts this entire combat system at risk.

The substances responsible for inciting trouble are known as free radicals. In stable molecules, electrons occur in pairs. If one of these partners is lost, the molecule becomes reactive. This new form is called a free radical. Free radicals try to become stable by stealing electrons from other stable molecules, and this launches a cascading process. Even though they're produced naturally by the body and are an essential part of the metabolic system, if the flow of free radicals isn't restrained it can alter metabolic activity and destroy healthy tissues. These effects can be felt in any area of the body.

Free radicals arise spontaneously within the body and are accelerated by various stressors, including air pollution, cigarette smoke, alcohol, high-fat diets, radiation, immoderate exposure to ultraviolet sunrays, toxic chemicals, illness, overexercise, and more. Living organisms have two principal means of protecting themselves from their harmful effects. One is via substances known as antioxidants. The other defense against free radicals is through enzymes. Each of these approaches is discussed below.

Direct Antioxidant Forces

Antioxidants act directly by stabilizing readily oxidizable substances, or indirectly by stimulating protective enzymes. There are many vitamins, minerals, phytochemicals, and other substances within food, such as fiber and resistant starch, that exhibit antioxidant activity. In addition, given sufficient amounts of precursor materials to work with, the body can manufacture some of its own antioxidants.

The behavior of antioxidants is intricate. Because oxidative reactions take place in a series of steps, antioxidants can intervene at several stages along the way. They can squelch reactions before they have a chance to begin, they can intercept their progress, or they can repair some of the damage after it occurs. Often they work more effectively in partnership than they do on their own, slowing down reactions sequentially; as one is used up another jumps in to take its place or revive it. This stepwise and interdependent entry of various elements to thwart oxidative damage supports the importance of a diverse diet, rather than focusing on single nutrients.

In addition to suppressing oxygen-induced reactions within the body, antioxidant compounds can inhibit toxic oxidation compounds from forming within foods during commercial manufacture or home preparation. Several oxidized products are mutagenic and carcinogenic in animal models, and oxidized fats have been mentioned in Chapter 2 as a potential factor in coronary heart disease. Repercussions in humans are virtually impossible to document. Nonetheless, limiting consumption of oxidized foods could be quite important, as once ingested, oxidized foods may react with other substances to affect fat and protein metabolism, the immune system, platelet activity, and more. In some foods, oxidation can be detected by their rancid taste; however, the condition isn't always sufficiently advanced to be noticed, and in many instances taste buds aren't keen enough to perceive oxidation changes.

Mounting a Defense. A number of vitamins function as antioxidants, most notably vitamins E, C, and beta-carotene. Their presence in foods protects the fatty components from oxygen damage. Similarly, their role within the body is to keep vulnerable tissues from being injured.

Vitamin E is soluble in fat and acts preferentially to inhibit free radicals in adipose tissue and the lipid-containing membranes of cells. It also safeguards plasma, red blood cells, and immune cells. Vitamin E's protective role in heart disease is widely acclaimed; vitamin E levels in the body compare so strongly with reduced deaths that many researchers consider them a better predictor than either cholesterol measures or blood pressure. The antioxidant activity of vitamin E in relation to cholesterol oxidation is discussed in Chapter 2. The results from a number of animal experiments and human epidemiological studies also suggest an anticancer role for vitamin E, and a tentative connection is proposed for protecting proteins in the lens of the eye against oxidation, thereby curbing cataract formation. Low vitamin E has also been linked to macular degeneration, a degenerative eye disease discussed in Chapter 2 in relation to diets high in saturated fat, and discussed in greater detail in Chapter 4, because of its strong inverse association with certain vegetables.

Vitamin C is the major water-soluble antioxidant. It's considered the most important antioxidant in extracellular fluids and has many antioxidant activities within cells as well. Among its roles, vitamin C protects against spontaneous DNA damage in human sperm. In this manner it could thwart genetic defects. Another environment where its antioxidant ability may be crucial is in the lens of the eye, serving to deter age-related cataracts. Numerous cancer investigations report significant protection by vitamin C. Among other things, it blocks the formation and action of N-nitrosamines, recognized cancer-causing agents formed from nitrates that occur in nature, including commonly eaten foods and beverages.

Vitamin C also safeguards cells by regenerating vitamin E and recycling it for continued radical-scavenging activity. Thus, an abundance of vitamin C in the diet can decrease the vitamin E requirement. This may somewhat account for the association of vitamin C with reduced heart disease in population studies where a direct mechanism hasn't been proved. (In a similar manner, vitamin E may be preferentially used in some oxidation reactions in order to conserve carotenoids, and vitamin C can be recharged by the protein glutathione, discussed in Protective Enzymes, on page 351.)

Note that despite widespread claims that vitamin C is harmless, supplemental megadoses of some vitamin C compounds can be detrimental. As you will read later in this chapter, excessive amounts of ascorbic acid, a form of vitamin C, can curtail the body's absorption of copper, a mineral of considerable value.

The term "phytochemicals" refers to a wide variety of substances produced by plants. Some of these compounds protect plants against insects or have other biological functions that may apply to humans, too. Some have antioxidant or hormonelike actions within plants that can be passed on to people who eat them. Of note here are the phytochemicals called carotenoids, which along with the related vitamin beta-carotene protect biological systems in an atypical way—by physically quenching singlet oxygen. Singlet oxygen, like free radicals, is a potentially damaging product generated by normal body activities. Carotenoids are the most efficient singlet oxygen suppressors, and therefore have a specialized function in the defense hierarchy.

Beta-carotene works in concert with vitamins C and E to protect immune cells from oxidative stress. It is the most well known carotenoid (of which estimates range from 500 to more than 700) and enjoys vitamin status because of the body's ability to convert it to vitamin A. However, beta-carotene isn't the most potent antioxidant in this family. Moreover, the specific antioxidant performance of many carotenoids is determined by their concentrations in different tissues. Overall, the liver, adrenal glands, and testes contain significantly higher amounts of carotenoids than the kidneys, ovaries, and adipose tissue. And while beta-carotene is the main carotenoid in the liver, adrenal glands, kidneys, ovaries, and adipose tissue, the carotenoid lycopene predominates in the testes. The protective carotenoids in the macula area of the retina are zeaxanthin and lutein.

Epidemiological studies indicate that beta-carotene could provide protection against cancers of the lung, stomach, colon, prostate, and cervix. A number of investigators report an enormous risk-reduction for lung cancer in people with high dietary beta-carotene intake. Interestingly, attempts to replicate this with beta-carotene supplements were ended when the reverse situation began to appear— that is, smokers taking synthetic supplements appeared to have an increased cancer outcome. Once again, this points out the crucial difference between isolated supplements and dietary sources. Perhaps it isn't the beta-carotene alone, but an association with other food factors that accounts for its protective effects. Prominent sources of all the carotenoids are presented in the tables on pages 381– 393, along with other phytochemicals that exhibit potent antioxidant activity.

The discussion so far has centered on the antioxidant powers of individual vitamins and phytochemicals. The mineral selenium should be acknowledged as well. In worldwide studies, dietary intake of selenium is associated with reduced cancer incidence, especially of the breast, colon, rectum, prostate, liver, lung, and leukocytes (cells found in the lymphatic and circulatory systems). Notably, the types of cancer for which selenium exhibits the strongest anticancer effect are those in which dietary fat is a suspected risk factor. Selenium also influences the metabolism and toxicity of a variety of drugs and chemicals.

In addition to direct antioxidant action, selenium both complements and conserves vitamin E. This explains, in part, the importance of this mineral in relation to the entire immune system. Another proposed route of protection is the presence of selenium as an enzyme cofactor, discussed below in Protective Enzymes.

★ THE IMMUNE SYSTEM SUMMARIZED ★

We talk about the body's immune system in a number of places within this and other Guidelines. Without getting too technical, just what is this marvelous infection-fighting system all about?

During immune response, especially in the early phase of infection fighting, certain white blood cells actually employ reactive oxygen molecules and free radicals as weapons against bacterial invaders. Although we have stated that free radicals can be quite damaging, in this case they're beneficial. However, during the killing of infectious organisms, free radicals may be overproduced and cause injury to the white blood cells, as well as neighboring cells and tissues.

Neutrophils make up one important group of white blood cells that act in this manner. When antioxidant nutrients are adequate, neutrophils do their job as intended and remain unscathed. But when there aren't enough antioxidants around, the neutrophils themselves are injured by the oxidative products they generate. In addition, the resulting free radicals can cause chromosomal damage to other cells they come in contact with.

White blood cells known as macrophages make up another division of infection fighters. Macrophages secrete numerous chemical mediators such as interferon, prostaglandins, interleukins, and tumor necrosis factor, discussed in Chapter 2. Oxidative damage caused by inflammatory conditions disturbs macrophage membrane receptors in cells and thus the ability of chemical mediators to perform.

Overall, deficiencies of some nutrients (mainly those that act as antioxidants) and imbalances or an excess of others (fats, for example) can impair the body's production of various immune cells or alter their capacity to properly recognize and respond to foreign invaders. The competence of macrophages, natural killer cells, B cells, and T cells, all of which enable the body to resist illness, can be affected. In the presence of antioxidant nutrients, these fighters all become more capable.

Protective Enzymes

Enzymes are made in the body by coupling designated amino acids, minerals, and vitamins. Their job is to stimulate specific chemical reactions within cells. A vast number of enzymes have been identified within the human system. Each one has a highly defined task in terms of the substrate it acts upon and the type of reaction it triggers. One critical role is guarding against the harmful effects of free radicals by serving as antioxidants. Certain enzymes can also detect the presence of abnormal DNA in cells and, under the right conditions, perform repairs before these renegade cells have a chance to duplicate.

The relationship between the mineral selenium and glutathione—a protein synthesized in the body from the amino acids cysteine, glutamic acid, and glycine—results in one of the most powerful antioxidant enzymes, glutathione peroxidase. In addition, glutathione is a critical component of the enzyme glutathione S-transferase. A member of a group called Phase 2 enzymes, glutathione S-transferase is one of the body's most important agents for reducing the activity of carcinogens and protecting against the proliferation of malignant cells.

Glutathione has been examined in relation to aging, with the general conclusion

351

Mentor

being that it is positively correlated with good health. In AIDS intervention trials, decreased blood levels of glutathione are associated with HIV infection. The cells that line the intestines use glutathione to defend against bacteria, toxins, and food antigens; diets lacking the essential amino acid precursors methionine and cystine—which are used to make cysteine—leave people susceptible to intestinal infections and chronic diarrhea. Ironically, these conditions further decrease the absorption of vital nutrients. In addition to defending against external toxins and improving immune function, glutathione stabilizes red blood cell membranes.

While the amino acids required to generate glutathione are essential for everyone, some people have a greater need due to circumstances that place a drain on body stores. Because of its role in reducing the activity of cancerous agents, exposure to chemical carcinogens increases glutathione demand. Similarly, people taking medication may use up their supply of glutathione to diminish the toxic effects of some drugs. Moreover, because heavier people generally have a higher proportion of body fat, they may use glutathione in greater amounts to fight adipose tissue oxidation.

Enzyme Building

Although glutathione is found in food, it may not survive digestion intact. Moreover, it appears to be used up rapidly and requires continuous replenishment. The most reliable approach is to supply the body with ample amounts of cysteine—the dietary amino acid whose absence limits glutathione synthesis—or consume its precursors, methionine and cystine. In order to transform these amino acids into the desired proteins, the diet must also have available supplies of vitamin B_6, choline, and folate.

Vitamin B_6 encourages the synthesis of cysteine from methionine. (B_6 is a cofactor for the neurotransmitters dopamine, norepinephrine, and serotonin, and thus also important for the brain and central nervous system.)

The methyl donor actions of methionine (and choline), mentioned earlier as lipotropic factors, are critical to glutathione synthesis. In addition, methyl groups have demonstrated protection against spontaneous and chemically induced liver cancer in rats. Human studies suggest that a methyl-deficient diet contributes to DNA abnormalities that result in loss of normal control over the genes associated with colorectal cancer. Dietary deficiencies of methyl donors may also increase tumors in the mammary glands, esophagus, and pancreas.

Since the B vitamin folate is an essential cofactor in the system that controls methyl group transfer, it, too, must be present for DNA integrity. Experiments showing a causative link between low folate intake and colon tumors in rats are most likely explained by its coworker action in methyl transfer.

When methionine is employed to make the amino acid cysteine, certain intermediary substances are produced. Of note is homocysteine. The accumulation of homocysteine in the blood has a damaging effect on blood vessels and is implicated in heart attacks and strokes. Since there is a continuous, dynamic flow between methionine and homocysteine, anything that creates interference can precipitate an unhealthy situation. Vitamins B_6, B_{12}, folate, and choline participate in the enzyme systems that facilitate this flow. If there is an inadequate supply of these vitamins, methionine production is curtailed and homocysteine builds up.

Interestingly, a fairly common genetic variant causes the folate-dependent enzyme in some people to be less efficient. Additional folate in their diets remedies the defect. Of added relevance, noted cancer researcher Bruce Ames believes that chromosome breaks in humans may be directly linked to low folate levels.

According to a meta-analysis of thirty-eight studies, in U.S. men aged forty-five years and older reducing homocysteine levels could conservatively lower the proportion of preventable deaths due to heart disease by 10 percent, or 35,000 lives saved per year. The estimate for women is a 6 percent decrease in coronary heart disease mortality, or 21,000 averted deaths. Some researchers believe that as many as 30 to 40 percent of heart attacks and strokes suffered by men in the United States each year are related to inadequate folate intake.

Apparently, many genetic factors determine how the body uses folate. For example, a genetic predisposition can depress production of an enzyme needed for normal neural tube development in the fetal stage. Increasing folate consumption during the very early stage of pregnancy can protect against such defects, which affect the brain and spinal cord. (For food sources, see page 357.)

Above we mentioned choline's participation in methionine regeneration, and earlier we spoke of its more widely acknowledged stature in liver protection, cell membranes, and nerve transmission. A lesser known function is choline's impact on an enzyme known as protein kinase-C (PKC), which in turn acts on insulin receptors, skin growth factor, and many proteins involved in the control of gene expression, cell division, and differentiation. When PKC doesn't function properly, cancers can develop. This may explain why animals fed a choline-deficient diet are much more likely to develop cancerous liver tumors.

A number of phytochemicals participate in antioxidant defense and chemoprotection by stimulating production and release of glutathione S-transferase and other Phase 2 enzymes. Various polyphenols, indoles, and thiosulfinates (organosulfides) are noteworthy for their glutathione-inducing capabilities. These phytochemicals are discussed in detail in Chapter 4. Of note here are the various additional roles of the thiosulfinates found in garlic and onions.

The thiosulfinates in the allium family, to which garlic and onions belong, are collectively referred to as allyl sulfides. These compounds are highly reactive: They change spontaneously into other organic sulfur compounds, which take part in further transformations. Early studies claimed that most of the protective powers of garlic were due to the allyl sulfide compound allicin that's present in the raw bulb and easily decomposed. A vast body of research now refutes this and documents the effectiveness of several allyl sulfides and their derivatives. Although they don't all act in the same manner or to the same degree, allyl sulfides display a remarkable range of biological effects.

Numerous studies indicate that allyl sulfides and their derivatives can inhibit activation of cancer-causing agents. Rodent experiments and studies using human cell cultures demonstrate protection against stomach, lung, colon, esophagus, breast, prostate, and skin cancers. Multicultural analysis shows a consistent correlation between garlic and onion consumption and decreased risk of gastrointestinal cancers. In controlled laboratory experiments, extracts of these compounds inhibit blood platelet aggregation and for many people effectively lower elevated blood pressure, plasma cholesterol, and blood sugar levels. Much of this activity is attributed to the effect of these organosulfides on cytochrome P-450 reactions.

Battalion P-450. A body of enzymes known as the cytochromes P-450 are collectively responsible for the bulk of activity in managing external toxins, including cigarette smoke, pharmaceutical drugs, pesticides, and food and chemical carcinogens. In cancer progression they're referred to as Phase 1 enzymes. Interestingly, while many P-450 enzymes afford protection, some act in opposition, activating carcinogens. Cytochromes P-450 also figure in the body's handling of fat-soluble vitamins, and the regulation of steroid hormones and eicosanoids.

The inhibition and stimulation of P-450 enzymes is a complex subject. Nutrients and food additives modify their activity and thereby mediate a number of hostile invasions. Cigarette smoke, chronic alcohol consumption, and protein-dominant weight-loss regimens that provoke ketone production all increase P-450 demand.

Cytochromes P-450 are dependent on adequate protein in the diet, whereas chronic high-carbohydrate diets decrease their activity. In rats, cholesterol and unsaturated fats in the diet induce P-450 enzymes, but whether this applies to humans isn't clear. In addition to the ability of certain natural chemicals within plants to activate cytochromes P-450, several vitamins and minerals exert their influence, including vitamin A, niacin, riboflavin, thiamin, vitamin C, vitamin E, folic acid, iron, copper, zinc, calcium, magnesium, and selenium.

Bring on the Metal. Among the dietary minerals, zinc is the most important coworker in enzyme systems. Zinc is required by more than seventy different enzymes, where its presence is greater than the rest of the trace minerals combined. Some of zinc's responsibilities have already been described in this chapter, including its affiliation with insulin (see Glucose Metabolism Needs Nutrient Helpers, on page 344) and its role in prostaglandin generation (see Fatty Acid Transformation Needs Nutrient Helpers, on page 345). Zinc's antioxidant strength is as a cofactor in the enzyme superoxide dismutase (SOD), one of the body's most important defenses against oxygen stress.

In addition, zinc participates in protein synthesis, making it crucial for growth and normal cell division, along with antibody and hormone production. Zinc intake is related to fertility, fetal health, labor and delivery outcome, appetite, growth, sexual maturation, bone formation, wound healing, and resistance to in-

The Healthiest Diet in the World

fection. It is found in particularly high concentrations in the prostate gland and semen, indicating a proportionally greater need in men compared with women.

Copper is another pivotal mineral in several enzymes. Normally cells produce energy by a process that depends on a copper-containing enzyme. When copper isn't available, cells compensate by switching to an alternative energy-generating system. In doing so, however, the cells compromise their ability to receive vital signals that tell them when and how to respond, and when to stop responding. This may explain the wide range of pathologies reported in copper-deficient animals—from heart muscle damage and depressed immune response to neurological problems.

Copper is required for infant growth and brain development; without adequate amounts, nerve cells in the part of the brain that governs learning and memory can't reach maturation. Copper-containing enzymes also influence the evolution of red and white blood cells, iron transport, bone strength, immune function, cholesterol and glucose utilization, and heart muscle contractions. Copper is a cofactor (along with zinc) in the potent antioxidant enzyme superoxide dismutase (SOD). Copper is also present in ceruloplasmin, a protein in the blood that transports copper to the tissues. Key functions of ceruloplasmin include its activity as an antioxidant and its ability to modulate the body's inflammatory system.

★ THE ANTIOXIDANT CAPACITY OF COMMON FOODS ★

USDA scientists have devised a sophisticated system for measuring antioxidant capacity that enables them to evaluate the relative ability of different foods to provide antioxidant protection. After analyzing a number of foods they concluded that "a balanced diet containing enough fruits and vegetables could be the most effective in protecting the body against various oxidative stressors" and "much more effective and also economical than supplementation of an individual antioxidant, such as vitamin C or vitamin E."

Using the procedure to assess teas, twenty-two different vegetables, twelve fruits, and five juices, they observed the following:

• Green and black teas showed higher antioxidant activity than all the fruits and vegetables examined.

• On a weight basis, the top eight antioxidant vegetables (in order, starting with the most potent) are kale, garlic, spinach, brussels sprouts, alfalfa sprouts, broccoli flowers, beets, and red bell pepper. The antioxidant rating of kale was three times that of the red pepper.

• Among the twelve fruits, strawberries ranked highest, followed in descending order by plums, oranges, red grapes, kiwi, pink grapefruit, white grapes, bananas, apples, tomatoes, pears, and honeydew melon. The antioxidant activity of strawberries was twice the capacity measured in oranges and red grapes, seven times higher than in bananas and apples, eleven times that of pears, and sixteen times more potent than the melon.

• The ranking of juices from high to low: grape, grapefruit, tomato, orange, apple.

Mentor

To establish an invincible antioxidant defense, all the nutritive elements presented above and others—some identified, others still outside scientists' grasp—must be present. Notable food sources are cited below in Dietary Sources of Nutrient Helpers. The culmination of this information brings us back to the Basic Steps of Guideline #3: Incorporate generous amounts of the food sources of nutrient helpers—fresh vegetables, legumes, whole grains, fruit, seeds, and nuts—into recipes, meals, and snacks, and for those so inclined, enjoy your eggs.

On top of this, steer clear of dietary schemes that overemphasize or severely restrict any of the three primary nutrients—carbohydrates, fat, and protein. An uncoordinated shift in balance puts extra demands on the nutrient helpers. If they aren't present in sufficient numbers, the entire defense strategy could topple.

Other Helper Activities

It isn't always possible to compartmentalize the role of nutrient helpers. In some situations what they do is evident, but how they do it isn't clear.

Lack of complete information about many food components prevents them from being considered nutrients. (For nutrient status there must be proof that a substance sustains or enhances physiological functions and/or prevents a disease.) Until further evidence is produced, they remain in a state of limbo. A term that has been applied to indicate their potential is "candidate nutrients." Among these candidate nutrients are four tocotrienols—chemical counterparts of the four tocopherols that collectively make up vitamin E.

Although tocotrienols have very little vitamin E activity, they curb cholesterol synthesis by obstructing an intermediary enzyme and inhibit certain cancer genes by blocking their attachment to cell membranes. While the impact of tocotrienols on human health is still uncertain, they can no longer be regarded as impotent incidentals in the vitamin E domain.

Foods that furnish tocopherols and tocotrienols are listed below.

Dietary Sources of Nutrient Helpers

The research advancing a protective as well as functional role for many substances found in food is impressive. Yet present knowledge isn't always sufficient to establish requirements or calculate the quantity of these supporting elements within individual foods. Overall, the volume of evidence currently on hand suggests that our health is best served by the conglomeration of helper nutrients imparted by eating a wide variety of fresh wholefoods. This way we're most apt to obtain the known, as well as the still to be isolated, factors that our natural food supply can contribute.

Following is a listing of where you can find the nutrient helpers introduced in this chapter. A number of these foods receive additional attention in other chapters.

Vitamin Helpers

Vitamin C. Vitamin C comes primarily from vegetables and fruit, especially citrus, broccoli, brussels sprouts, cabbage, cauliflower, dark leafy greens, kiwis, papaya, peppers, potatoes, strawberries, and vine-ripened summer tomatoes.

Vitamin E. Nuts, seeds, and their oils contain the active alpha-tocopherol form of vitamin E. Wheat germ, avocado, and cooked greens are also good sources. Foods that supply other tocopherols or related tocotrienols include soybeans, whole-grain barley, buckwheat, rye, wheat bran, and, of course, products made from these ingredients.

Beta-carotene. Beta-carotene is amply supplied by apricots, broccoli, cantaloupe, carrots, dark leafy greens, mangoes, peaches, papaya, parsley, pumpkin, red peppers, sweet potatoes, and winter squash.

Thiamin, Niacin, and Pantothenic Acid. Legumes, nuts, seeds, brewer's yeast, whole grains, and especially wheat germ all furnish substantial amounts of the B vitamin thiamin. Niacin is similarly found in legumes, nuts and seeds (especially peanuts, almonds, and sunflower and sesame seeds), brewer's yeast, wheat germ, and whole grains, as well mushrooms. Pantothenic acid is widely available—the name comes from "pantos," which means everywhere. Prominent sources include sunflower seeds, nuts (particularly pecans, peanuts, cashews, hazelnuts/filberts, pistachios), legumes (with highest amounts in black-eyed peas, lentils, split peas, and limas), kasha, quinoa, soy flour, avocado, acorn squash, broccoli, corn, escarole, mushrooms, parsnips, potatoes, snow peas, sweet potatoes, wakame seaweed, egg yolk, yogurt, cheese, and brewer's yeast.

Vitamin B$_6$. Foods particularly rich in vitamin B$_6$ are bananas, avocado, acorn squash, brussels sprouts, carrots, green peas, potatoes, sweet potatoes, cooked spinach, wheat germ, kasha, millet, brown rice, wild rice, sunflower seeds, hazelnuts/filberts, walnuts, peanut butter, soy products, legumes (especially lentils, navy beans, and lima beans), flaxseed, and brewer's yeast.

Folate. Folate isn't too difficult to obtain through diet if vegetables and fruits are eaten regularly. Dried beans are particularly well endowed. Other good sources include artichokes, asparagus, avocado, bean sprouts, beets, broccoli, brussels sprouts, dark leafy greens, okra, orange juice, wheat germ, and brewer's yeast. It is inhibited, however, by alcohol consumption. In our opinion, the move to fortify grain products with folate is a less desirable way to obtain this vitamin. We share the concerns of many health professionals that addition of folate in this manner could lead to imbalances in overall B vitamin intake and mask certain anemias, particularly in the elderly. As always, eating foods inherently rich in nutrients is the best way to maintain ample reserves while avoiding extremes caused by artificial supplementation.

Biotin, Lecithin, and Choline. Because the databases that nutritionists rely on to quantify nutrients in food don't include data on choline (or lecithin) and are sporadic regarding biotin, their presence in food is difficult to pinpoint. It is widely acknowledged that egg yolks and soybeans are excellent sources of biotin and lecithin. (Most dietary choline is obtained from lecithin.)

In addition, for choline we recommend legumes in general, whole grains, wheat germ, brewer's yeast, and possibly various nuts and seeds, including Brazil nuts, pumpkin seeds, sunflower seeds, sesame seeds, peanuts, and flaxseed. Cauliflower, cabbage, and kale also appear to be relatively good sources. Moreover, if the body is given an adequate supply of methionine, folate, and vitamin B_{12}, it can manufacture its own lecithin. Foods that furnish folate and methionine are listed on pages 357 and 360. Vegetarians can easily take care of vitamin B_{12} needs by eating even small amounts of eggs or dairy products. Vegans are generally advised to take a B_{12} supplement, as plant foods aren't a reliable source of this vitamin.

Biotin is found in ample amounts in most nuts, and is particularly abundant in peanuts, almonds, and hazelnuts/filberts. Other good sources include wheat germ, whole grains, artichokes, avocado, carrots, mushrooms, sweet potatoes and yams, Swiss chard, tomatoes, bananas, soy milk, goat's milk, yogurt, various cheeses, and egg yolks. Lesser amounts are provided by most vegetables and fruit.

Mineral Helpers

Chromium. Chromium is a difficult nutrient to locate in food. Analytical methods introduced in the 1980s provide an accurate method of detection, but there are still no comprehensive databases. Moreover, not all ingested chromium is in a biologically active form. Chromium is found in wheat germ and bran, but to some extent, chromium levels in cereals, as well as many other foods, appear to be a result of processing rather than intrinsic to the foods themselves. For example, canned fruits and vegetables (especially pineapple and tomatoes) exhibit high levels of chromium. Since processed foods are prepared in stainless-steel vessels, which contain chromium, this appears to be a case of good contamination. (The body is able to convert this inorganic chromium to a usable form.) Likewise, cooking in stainless-steel pots may confer a chromium advantage, especially when the food is acidic.

Modest amounts of chromium are found in many commonly consumed fruits, vegetables, legumes, and whole grains. Thus, diets that emphasize these food groups are more apt to meet chromium needs. In addition to canned pineapple and tomato, foods predicted to deliver chromium in somewhat higher concentrations include broccoli, brussels sprouts, corn, cucumber, mushrooms, onions, peas, potatoes, tomatoes (fresh), lettuce, apple (skin), cantaloupe, papaya, pears, prunes, beer, wine, dark molasses, and brewer's yeast.

Because chromium is hard to obtain, lowering the demand is a prudent strategy. Concentrated sugars and other foods with a high G-Force all increase the need and prompt urinary chromium loss. Richard Anderson, a biochemist at the U.S. Department of Agriculture's Human Nutrition Research Center who has done extensive research on chromium, says the best way to enhance the body's chromium supply is to limit simple sugars, which cause the body to excrete large amounts of the mineral.

Zinc. Zinc is found in association with protein foods. Consequently, vegetarian diets often contain less zinc than meat-based diets. The best sources for nonmeat eaters are wheat germ, seeds such as pumpkin seeds, sunflower seeds, sesame seeds (and tahini), brewer's yeast, nuts, roasted soybeans (soy nuts), and sprouted seeds. Other reliable sources include legumes, whole grains, hard cheese, and egg yolks.

Although the fiber and phytate in grains can inhibit zinc absorption, cooking, including baking, tempers this problem. On the other hand, the antagonistic effect of phytate is exacerbated by the simultaneous presence of high amounts of calcium. In fact, high calcium intake in general can reduce zinc absorption by as much as 50 percent, creating a potential problem for those who follow the popular trend to boost their diets with calcium supplements. Of additional note is the fact that zinc requirements are elevated by diets that contain a lot of protein and phosphorus, both of which promote urinary zinc excretion.

Magnesium. Magnesium is found in a wide variety of foods and beverages. It is particularly bountiful in flax, pumpkin, sunflower, and sesame seeds. Nuts are another excellent source, with highest measures in almonds, Brazil nuts, cashews, hazelnuts/filberts, and pine nuts, and very respectable amounts in peanuts, pecans, pistachios, and walnuts. Legumes provide notable amounts, particularly the various soy-based foods. Whole grains provide lesser but still significant quantities, especially wheat germ. Vegetables that offer a particularly good supply of magnesium include the seaweeds, spinach, Swiss chard, beet greens, cactus (nopales, prickly pears), artichokes, okra, acorn squash, corn, green peas, yuca, and sprouted beans and seeds. Beverages offering magnesium include coffee, tea, and cocoa.

Processing is particularly detrimental to magnesium. For example, the refining of whole wheat and brown rice can reduce the magnesium content of these grains by more than 80 percent. Moreover, magnesium absorption can be hindered by consuming excessive amounts of protein, phosphorous, and calcium. (The mineral phosphorus is considerably in excess of requirements when animal foods abound. Phosphorous intake is also increased by soda consumption. Calcium intake from food is modest in most people's diets; however, the popularity of calcium supplements may compromise magnesium absorption.)

Selenium. A number of factors influence the levels of selenium in food, including the selenium content of the soil in which crops are grown and, where animal foods are concerned, the levels in livestock and poultry feed. As a result, the data in food tables aren't always reliable. The most abundant and dependable food source is Brazil nuts, which are grown in a region of Venezuela where the soil is rich in selenium. Just one Brazil nut provides twice the highest U.S. Recommended Daily Allowance of selenium (which is 70 mcg for men), while two nuts surpass potent 200 mcg selenium supplements. Other common foods likely to confer selenium at substantial levels are egg yolks, sunflower seeds, wheat germ and bran, whole wheat products, brown rice, oats, and oat bran; lesser but still significant amounts come from other nuts, soy products, legumes, and mushrooms. Meat, fish, and cheese are also potential selenium sources.

Copper. Compared to other minerals, copper is only needed in minute amounts. However, because zinc and copper compete for absorption, a deficiency can be provoked by taking high doses of supplemental zinc. Excessive intake of ascorbic acid also depresses copper availability. According to food surveys, a majority of Americans consume less than the suggested minimum of copper, although with a reasonably diverse diet it isn't hard to meet needs.

Prime sources include most nuts and seeds, with the highest amounts in Brazil nuts, cashews, hazelnuts/filberts, pecans, pistachios, sesame seeds (tahini), sunflower seeds, walnuts; wheat germ and bran; whole grains, including buckwheat, rye, wheat, brown rice, and whole-grain cornmeal and barley; legumes; dried fruit.

The best sources among vegetables and fresh fruit are asparagus, avocado, bananas, beets, mushrooms, parsley, and canned tomatoes.

In the animal kingdom, oysters and organ meats (especially liver) are the significant contributors. Copper is also found in cocoa and chocolate.

Amino Acid Helpers

While glutathione is said to be in a number of vegetables and fruits, it may not survive ingestion intact. For the body to build its own supply of glutathione, it requires foods containing the precursor sulfur-containing amino acids methionine, cystine, and cysteine.

Sulfur-containing amino acids are plentiful in nuts and seeds such as sunflower, sesame, and pumpkin seeds and Brazil nuts, almonds, and pine nuts, and in lesser but still substantial amounts in pistachios, walnuts, cashews, and peanuts. Wheat germ is another excellent source. Legumes are generally deficient in this area, although soy foods make a notable contribution, especially soy flour and soy nuts, while lentils and dried peas add to cystine intake. Many whole grains are also a good source of cystine, particularly wheat, rye, quinoa, and oats. Cheeses are well endowed with methionine, and eggs are another reliable source.

Data on cysteine content of foods aren't available, but it's presumed to parallel cystine content. Additional foods that make a notable contribution to sulfur intake include garlic, onions, asparagus, cabbage, brussels sprouts, broccoli, cauliflower, and most dark leafy greens.

Eggs

Eggs can make a valuable contribution to some of the most important nutrient helpers. The criticism against eggs stems from their high cholesterol content, although no direct link between heart disease and egg consumption has ever been validated.

Unless you have a genetic condition that interferes with cholesterol metabolism, eating four to six eggs a week shouldn't create any problems. In the span of twenty years (1972 to 1992), average yearly egg consumption in the United States decreased from 268 per person to 180. Thus we have gone from eating a reasonable 5 eggs a week down to a mere 3.5. Naturally, these figures don't represent individual intake, and within this national average some people exceed this amount, while others eat no eggs at all. In fact, many people can eat more than the amount just suggested without exhibiting any adverse effects on blood cholesterol levels.

Egg yolks are the richest source of lecithin and choline. They're also a primary source of biotin and offer a respectable amount of pantothenic acid, which is conveniently found in a number of foods. The yolks are regarded as a good source of selenium, although this may vary with the hen's diet, and offer modest amounts of zinc. In addition, the sulfur-containing amino acids can be obtained by eating eggs.

Eggs yolks contain two important carotenoids, lutein and zeaxanthin, whose roles are discussed in Chapter 4. They contain modest amounts of vitamin K, although this, too, can change according to what the hens are fed.

The protein content of eggs is particularly noteworthy. One way in which the protein value of foods is determined is based on their assortment of amino acids. A number of terms are used to describe their worth, including "biological value," "protein efficiency ratio," and "net protein utilization." What they all boil down to is this: Our bodies need a certain amount of each amino acid in order to build protein. If one is lacking, this process slows down or ceases altogether. While these amino acids can be combined from many different sources, individual foods that have the right proportion of the amino acids that must be supplied by the diet have the highest biological value. Because the amino acids in eggs come closest to matching the ideal usable pattern, egg protein is considered the model for rating all other foods.

Garlic

Garlic (*Allium sativum*) has been used in food preparation and as a popular folk medicine for centuries. In assessing the nutritional role of garlic, it's important to distinguish between what is known and what may simply be legend. There's nothing wrong with enjoying garlic solely for its culinary excellence; however, if nutritional benefits are anticipated, it's important to determine which results are attainable when garlic is eaten in reasonable amounts, in food rather than as a supplement.

A breakdown of the nutrients in 100 grams of garlic, a standard comparative measure, reveals notable amounts of many nutrients. These include thiamin, riboflavin, vitamin B_6, vitamin C, calcium, chromium, copper, iron, manganese, phosphorous, potassium, selenium, and zinc. But since a single clove of garlic weighs only 3 to 5 grams, the actual contribution of dietary garlic to nutrient intake is really too small to be highly significant. This doesn't mean that eating garlic is without value. In easily consumed amounts, the thiosulfinates in garlic—collectively referred to as allyl sulfides—have many documented effects.

Trials using as little as 3 to 10 grams of fresh garlic or its extracted equivalent on a daily basis have lowered cholesterol an average of 6 to 12.6 percent, LDL cholesterol 4 to 16 percent, and triglycerides anywhere from 13 to 30 percent in subjects who started out with high blood levels. Similar quantities have lowered systolic and diastolic blood pressures by as much as 6.7 percent and 7.9 percent, respectively. When consumed in feasible amounts, garlic also diminishes blood platelet clumping, thereby reducing the risk of blocked arteries.

Multicultural studies reveal an association between garlic-eating groups and decreased risk of gastrointestinal cancers. In comparison studies of people in various communities of Shandong Province of the People's Republic of China, where gastric cancer is especially high, a significant reduction in incidence parallels increased consumption of garlic, as well as other allium vegetables (scallion and Chinese chive). Residents in Cangshan County, who consume an average of 20 grams of fresh garlic per person daily, have a stomach cancer mortality rate of about 3 per 100,000 people. In Qixia, where residents rarely consume garlic, the stomach cancer mortality rate is 40 per 100,000 people. Moreover, the county in northern China with the lowest stomach cancer mortality is well known for its garlic production. In laboratory experiments, garlic powder added to the diets of rats blocks the formation and action of N-nitrosamines, recognized carcinogens mentioned above in the discussion of vitamin C.

Thiosulfinates in garlic are also responsible for its historically touted antimicrobial action. A protective role against bacteria and fungus in the digestive tract and skin are clearly established (particularly for the allyl sulfide allicin), and studies on blood-borne microorganisms, although few, are encouraging. Several compounds in garlic are credited with stimulating the immune system, even at low doses. In a comprehensive review of foods associated with low incidence of precancerous colon polyps, garlic was cited as significant. (A similar role for other allium vegetables couldn't be determined from this study due to the nature of the food questionnaire used.)

Although large quantities of garlic can modestly reduce blood sugar, it still hasn't been determined whether consistent consumption of garlic at dietary levels has a notable hypoglycemic influence.

There have been caveats concerning garlic, but they're relevant to therapeutic pharmacological doses, not what you would expect to get through normal food use. Several human studies have shown that as much as 15 to 20 grams (4 cloves) of uncooked garlic can be eaten daily without adverse effects. The main concern is in regard to the compound allicin. Excessive amounts of allicin can cause abdominal irritation, particularly when raw garlic is eaten on an empty stomach. Since cooking converts allicin into other organosulfides, a larger quantity of cooked garlic can be safely consumed.

The impact of cooking is a controversial topic. Garlic's attributed health benefits are conferred by a number of constituents. To determine which out of something like one hundred different compounds is the active ingredient in any situation is extremely difficult. Because heat and air contact alter many of its volatile elements, in raw garlic you get one thing, garlic cooked in a liquid medium yields another, and garlic cooked in oil still another. Thus, each way you prepare it, you create a different kind of chemical. Since we have no clear answers, the best strategy is to employ many different modes of preparation. Likewise, it's a good idea to choose as many varieties of garlic as you can find.

Packaged (prechopped) garlic preparations have been implicated in cases of food poisoning. This has no bearing on fresh garlic use, but people who view these products as a convenient alternative should be aware of the dangers. If the product isn't acidified to inhibit bacteria growth, it requires pressure retorting (as used by the canning industry) to insure safety. Although oil-packing is less chancy than water-packing, neither method is risk-free. Attempting to duplicate these products at home isn't advisable.

Other health problems related to the use of garlic are topical. Some people who frequently handle the cloves experience localized skin allergies. And burns have been evidenced when crushed garlic remains in contact with the skin for several hours.

Onions

Onions, along with scallions, leeks, chives, and shallots, belong to the allium family of vegetables that encompasses garlic. There is speculation that their botanical name derives from the Celtic word "all," which means pungent. Indeed, the odorless constituent of garlic known as alliin, which is transformed into the odorous allicin when the clove is cut or crushed, is chemically identical to the compound that causes your eyes to tear while cutting onions.

Because of the similarity in organosulfides, many of the same health effects apply to all the allium vegetables, although among them certain active allyl compounds are structurally a bit different. What makes onions especially valuable is

363

that they're already very popular and the potential to consume even more is easily fulfilled.

Conclusions drawn from studying the dietary habits of various people point to a particularly protective role for onions against stomach cancer. In the United States, a county in Georgia famous for Vidalia onions has a stomach cancer mortality rate among whites that is about one-third the national level and one-half the state level. Among Japanese in Hawaii, those eating onions twenty-one times or more per month are three times less likely to develop stomach cancer than those eating onions eight or fewer times. In Linqu County of Shandong Province, China, where stomach cancer prevails, in addition to garlic, scallions and Chinese chives were independently connected to risk reduction. And in the Netherlands Cohort Study on diet and cancer, which began in 1986 with 120,852 men and women aged fifty-five to sixty-nine years, follow-up after 3.3 years indicated half the frequency of stomach cancer in subjects consuming half an onion or more a day compared with those who didn't customarily eat onions. These observations have been corroborated by laboratory testing of hamsters and mice, where tumor formation by known gastric carcinogens was inhibited by onion extracts. While stomach cancer mortality has gone down more than 50 percent in the United States since 1960, it's still among the top ten causes of cancer deaths for African Americans, Native Americans, Asians living in the United States, and Hispanics.

In the famous Seven Countries Study (discussed on page 325) the intake of flavonoids (phytochemicals found in various plant foods) was deemed a significant protective factor against coronary heart disease. While the main sources of flavonoids differed largely in the populations studied, onions were among the most important sources in the United States, Finland, former Yugoslavia, and Greece. In addition, tests run on extracts from onions demonstrate their ability to reduce platelet stickiness, which adds to their heart-protective potential.

In Chapter 4, we talk about the importance of variety, achieved not only by eating all different kinds of vegetables and fruits, but also by eating different varieties of particular vegetables and fruits. There are many types of onions to try, some sharp like common yellow cooking onions, some more mellow (for example, red Bermuda, white pearl, and Spanish onions), others almost sweet, such as Vidalias, Walla Wallas, Maui onions, and Sweet Imperials. Scientific analysis reveals diverse chemical constituents in each, supporting the value of real variety.

Mushrooms

Mushrooms furnish riboflavin, niacin, biotin, pantothenic acid, potassium, chromium, copper, and selenium. Judging from their historical use, they're likely to contain elements that we're currently unaware of or lack the capability to quantify. One distinctive quality is their ability to amplify other food flavors.

Cultivated white mushrooms have been joined in the culinary arena by a variety of more exotic species that are being marketed in both fresh and dried forms.

Meaty (and mammoth) portobellos, tender porcinis, earthy creminis, woodsy shiitakes, oyster mushrooms (named for their fluted shell shape and briny flavor), delicate enoki mushrooms with long stems and tiny button caps, dainty straw mushrooms, and highly prized chanterelles and morels (the favorite foraged mushrooms in Europe) appear on many restaurant menus and are increasingly available for home cooking.

In addition to using cultivated white mushrooms in our cooking, we offer a number of recipes that provide an opportunity to appreciate the more pronounced flavors of some of the so-called wild varieties. (This is really a misnomer; many commercial offerings of wild mushroom varieties are, in fact, cultivated, rather than gathered in their natural habitat.) Note that if you don't have access to any of these mushrooms, the ubiquitous white mushrooms sold in supermarkets can be used in their place. Their flavor may be less distinct, but they're still nutritionally replete.

CHAPTER 4

A Foundation of Vegetables (and Fruit)

In Chapters 1 and 2, you read how there are various opinions regarding the ideal balance of nutrients. Health professionals have hotly debated how much carbohydrate—and thus how much bread, pasta, and cereal—we should eat, and how much fat, reflected not only in our choice of oil, butter, margarine, and the like, but also how much dairy, eggs, meat, and nuts we ought to consume. When it comes to vegetables, however, widespread consensus is reflected in the first recommendation set forth by the American Cancer Society in their 1996 guidelines:

"Choose most of the foods you eat from plant sources."

Although grain foods form the base of the USDA Food Guide Pyramid, for many people they really don't offer a sound foundation. Vegetables, on the other hand, do. With few exceptions, people can indulge in vegetables and reap numerous returns. Fruit, too, yields many rewards, but as we have said, because it can disrupt blood sugar, some restrictions may be required.

The USDA pyramid advises three to five servings from the vegetable group. This is quite modest compared to the actual amount people could be eating. The pyramid advises two to four servings of fruit, which is sufficient. With adequate vegetables in the diet, fruit actually diminishes in importance.

Despite widespread promotion of these guidelines, the USDA notes that "Americans of all ages eat fewer than the recommended number of servings of . . . vegetables and fruits, even though *consumption of these foods is associated with a substantially lower risk for many chronic diseases, including certain types of cancer*" [emphasis ours]. And while the importance of eating vegetables and fruit is nothing new, for a surprising number of people modifying their diet in this way is revolutionary.

Interestingly, people may not even be aware of their own deficiency. A study done in Scotland found that among respondents who ate less than two portions of fruit or vegetables a day, 55 percent thought they were already eating enough.

How Much Vegetables (and Fruit) Is Enough?

Use of the term "servings" as a guideline is confusing to many. The USDA considers a serving of vegetables as 1 cup uncooked leafy greens, 1/2 cup of other vegetables—cooked or chopped raw—and 3/4 cup vegetable juice. One medium-size fruit, 1/2 cup chopped raw, cooked, or canned fruit, and 3/4 cup fruit juice constitute a serving in this category.

In other countries more precise figures have been suggested. For example, in Scotland and Great Britain a minimum goal is about 400 grams (14 ounces) of fruit and vegetables a day. This approximates the lower limit of the world population goal introduced by the World Health Organization.

When translated into weights, a "serving" by U.S. standards covers a wide range depending on the particular food chosen:

1 cup of greens = about 2 ounces
1/2 cup chopped mushrooms = 1.5 ounces
1/2 cup chopped broccoli, cauliflower, or green beans = 2 ounces
1/2 cup diced potatoes, carrots, radishes, or asparagus = 3 ounces
1 medium peach = 4 ounces
1/2 cup fruit varies from 2 ounces for berries to 6 ounces for apples and pears

Using an average figure of 2.85 ounces per serving, a combined intake of the daily minimum three vegetables and two fruits comes to 14.25 ounces, or a few ounces shy of 1 pound. The higher recommendation of five vegetables and four fruits per day is just over 1 1/2 pounds. This means achieving the lower goal of the U.S. guidelines would about match the World Health Organization's minimum target.

Although a slice of tomato on a sandwich or a few mushrooms tossed into a casserole don't qualify as a "serving," they can bolster daily totals. Over the course of a week, if you don't personally go through a combined amount of at least 6 pounds of vegetables and fruit (with most of the weight given to the former), you aren't eating enough of these foods.

Picking Vegetables and Fruit

In Scotland the guidelines for vegetables exclude potatoes. This isn't because potatoes aren't a good food to eat. It's meant to foster diversity in a country where few other vegetables are enjoyed. The intended message is extremely important: Different types of vegetables and fruit have diverse nutritional characteristics. It takes a range of these foods to fully obtain their offerings.

The form in which vegetables and fruit are consumed also matters. While fresh and frozen products are nutritionally comparable, canned versions often aren't. In addition to the destruction of certain constituents imposed by the canning

Mentor

Six pounds of produce a week sounds like a lot.
How can people fulfill this guideline?

"Adding more vegetables (and fruit) to your day is actually the simplest Golden Guideline of all to follow. Because so much produce (including most vegetables) can be eaten raw, it provides an almost instant snack. Another fundamental way to increase consumption is to simply take larger portions.

"When the actual servings of vegetables (and fruit) don't measure up to prescribed or personal goals, you may be able to meet the mark by paying attention to opportunities to add them in smaller increments. How can you do this? Whenever you eat a sandwich, make sure to include lettuce, tomato, sprouts, and the like. Although less common, sliced cucumbers and thin slices of raw beets are both nice in sandwiches. When preparing sandwich fillings, add chopped celery, sweet red and green pepper, cucumber or similar vegetables. Always include raw vegetable sticks (and fresh or dried fruit) in lunch boxes.

"Liven up pizza and pasta by topping with artichokes, onions, peppers, mushrooms, broccoli, shredded greens, and such. 'Chips and dips' may rhyme, but vegetables and dips are sublime (and better for you). Eating out? Don't forget to eat the garnish.

"Instead of jelly, pair nut butters (peanut, almond, cashew) with sliced pears, apples, bananas, or berries. Snack on dried fruit instead of candy. Remove thin slivers of peel from (organic) oranges, lemons, and limes, mince, and toss into salad dressings, vegetables, beans, grains, soups, blender shakes, and the batter for pancakes and baked goods.

"If you bake, stir berries, corn kernels, or shredded zucchini, carrots, pears, or apples into favorite muffin recipes."

process itself, canned vegetables are inclined to contain excess amounts of salt, while canned fruits parallel this with too much sugar. If the liquid medium is discarded, along with it goes water-soluble nutrients. (As discussed in Chapter 3, canning can have a favorable effect on chromium intake, imparting significant amounts of this mineral to canned tomatoes, mushrooms, and pineapple.)

What about the precut and bagged vegetables and fruit that have begun to proliferate? A big plus is that many people see them as terrific time-savers, and as a result of this convenience eat more of these foods. From a nutritional standpoint their impact is controversial. The longer produce sits, and the more exposed surfaces there are, the more potential there is for nutrient loss.

Although special plastic packaging in which some precut vegetables are placed takes advantage of a technology that slows down nutrient loss, if this "modified atmosphere packaging" isn't used, or if sellers use the appearance of freshness they lend to extend selling time, nutrients could diminish. Another concern is the FDA-sanctioned washing of precut produce in a chlorine bath. According to an FDA spokesperson, "The Food and Drug Administration allows washing of fresh-cut products with chlorine solution, but the chlorine solution is to be rinsed off with potable water. I do not think that all companies wash their fresh-cut

There's No Such Thing as Too Many Vegetables
(but Fruit Is Another Story)

"When working with clients, I provide them with the 'Picking Vegetables' list below and tell them to eat as much and as many as they possibly can. Vegetables don't contain significant amounts of protein; they're fat free, with the exception of avocados and olives (which are actually fruits); and they're low in glucose-raising carbohydrates, excluding tubers such as potatoes, rutabagas, turnips, parsnips, carrots, and beets, as well as winter squash and corn. Consequently, unlike meat, eggs, dairy foods, oils, grains, nuts, seeds, and concentrated sweets—each of which can dramatically influence fat, carbohydrate, or protein intake—vegetables can rarely be eaten in excess. (Possible exceptions to this might be people with specific allergies or rare metabolic conditions.)

"Next I give them the 'Picking Fruit' list and, depending on their health issues, suggest they eat from one to four servings, while defining just how much 'a serving' is. I want to reiterate that fruit, because of its high sugar content, can create problems for people with varying degrees of carbohydrate intolerance. People who choose to restrict their carbohydrate intake can actually skip fruit altogether, so long as they compensate with more vegetables."

products with chlorine solution. This wash is not indicated on the label, because the chlorine is rinsed off with potable water."*

Give priority to products of sustainable agriculture, emphasizing locally grown and organically raised produce. Locally grown and organically raised vegetables and fruit are healthier in many ways. They are free of applied pesticides, herbicides, and fungicides, safer for farm workers, and contribute to a cleaner environment and stronger local economy. Compared with foods from afar, the harvest of locally grown and organically raised produce is bound to be fresher and, if properly handled, retain high nutrient levels. On the other hand, it must be acknowledged that long-distance shipping allows a much greater variety than most communities could provide for themselves on a year-round basis, and this, too, is something to take advantage of.

Mix It Up: Vegetable Soup (and Fruit Salad)

To successfully fulfill Golden Guideline #4 you may need to expand your routine diet. Moreover, it is important to pursue variety not just in terms of different kinds of vegetables and fruit, but also by choosing different varieties of a particular item. For example, when shopping for potatoes, consider red bliss, Yukon Gold, yellow Finns, russets, burbanks, etc. Hungry for an apple? Don't stick with just red delicious or macs, try a winesap, empire, fuji, gala, Granny Smith, mutsu, or Northern spy. And when it comes to oranges, navels, clementines, blood red, and valencias all have their own unique tastes.

* Personal E-mail communication with Alley E. Watada, February 21, 1997.

Be adventurous. If you encounter an unfamiliar vegetable or fruit at the market, give it a try.

Beans Are Vegetables (Sometimes)

Legumes, which many people know as "beans," are vegetables. In fact, dried beans are the mature seed of a vegetable plant, capable of spawning more of the same. However, because their nutritional makeup is different from other vegetables, they don't fulfill this Guideline other than in the young stage (fresh peas, green soybeans) or in sprouted form (as bean sprouts). Legumes receive tribute in the two following chapters.

Juicy Prospects

Many people drink their fruit (and sometimes their vegetables) instead of eating them. Considering it takes three oranges or about a pound of carrots to fill an 8-ounce glass with juice, this certainly seems like a way to satisfy needs quickly. Too quickly, perhaps!

While most of the nutritional virtues of the original food source are maintained in liquid form, there are two critical differences. The first is that juice lacks the fiber of intact produce. The second is that the amount of fruit sugar in an 8-ounce serving of juice is about triple what you get from an average piece of fruit. The combination of these two factors speeds up delivery of glucose into the bloodstream. This can have a disruptive effect on blood sugar and insulin levels.

Because it lacks the fiber of vegetables and fruit, it's easy to drink juice in great quantities. As a result, calories mount up fast, and hunger is satisfied quickly but rarely sustained. In this manner juice can crowd out the intake of other nutrients and simultaneously stimulate weight gain.

In a study of 168 two- to five-year-olds, high body mass and short stature coincided with juice consumption. A third of the children drinking more than 12 ounces of fruit juice per day were in the group with the highest body mass index (considered the most accurate measurement of leanness and obesity). Only 9 percent of the children drinking less juice fell into this category. More than 40 percent of these high juice-drinking preschoolers were also among the shortest, compared with just 14 percent of children drinking lesser amounts. Note that 12 ounces of juice just satisfies the two recommended servings (3/4 cup each) of fruit or juice promoted in the USDA pyramid.

Although juice is certainly healthier than juice drinks, soda, sweetened iced tea, and similar "soft drinks," children filling up on a lot of juice may be missing other nutritious foods and essential nutrients that promote optimum growth and a more healthy weight status. Therefore, kids should be encouraged to eat whole fruit and satisfy their thirst with water.

★ ONE CANNOT LIVE ON VEGETABLES AND FRUIT ALONE ★

People often confuse a vegetarian diet with eating vegetables and fruit. *Vegetables and fruit are an essential part of everyone's diet.* But despite their numerous assets, vegetables and fruit don't contain a complete selection of nutrients necessary to sustain life.

A minimum of 10 percent of calories must come from fats, which are found in very few fruits and are almost insignificant in vegetables (see Chapter 2 for more details).

Protein needs vary with age. The general recommendation for adults is to consume at least 10 percent of daily calories as protein. A generous upper limit is 25 percent of daily calorie intake. Protein accounts for a smaller percent of overall calories for children. Advice on how to best apportion protein can be found in Chapter 6. Protein is available primarily from legumes, eggs, dairy products, nuts and seeds, and animal flesh.

A Historic Perspective

Biochemistry is the science that applies theories derived from biology, chemistry, and physics to living systems. Where humans are concerned, biochemistry and nutrition—the process by which we take in and utilize food matter—are intimately connected. College-level courses in biochemistry were first introduced in this country during the late 1930s. Extraordinary advances in technical capability since then have resulted in frequent additions to our knowledge. While for a time breakthroughs in nutrition seemed to be at a standstill—indeed some academicians felt what we knew was all there was to know—once again scientific discoveries pertaining to the composition of food and how our bodies profit or suffer from what we eat, seem to be hurtling forward at an impressive pace. Consequently, some of what we have relied on for decades may be obsolete, and what we are still in the process of finding out is sometimes prematurely mistaken for fact.

What Has Been Known for Decades

Vitamins are essential micronutrients involved in fundamental functions of the body, such as growth, metabolism, and maintenance of health. Because these substances must be supplied in food, their discovery was a result of their absence in some people's diets.

Most people are aware that vegetables and fruit are important sources of vitamins. However, many are surprised to learn that this knowledge wasn't gained until the 1880s, when the connection was made in Japan between a disease known as beriberi and the ability of certain foods to eradicate it. Another twenty years passed before a Polish biochemist named Funk pinpointed the lack of a single substance (found in whole-grain rice but missing in refined, polished rice) as the cause of beriberi. Because of its chemical structure—as an amine—and the fact that it was vital for life, Funk named his discovery "vitamine."

Soon after, a previously unrecognized substance in milk was identified as essential for the normal development of rats, and yet another, found in egg yolks, was similarly required to sustain life. Thus began the alphabetic naming of vitamines—A, B, C, and so on. (When scientists discovered that not all were structurally amines, the "e" was dropped and "vitamin" became the operative word.) Later, when it became easier to isolate and analyze these elements, scientists realized that each of these vitamins was actually composed of several related compounds. This helps explain the sometimes disparate functions ascribed to what was originally thought to be just one vitamin.

The more we're able to break down and analyze the various components in food, the more we discover regarding the mineral value of vegetables and fruit. Historically, knowledge of the requirement for minerals evolved from the recognition that they were present in body tissues and fluids. The invention of analytic techniques enabled scientists to detect their presence in food, isolate and examine them, quantify their levels, and come to conclusions regarding how much of each appears to be required to prevent body stores from running down.

It's interesting to note that in the *Textbook of Biochemistry* employed in 1966 by Cornell University in the introductory biochemistry course, minerals are covered in 10 pages (out of 633). Twenty-five years later we find this statement in the beginning of the first of two chapters on minerals (filling 84 out of 498 pages) in *Advanced Nutrition and Human Metabolism*: "The importance of minerals in normal nutrition and metabolism cannot be overstated, despite the fact that they constitute only about 4% of total body weight." As you can see, a lot was learned during that quarter century. And more has emerged since.

Beyond supplying a variety of vitamins and minerals, an additional use for fruit as a source of quick energy (resulting from its high sugar content) has also been long acknowledged.

This about covers what was accepted as the worth of vegetables and fruit for many years.

What Has Been Learned

Although the word "vitamins" was only inaugurated in 1912, just a few decades later it was presumed that their discovery and activity was fully known. The most important thing that has been learned since this pompous assumption is something quite rudimentary: The premise was wrong! We still don't know all the varied ways in which vitamins act. Moreover, many constituents within food that are still considered incidental may indeed be necessary—which could eventually elevate them to vitamin (or other nutrient) status.

The "Koagulations" Vitamin: Vitamin K

One of the most neglected vitamins has been vitamin K (alternately known as phylloquinone). It was discovered in 1929 as the factor necessary for blood clotting, and this was accepted as its sole function for more than fifty years. Even now, despite the initial discovery in the late 1970s that vitamin K is a component of three proteins that influence calcium levels in bones, recommendations for vitamin K intake are still based exclusively on blood needs. The significance of vitamin K's participation in bone integrity—and therefore osteoporosis—is unclear (see Osteoporosis, on page 405). What is clear, however, is that recommendations for one purpose (blood clotting) may not adequately cover other uses (such as bone status).

The first time a recommendation for dietary intake of vitamin K was issued in a specified amount was the 1989 U.S. Recommended Dietary Allowances (RDA), which are drawn up by the National Academy of Sciences. Prior to this a range was suggested and it was assumed that bacterial synthesis in the colon enabled most people to cover their needs, making actual food sources inconsequential. The belief that a "normal diet" contributes more vitamin K than most people need has been widely accepted, but we now have reason to suspect that this assumption may not be correct.

In 1996, researchers at the U.S. Agricultural Research Service initiated a pilot study with healthy young men and women, using a newly developed blood test to measure changes in one of the bone-related proteins. When the subjects consumed four times the RDA for vitamin K, their blood profiles relative to this protein significantly improved compared with when they consumed the RDA. This increased retention points to a potential use that is worthy of investigation.

In 1995, yet another vitamin K–dependent protein was revealed, this one related to an enzyme group involved in cancer progression. Since the task of this and other vitamin K–dependent proteins found in the liver, kidneys, lung, skin, spleen, placenta, reproductive organs, vascular tissue, and other sites has yet to be determined, what we have learned to date about vitamin K may be just a small percentage of what we may someday know.

Friendly Fiber Revisited

Vegetables and fruit furnish both water-soluble and water-insoluble fibers. The significance of this is explained in Chapter 1.

Although the concept of fiber—or indigestible matter in foodstuffs—was introduced in Germany during the 1850s, its applications were limited to animals. It wasn't until one hundred years later that the actual composition of fiber was even considered, and we are still in the process of creating more sophisticated ways of discerning the different types of fiber in most foods.

It was about the same time—the mid-1950s—that a role in humans was assigned to fiber. Quite simply, it was thought to relieve constipation. Not until the 1970s did the possibility of a more active part in human nutrition gain serious attention. Nutrition researchers admit now that we still have much to discover about this important food constituent, and fiber is currently one of the most prolific topics of research. Much of what we have learned to date is covered in Chapter 1. The health-protective influence of vegetable and fruit fibers is also noted later in this chapter in How Vegetables (and Fruit) Influence Your Health. The fiber contribution of various vegetables and fruit is provided in the table Fiber Content of Some Common Foods, on page 296. Most vegetables and fruit have some bearing; among the most impressive vegetables are acorn squash, artichokes, brussels sprouts, green peas, jicama, nopales (cactus), and parsnips; in the fruit category, apples, bananas, berries, cherries, dried fruit (apples, apricots, dates, figs, peaches, pears, prunes, raisins), fresh figs, kiwis, nectarines, oranges, and pears are all excellent choices for fiber.

May the G-Force Be with You

The G-Force, our new term for a way of looking at how food intake is reflected in blood sugar levels and what this may mean to your health, was covered extensively in Chapter 1. The influence most vegetables have on G-Force is insignificant, excepting potatoes, rutabagas, turnips, parsnips, carrots, beets, winter squash, and corn.

Fruit presents a different picture. Fruit is often promoted as a healthful appetite suppressant—a means by which "dieters" (translated as people attempting to lose weight) can control calorie intake. Is the notion that fruit is a prudent asset to weight loss based on sound science? Perhaps not.

Fructose, the principal sugar in fruit, doesn't immediately elevate blood glucose levels the way other sugars do, because it follows a different metabolic path. Nonetheless, high levels of fructose impact on how the liver handles carbohydrate storage, hormone release, and the disposition of ingested fats. Glucose tolerance, insulin resistance, blood triglyceride levels, and the proportion of LDL and HDL lipoproteins are all adversely affected by this. The situation is magnified by the combined force of fructose accompanied by other sugars in the diet.

Therefore, another thing we have learned is that although most vegetables can be consumed without any apparent need for limits, fruit eaten without restraint can provoke an unexpected and possibly unhealthy outcome.

What the Future Holds

Until the early 1990s, the word "phytochemical" was practically unknown outside the nutrition research arena. But within a few years, phytochemicals became a popular nutrition topic. As a result, the connection between foods and health has moved onto a more sophisticated plane.

Phytochemicals is the name (derived from *phyton*, the Greek word for plant) given to a vast and complex group of substances found in just about every plant, including vegetables, fruit, legumes, and grains. Phytochemicals are thought to be the key to why so many plant foods seem to reduce the risk of cancer, as well as other degenerative illnesses. Although most of the research only began in the late 1980s, there already appear to be thousands of different phytochemicals, and new ones are being discovered at a brisk pace.

Phytochemicals aren't classified as nutrients, for unlike vitamins and minerals, their absence from the diet hasn't led to any documented deficiencies. Consequently, they aren't deemed necessary for normal body activities. Nevertheless, it appears that quite a lot of these food constituents play a critical role in human health. We feel so strongly about the importance of phytochemicals that we include an extensive discussion and table outlining currently presumed functions and food sources below.

Keep in mind that most of the investigation into the actions of phytochemicals involves animals. Such studies greatly enhance our knowledge; however, due to species differences, caution must be used in applying the results to humans. Still, what has been seen is impressive. As you read about their potential, remember that what we thought we knew decades ago and what we now feel fairly certain about are still subject to change. What we are only on the brink of discovering is certain to be revised for years to come.

The discovery of phytochemicals teaches us some very important lessons:

• It is proof of how much we still have to learn about the contribution of various foods to human nutrition and health.

• It could alter many of our prior assumptions about what to consider a "nutrient," and how specific food constituents act within the body.

• It supports the theory that food is the best insurance for good health, rather than nutritional supplements, which may be lacking some of the most important components. (We can't create a pill for an unknown factor!)

Individual Foods vs. Overall Diet

Does the investigation of phytochemicals in food suggest anything more than the importance of eating plant foods? All this research certainly affirms the recommendation already touted by every health agency—to eat a plant-based diet. If the research does nothing but provide us with a better understanding of why, that is worthwhile.

But the researchers seem to be saying something more profound. Many contend that some foods, because of their distinctive chemical constituents, warrant a special place in the diet, or perhaps in the diets of people at high risk for certain diseases. It is the unique character of individual foods that has given them a new and special designation as "functional foods." The implication is that when incorporated into the diet, these functional foods can confer health benefits not easily duplicated by other foods. For example, although oranges make a health contribution in terms of vitamin C content, this doesn't qualify them as "functional foods," since many other foods provide vitamin C as well. However, the unique flavonoids in citrus fruit do perhaps win them this designation.

In order to ultimately promote individual foods based on their distinguishing phytochemical content, we must not only determine that these compounds are useful and present, but we must also assure that they're available in amounts sufficient to have a notable effect when these foods are consumed in quantities compatible with a practical and overall sound diet. The argument to consume plant-based foods for their phytochemical potential is a good one. But it shouldn't create the impression that they have magical qualities that will overshadow the effects of an otherwise poorly chosen diet.

Feasting on Phytochemicals, Fiber, Phylloquinone, and More

You don't have to memorize a long list of phytochemicals to add more to your diet. As you can see from the table Phytochemicals: Which, What, and Where, on pages 381–393, they're plentiful in foods that are already familiar. Good places to find other essential nutrients in vegetables and fruit are noted throughout this chapter. In Chapter 1, you'll find a list of vegetables and fruit that offer the most fiber.

"In Nikki's Kitchen" is designed to increase your enjoyment of vegetables and fruit, but you can certainly start without a pot, stove, or cookbook, by grabbing a carrot, a stalk of celery, or an apple. You can also up your intake by creatively slipping more vegetables and fruit into favorite dishes as described earlier. To expand your diet, seek out the items in Picking Vegetables and Picking Fruit above whose names caused you to say "Huh?"

How to Make the Most of Vegetables

"People often ask me if they should be eating most of their vegetables raw. While raw vegetables get the bulk of credit for cancer protection, cooking occasionally makes nutrients *more* available. Therefore, I think a smart strategy is to enjoy them both raw and cooked.

"An important role of fat is to assist in the absorption of fat-soluble vitamins. In order for foods containing vitamin K or various carotenoids to achieve their full potential, they must be accompanied by fat. (Specific amounts haven't been determined.) If fats are avoided in cooking, you can drizzle a little oil on greens, tomatoes, and the other vitamin K– and carotenoid-rich foods listed in this chapter, or integrate these foods into meals that provide healthy fats in another dish."

The Phytochemical Phenomenon

Phytochemicals contribute to the color, flavor, and odor of plants. There may be hundreds of them in a single food. Scientists also believe that phytochemicals are responsible for many of the health-promoting qualities of vegetables and fruit.

Because research is still in its infancy, classifying phytochemicals by type and function and confirming the foods that contain them is a frustrating experience. In the accompanying table, we have done our best to divide phytochemicals by family classes and subclasses, report on what researchers have discovered thus far in terms of their potential to protect health, and cite some prominent food sources. The current state of phytochemical data reminds us of the computer industry: As soon as you master a program, someone upgrades it! Likewise, constant updating is necessary to keep any phytochemical database fully current. Don't let yourself be distracted by each innovation. There is already an ample choice of foods to cover our needs. Everything else just increases the incentive.

The emerging knowledge about phytochemicals clearly illustrates why nutritional supplements can't be relied on for perfect health. Quite obviously, many potentially beneficial elements in food haven't yet been identified; furthermore, many of the known protective factors have yet to be extracted and/or reproduced in a laboratory. Moreover, even when we do have the ability to manufacture substances like phytochemicals in concentrated supplement form, deciding what dose is needed to be effective, how much may have harmful side effects, and in what combination these substances are most effective is a long way off. Nonetheless, "phytamin" pills are already on the market, claiming to do the job.

The synergistic effect phytochemicals have on each other and on other food constituents, as well as the inhibiting effect that can result when they're consumed out of balance, offers even more reasons to eat as wide an assortment as possible of plant-based foods, including vegetables and fruit, along with grains,

377

Mentor

legumes, and nuts. In the words of Mark Messina, Ph.D., former program director of the National Cancer Institute's Diet and Cancer Branch, "We have to focus not on macronutrients or micronutrients, not even on phytochemicals, but on our foods."

Chemoprotection and Phytochemicals

There are several different stages in the development of cancers, and aggravation or intercession at any one of them can influence the course the disease takes. The objective of chemoprevention is to block one or more of the mechanisms that create cancer cells and allow them to grow. A great deal of research is being done to determine if phytochemicals in commonly eaten plant foods can act in a preventive manner.

- Many phytochemicals are potent antioxidants and in this way protect the cells from harmful damage caused by oxidation.
- Phytochemicals may also act by:
    Directly inhibiting the formation of carcinogens
    Working indirectly to stimulate the production of enzymes that detoxify carcinogens
    Preventing carcinogens from reaching target tissues or organs
    Acting on cells that have already been exposed to carcinogens, suppressing or even shrinking tumor development

At every step along the road to malignancy, plant chemicals have a tendency to reduce the likelihood of transition to the next stage. Not all do this equally, but the overall effects of these compounds is to slow down or reverse the progress.

The cancer-protective mechanisms attributed to specific phytochemicals are outlined in the table starting on page 381. Some of the most studied phytochemicals are elaborated on below.

Flavonoids and lignans have been credited with inhibiting estrogen synthesis in fat cells to a degree equal to drugs used in cancer chemotherapy. In postmenopausal women, fat tissue is the most important site of estrogen synthesis and estrogen is deemed one of the most important risk factors for breast cancer.

Indoles strongly influence the Phase 1 enzymes that alter estrogen potency, thereby reducing the risk for breast and endometrial cancers. The isothiocyanate sulforaphane is a very potent inducer of Phase 2 enzymes that block mammary tumor formation. As the table Phytochemicals: Which, What, and Where indicates, many other phytochemicals are capable of inducing Phase 1 and Phase 2 enzymes. Although numerous vegetables and fruits provide these phytochemicals, the most notable are the cruciferous vegetables of the Brassica family (bok choy, broccoli, brussels sprouts, cabbage, cauliflower, collard greens, kale, mustard greens).

The powerful antioxidant effect of various polyphenols and terpenes is another mechanism by which phytochemicals may reduce cancers.

Carotenoids are the source of yellow-to-red pigmentation in plant cells. Beta-carotene is historically the most well known carotenoid; however, more than six hundred have been identified, of which at least fifty are presumed to be absorbed and metabolized. So far the role of just a few is understood in relation to human nutrition. Each one seems to be specific in the cells it protects. However, their activity is thought to be enhanced when they're mixed, as in a varied diet. Although they are found in many foods (see the table on pages 381ff.), carrots, tomatoes, and green leafy vegetables are the main sources in the North American diet. Evidence strongly supports a role in reduced risk of lung and other surface tissue (epithelial) cancers.

Another way phytochemicals may help battle cancer results from their effect on blood cell growth, or angiogenesis. Angiogenesis refers to the formation of new blood vessels, a process essential for normal reproductive function, growth, and wound repair. However, in some disease states angiogenesis becomes uncontrolled, wreaking havoc. For example, formation of new blood vessels is critical for tumors to grow. Cancerous tumors actually stimulate angiogenesis, causing rapid growth and spin-off cells that slip into the bloodstream and establish secondary tumors or metastases. On the other hand, a malignancy that can't induce new blood vessels is unable to survive. Because tumors are fast growing, anything that interferes with angiogenesis has the potential to starve the cells and halt tumor growth. Drugs that inhibit angiogenesis are being used to treat cancer. Some phytochemicals exhibit antiangiogenic properties, including isoflavones, found in cruciferous vegetables, and lignans, most prominent in soybeans but also derived from a number of vegetables and fruits. One good lignan source, seaweed, popular in nonwestern diets, could easily be incorporated into our meals as well (see the recipes for Orange-Arame Salad and Sea Vegetable Topping).

Phytochemicals and the Heart

A number of phytochemicals appear to reduce the risk of coronary heart disease by suppressing total cholesterol production (certain polyphenols and triterpenes) and via antioxidant capability, preventing the oxidation of LDL cholesterol, which damages artery walls. Some phytochemicals protect against heart attacks and strokes by reducing blood platelet aggregation, which might otherwise lead to dangerous blood clots. The polyphenols classified as flavonoids and phenolic acids, as well as thiosulfinates, act in this manner. Many researchers have declared the ability of flavonoids to inhibit platelet activity more profound than that of aspirin, which is recommended as a safeguard by numerous physicians. Another mode of flavonoid action is the strengthening of vascular tissue, thereby improving circulation. In addition, phytochemicals (flavonoids and catechins) help regulate blood pressure.

Evidence strongly suggests that carotenoids decrease the risk of coronary heart disease in a manner separate from their antioxidant effect. Animal experiments show that certain carotenes reduce lesions on arterial walls. Another mechanism that has been proposed to explain how carotenoids might work is by helping to relax the arteries.

Other Protective Paths

Phytochemicals exhibit the potential to act against many perplexing and debilitating health conditions. For example, because of their ability to alter enzyme production, flavonoids could help subdue many inflammatory ailments, including arthritis, fibromyalgia, asthma, and colitis, among others. Their influence on estrogen metabolism is being investigated in relation to enhanced bone strength. Their inhibitory effect on tyrosine protein kinase, an enzyme connected to retroviral gene expression, makes them a candidate for study in the fight against HIV/AIDS.

The protection afforded by certain vegetables against degenerative eye diseases is discussed later in this chapter. Credit goes to the specific carotenoids lutein and zeaxanthin.

Uncontrolled angiogenesis (discussed above in Chemoprotection and Phytochemicals) is also a factor in rheumatoid arthritis and diabetic retinopathy. Cruciferous vegetables, soy products, and seaweeds are among the foods containing antiangiogenic isoflavones and lignans.

PHYTOCHEMICALS: WHICH, WHAT, AND WHERE

The actions of phytochemicals, as outlined below, are based on credible (peer-reviewed) published research, mostly using rodents and other small animals fed either specific foods or phytochemical extracts. This research doesn't guarantee these effects in humans at levels consumed in foods, nor are the presumed actions cited here all-inclusive. At this time, information comparing absorption or performance of phytochemicals among various food sources is unavailable.

Phytochemical	Presumed Action	Food Sources
INDOLES	Indoles promote production of enzymes that detoxify and/or remove carcinogens; stimulate enzymes that alter estrogen potency, offering protection against estrogen-related cancers of breast, endometrium, and uterus; show protection against lung, stomach, and liver cancers in animal studies.	cruciferous vegetables of the Brassica family (bok choy, broccoli, brussels sprouts, cabbage, cauliflower, chard, collard greens, kale, mustard greens)
POLYPHENOLS	Polyphenols are the most widely distributed group of phytochemicals, appearing in every plant family. They are active antioxidants. Various polyphenols block cancer at the initiation stage, preventing damage to DNA; others inhibit activity of enzymes involved in cancer promotion and progression. Their anticancer potential has been associated with colon, esophagus, lung, liver, pancreas, mammary, and skin cancers in particular. Polyphenols also inhibit coronary heart disease.	see below

The Healthiest Diet in the World

Phytochemical	Presumed Action	Food Sources
Catechins (Flavanols)	Catechins, in general, are potent antioxidants, protecting unsaturated fats in particular; protective effect against lymphomas caused by radiation; protect skin from damage by ultraviolet rays; antimutagen; deactivate carcinogens; inhibit tumor production in skin, lungs, esophagus, stomach, colon, liver, pancreas, and breast; influence estrogen and testosterone metabolism; suppress excessive elevation of blood cholesterol, especially LDLs; help prevent rise in blood triglycerides by interrupting the absorption of fats; inhibit activity of vasoconstrictive enzymes and in this way may prevent or even reduce high blood pressure; inhibit growth of bacteria that cause dental plaque and cavities; inhibit enzyme required by HIV virus to initiate AIDS.	see below
Catechin/Epicatechin	as above	apples, avocado, bananas, cherries, cranberries, figs, millet, peaches, plums, grapes, raspberries, strawberries, tea (green, oolong, black), wine
Epicatechin Gallate	as above	avocado, green tea
Epigallocatechin	as above	apples, green tea, wine
Gallocatechin	as above	apples, green tea, grapes, raspberries, wine
Theaflavins and Thearubigens	as above	black tea (produced from catechins during manufacture)

Phytochemical	Presumed Action	Food Sources
Flavylium compounds (sometimes classified as Flavanols)	The flavylium class of polyphenols scavenge free radicals, exhibiting potent antioxidant activity in lung tissue; decrease tumor growth; reduce elevated blood cholesterol and curb oxidation of LDL cholesterol; enhance activity of vitamin C; strengthen collagen tissue and vascular walls; improve peripheral circulation; have a positive effect on eyesight, especially in regard to diabetic retinopathy; prevent blood cell clumping.	see below
Anthocyanins and Anthocyanidins	as above	apples, apricots, asparagus, bananas, bilberries, blackberries, blueberries, cherries, corn, cornmeal, cranberries, currants, eggplant, figs, kidney beans, lima beans, mangoes, millet, mung beans, oats, olives, peaches, peanut skins, plums, pomegranates, raspberries, red cabbage, red grapes (also grape juice and raisins), red onions, red wine, rhubarb, rice, rye, soybeans, straw-berries, wheat
Proanthocyanidins	as above	apples, avocado, bananas, blackberries, cornmeal, figs, grapes, millet, oats, peaches, plums, raspberries, wine

Phytochemical	Presumed Action	Food Sources
Flavonoids	The flavonoid category of polyphenols are antihistamines; anti-inflammatory; anti-infectious against bacteria and viruses, even in the small quantities found in food; scavenge free radicals; inhibit oxidative changes in LDLs that lead to atherosclerosis; decrease blood platelet stickiness; decrease blood pressure; block enzymes that produce estrogen and reduce risk of estrogen-induced cancers.	see below
Flavanones	In general, flavanones protect cells from oxidation damage; reduce risk of breast cancer; slow growth of breast cancer cells; decrease tumor size.	see below
hesperetin/hesperidin	as above	grapefruit, lemons, oranges, tangerines, tomatoes
naringenin	Inhibits enzymes that influence drug metabolism and can thus alter the effect of certain drugs (e.g., inhibits certain calcium channel blocker drugs).	grapefruit, lemons, limes, oranges, tomatoes
Flavones	In general, flavones decrease platelet stickiness; in animals, inhibit tumor growth in extremely low concentrations; activate cancer-fighting enzymes in esophagus and pancreas; protect cells from damage by transforming carcinogens into nontoxic products.	see below
apigenin	Inhibits conversion of androgens to estrogens.	barley, buckwheat, celery, chamomile, endive, grapefruit, honey, lemons, millet, oats, oranges, parsley, soybeans, wheat

Phytochemical	Presumed Action	Food Sources
luteolin	as for flavones	artichokes, barley, buckwheat, celery, lemons, oats, parsley, red bell peppers, sesame seeds, wheat
nobiletin	In animals, suppresses growth of all types of breast cancer cells, as well as reducing effects of carcinogens in lung and liver.	oranges, tangerines
tangeretin	Blocks entry of cancer cells into normal tissues; in animals, suppresses growth of all types of breast cancer cells and shows protective effect in lung and liver; inhibits invasive tendency (metastases) of malignant tumors in mice.	oranges, tangerines
Flavonols	In general, the flavonoids known as flavonols are free-radical scavengers (antioxidants); protect LDL cholesterol against oxidation; decrease platelet stickiness; may inhibit colon cell proliferation.	see below
kaempferol	as above	apricots, bananas, blueberries, bok choy, cranberries, currants, endive, fennel, garlic, grapefruit, kale, leeks, lima beans, mangoes, millet, peaches, red raspberries, strawberries, sweet potatoes, tea (black, oolong, green), wine
myricetin	as above	blueberries, cranberries, grapes, tea (black, oolong, green), wine

Phytochemical	Presumed Action	Food Sources
quercetin	Reduces inflammation and allergies; inhibits absorption of carcinogens from digestive tract; inhibits oxidation of LDL; inhibits experimentally induced skin and lung cancers; inhibitory action on growth of human leukemia cells and squamous cell cancers of head and neck.	apples, apricots, bananas, barley, blackberries, blueberries, broccoli, brussels sprouts, celery, cherries, cranberries, currants, fennel, grapefruit, grape skins, green beans, honey, kale, kidney beans, lemons, lettuces, mangoes, millet, mung beans, onions, parsley, parsnips, peaches, pears, potatoes, radishes, red bell peppers (capsicum), red raspberries, red wine, strawberries, tea (black, oolong, green), tomatoes
rutin	as for flavonols	asparagus, buckwheat, capers, coriander, currants, honey, tea (green, oolong, black)

Phytochemical	Presumed Action	Food Sources
Isoflavones	The polyphenols called isoflavones inhibit activity of enzymes involved in the conversion of normal cells into cancerous cells; block estrogen from entering cells, possibly reducing the risk of breast, ovarian, cervical, endometrial, and prostate cancers; may also inhibit lung and colon tumors; the isoflavone derivative ipriflavone protects bone mass in several experimental models of osteoporosis; in postmenopausal women with low estrogen, isoflavones have an estrogenic effect, thus their real value may be an ability to properly balance estrogen activity.	see below
Daidzein		soy products, kudzu
Genistein	Antiangiogenesis (inhibits new blood vessel formation and may thereby suppress tumor growth, rheumatoid arthritis, and diabetic retinopathy); antiestrogen; influences steroid hormone metabolism; inhibits enzymes that promote tumor initiation, particularly in the breast, brain, and prostate.	cruciferous vegetables (bok choy, broccoli, brussels sprouts, cabbage, cauliflower, chard, collard greens, kale, mustard greens), soy products
Lignans	The polyphenols known as lignans exhibit antiestrogenic or estrogen-balancing activity; associated with reduced incidence of breast cancer; antiangiogenesis; inhibit enzymes that promote tumor formation and malignant cell proliferation; potent antioxidants; help regulate cholesterol metabolism in rat studies.	flaxseed, sesame seeds, other oilseeds; soybeans; lignan precursors also found in a variety of plants, including whole grains, legumes, vegetables, fruit, seaweeds

Phytochemical	Presumed Action	Food Sources
Phenolic acids and other polyphenol compounds (many are precursors of lignans)	In general, this group of polyphenols shows promising antioxidant activity; blocks tumor initiation and growth at many sites, including skin, breast, lung, colon, and stomach; exhibits blood sugar–lowering capabilities.	various phenolic compounds have been found in herbs and spices, including sage, rosemary, marjoram, basil, oregano, thyme, parsley, celery, cardamom, ginger, nutmeg, cinnamon, allspice, cloves, cumin, fennel
Caffeic acid	Prevents certain procarcinogens from becoming carcinogenic, including nitrates and aflatoxins; assists in production of enzyme that enhances excretion of carcinogens.	apples, basil, citrus fruits, green coffee beans, garlic, pears, potatoes, radishes, soybeans, sunflower seeds, thyme
Capsicum (capsaicin)	Antioxidant (scavenges free radicals, thereby inhibiting cellular destruction); analgesic; antiplatelet aggregant; anti-inflammatory; cardiotonic; antiulcer; induces sweating; inhibits formation of carcinogens.	cayenne, chile pepper, red bell pepper
Chlorogenic acid	Prevents formation of carcinogenic nitrosamines; inhibits tumor promotion; anti-inflammatory.	blueberries, coriander leaf (cilantro), potatoes, sunflower seeds, tomatoes
Curcumin	Antimutagen; anti-inflammatory; cholesterol-reducing effect in rats; blood sugar–lowering effect in human studies; inhibits initiation and promotion of skin, breast, colon, and gastrointestinal cancers in rodents.	curry powder, ginger, some prepared mustards, turmeric

Phytochemical	Presumed Action	Food Sources
Ellagic acid	Antioxidant; prevents certain procarcinogens from becoming carcinogenic; inhibits activity of compounds that initiate cancer and prevents tumor growth; in animal studies, exhibits potent activity against skin, lung, esophageal, small intestine, liver, and pancreatic tumors; reduces genetic damage caused by tobacco smoke and air pollution.	apples, blackberries, cranberries, grapes, pears, plums, pomegranates, raspberries, strawberries, tea, walnuts
Ferulic acid	Binds to nitrates and prevents them from becoming cancer-causing nitrosamines; antiestrogenic; anti-inflammatory; antioxidant; dilates arteries; reduces platelet stickiness.	fruit, sesame seeds, soybeans, whole grains
TERPENES		
Carotenoids	Carotenoids are the most well known of the phytochemical family known as terpenes.	see below
Carotenoids	Carotenoids are yellow-to-red-colored compounds synthesized in plant cells. Over 600 have been identified, and while at least 50 are presumed to be absorbed and metabolized by humans, so far the role of just a few is understood. Each seems to be specific in the cells it protects; however, their activity is thought to be enhanced when mixed, as in a varied diet. Evidence especially supports a role in reduced risk of lung and other surface tissue (epithelial) cancers. Specific carotenoids (listed below) also act as protective agents against cataracts, macular degeneration, and heart disease.	see below
Carotenes	Carotenes in general are antioxidants. While some are precursors of vitamin A, carotenes also have direct actions on the body.	see below
alpha-carotene	Antioxidant; suppresses tumor growth; vitamin A precursor.	carrots, pumpkins

Phytochemical	Presumed Action	Food Sources
beta-carotene	Antioxidant; vitamin A precursor.	apricots, broccoli, cantaloupes, carrots, dill, leafy greens, leeks, mangoes, parsley, pink grapefruit, pumpkins, red peppers, sweet potatoes, tomato products, winter squash
lycopene	Exceptionally potent antioxidant; inhibits growth of cancer cells at many sites, including lung, breast, endometrium, mouth, esophagus, stomach, colon, rectum, prostate; suppresses growth stimulated by insulinlike growth factor and this is protective against breast and endometrial cancers; reduces oxidative damage to skin from ultraviolet rays, thereby reducing risk of photodamage due to sunburn and skin cancer; suspected role in protecting LDL cholesterol from oxidation and reducing heart disease.	dried apricots, guavas, pink grapefruit, tomato products, watermelons
Monoterpenes	In general, the carotenoids called monoterpenes are also antioxidants, and stimulate removal of carcinogens by the liver.	carrots, cruciferous vegetables, squash, tomatoes, as well as foods below
limonene	Stimulates production of enzymes that detoxify carcinogens and enhances their removal; in animal studies, stops growth of cancerous tumors in breast and lung, and causes existing breast tumors to regress.	caraway seeds, cardamom, citrus peel, coriander, fennel seeds, garlic, mint, nutmeg, thyme
perillyl alcohol	Prevents cancerous tumors from forming in mammary glands, lung, stomach, liver, and skin of mice; causes regression of malignant pancreatic tumors in laboratory animals.	cherries

Phytochemical	Presumed Action	Food Sources
Xanthophyll	This group of carotenoids is protective against cancers and age-related macular degeneration.	see below
beta-cryptoxanthin	Antioxidant; blocks development of tumors in cervical and uterine tissues; may afford protection against UV-induced skin cancers; vitamin A precursor.	mangoes, oranges, papayas, peaches, prunes, tangerines, winter squash
lutein	Exceptionally potent antioxidant; protects against lung, breast, uterine, prostate, and colorectal cancers; decreases risk of age-related macular degeneration.	most abundant in kale, spinach, and other dark leafy greens (amaranth leaves, beet greens, chicory, collards, mustard greens, Swiss chard, turnip); notable amounts in broccoli, brussels sprouts, celery, corn, dill, endive, green beans, green peas, leaf lettuce, leeks, lima beans, okra, parsley, pumpkins, prunes, red peppers, romaine lettuce, scallions, strawberries, summer squash, sweet potatoes, watercress, winter squash
zeaxanthin	Antioxidant; destroys free radicals in blood and body fluids; decreases risk of age-related macular degeneration.	apricots, corn, green peas, oranges, papaya, peaches, prunes
Triterpenes	A less well known, but important category of terpenes with antitumor activity.	see below

Mentor

Phytochemical	Presumed Action	Food Sources
Soyasaponins	Interfere with DNA replication in tumor cells, preventing cancer cells from multiplying; may block cell receptors for estrogen, thereby inhibiting breast, cervical, uterine, and other estrogen-related cancers; bind with bile acids and cholesterol in colon, with possible protective effect against colon cancer; potent antioxidant; inhibitory activity against HIV virus and Epstein-Barr virus infections; antitumor; hypolipidemic (decrease blood fats).	soybeans and other legumes, including kidney beans, chickpeas, mung beans, peas
Glycyrrhizin	Antitumor promoter; suppresses transformation of estrogen into more cancer-stimulating form, or possibly prevents estrogen from binding at specific sites; increases interferon activity; antiulcer activity; anti-inflammatory.	licorice root
THIOSULFINATES (Organosulfides)	The compounds in this family all support the production of enzymes that deactivate various cancer-causing compounds and are capable of suppressing tumor initiation and tumor progression.	see below
Allyl sulfides	Inhibit cancer-causing chemicals; increase production of enzymes that protect against initiation and proliferation of cancer cells; observational studies in humans suggest a protective effect against stomach cancer, while animal studies indicate inhibition of tumor growth in skin, stomach, lung, liver, esophagus, and colon; antimicrobial; inhibit platelet aggregation.	allium vegetables (chives, garlic, leeks, onion, scallions, shallots)

Phytochemical	Presumed Action	Food Sources
Glucosinolates	The phytochemicals in this group stimulate production of enzymes that increase the ability of the liver to detoxify carcinogens and protect against cell mutation. Adverse effects have also been attributed to glucosinolates, including increased pancreatic cancer in some rodent studies, and in large concentrations a negative impact on the goiter (although these goitrogenic phytochemicals are heat-sensitive and thus diminished or destroyed by cooking).	cruciferous vegetables (arugula, broccoli, brussels sprouts, cabbage, cauliflower, chard, collard greens, horseradish, kale, mustard greens, radishes, watercress)
Dithiolthiones	In rat studies, afford protection against cancers of lung, trachea, stomach, colon, breast, skin, liver, and bladder.	Brassica family of cruciferous vegetables (bok choy, broccoli, brussels sprouts, cauliflower, collards, chard, kale, red and green cabbage
Isothiocyanates	In animal experiments, inhibit tumor growth in the esophagus, mammary gland, liver, lung; may blunt the effect of at least one carcinogenic compound in cigarette smoke.	Brassica vegetables (see above), kohlrabi, mustard greens, radishes, rutabaga, turnips, watercress
sulforaphane	Exceptionally potent isothiocyanate inducer of enzymes that increase ability of liver to detoxify carcinogens and protect against cell mutation.	Brassica vegetables (with highest amounts in broccoli), horseradish, mustard greens

393

Mentor

Herbs and Spices: Health-Enhancing Flavorings

Most herbs and spices appear in folk remedies that purport to have healing powers. Modern scientific methodology has made it possible to analyze many of these flavor-enhancing plants, and to an impressive extent, the health claims are well founded.

Although only eaten in small amounts, several herbs and spices exhibit antioxidant potential and promote activity of Phase 2 cancer-protective enzymes. Included in this list are oregano, rosemary, dill, celery seed, citrus peel, fennel, cardamom, coriander, mint, nutmeg, thyme, sage, and caraway.

A potent antioxidant phytochemical known as curcumin has been documented in turmeric, an ingredient in curry powder that is consumed in quite large quantities by many nationalities. One of the ways curcumin acts is to block the mutagenic effects of a chemical that is concentrated in a type of cigarette known as "bidi," commonly smoked in India, where turmeric is a popular seasoning. It has been linked to lower rates of colon cancer, and there is some speculation that it might help offset exposure to sunlight. In Thailand, where turmeric is used in many traditional foods, there is a very low rate of skin cancer.

A huge body of research in this area has been compiled by Dr. James Duke, a retired USDA botanist. Before leaving the agency in 1995, he established the Phytochemeco Database—a list of all the known chemical compounds in more than one thousand edible plants, including most herbs and spices. He continues to update his work by reviewing articles in scientific journals every month. The objective of this mammoth undertaking is to help scientists figure out the most promising compounds to study for disease protection. What Duke has determined from his decades of research is that many popular seasoning ingredients are significant sources of cancer-fighting compounds.

Other popular flavoring ingredients that have been promoted for their medicinal qualities are garlic and onion (covered in Chapter 3), along with ginger and an assortment of hot peppers. Another less common, but quite interesting, candidate is licorice. These three foods are discussed below.

What's So Hot About Hot Peppers?

Capsaicin is the chemical in peppers that makes them taste hot. It acts as an antioxidant, an anti-inflammatory, and to inhibit blood platelet aggregation. Of considerable surprise to many people is the fact that it is considered useful against ulcers (perhaps due to an antibacterial action) and can topically serve as an analgesic (i.e., pain reliever).

Some concern has been voiced as to whether capsaicin might actually be a cancer promoter. A connection made in Mexico between stomach cancer and hot pepper consumption has been widely criticized. However, this doesn't rule out the possibility. In the United States, stomach cancer is among the top ten causes of cancer deaths among Hispanics, Asians, Native Americans, and African

Americans, but not among Whites. Indeed, there are many dietary and genetic factors to consider—relative intakes of spicy foods being among them.

Until further information is available, the best advice is to partake of chile-laden foods in moderation.

Ginger

Gingerroot has been used for thousands of years to treat a variety of conditions, including stomachaches, diarrhea, constipation, nausea, motion sickness, colds, flu, and many other ailments.

Many of ginger's pharmacological properties stem from its effect on prostaglandins, such as its profound ability to reduce blood platelet stickiness, which is considered more powerful than that of aspirin. Compounds found in ginger similarly reduce the inflammatory process. Clinical trials conducted by Danish researchers on patients suffering from muscle pain, osteoarthritis, and rheumatoid arthritis substantiate this. They found that an average of 5 grams of fresh ginger (which is approximately a $^1/_2$-inch piece or half a tablespoon minced) or 1 gram of dried ginger powder (1 teaspoon), when taken daily, greatly reduced pain for more than half of the osteoarthritis patients and almost 75 percent of the rheumatoid patients, with no notable side effects.

Ginger also demonstrates antioxidant activity. Twelve different compounds found in ginger exhibited greater potency in laboratory tests than vitamin E (alpha-tocopherol).

The spicy flavor of both the fresh root form and the dried powder is a culinary asset. It teams up especially well with beans (where it has the added value of reducing flatulence). Root vegetables make another good partner, as many of our recipes illustrate. Another favorite application is in beverages (such as ginger tea).

Licorice

Glycyrrhizin, a potent chemical found in licorice root, is deemed an antitumor agent, particularly in cases where estrogen acts as a promoter, such as in the colon and breast. It is also considered to have antiulcer and anti-inflammatory activity.

The health benefits of licorice have been recognized in China for more than five thousand years, where it is a popular remedy for relieving congestion of colds and flu, and soothing the pain of sore throats and ulcers.

People in the United States who want to try out its effects won't find it easy at this time, since real licorice (the only kind that contains the critical phytochemical) isn't found in most licorice-flavored foods, including the candy that goes by the same name. It is more common for manufacturers to employ anise oil or a synthetic substitute. Although anise, fennel, and licorice all have a similar flavor, only licorice contains glycyrrhizin.

Before setting off to search for real licorice, its potentially harmful effects should be noted. One that is well documented is licorice's ability to dramatically raise blood pressure. Glycyrrhizin is structurally similar to a hormone in the body called aldosterone that regulates sodium and water balance. Eating too much licorice can trick the body into performing the natural task of aldosterone, which is to conserve water and sodium, and excrete potassium. The initial side effect is a headache; if enough is eaten, it can cause blood pressure to soar. Thus, anyone with high blood pressure should be cautious when it comes to licorice, satisfying their taste buds with harmless anise oil.

Going Organic

Concern about pesticide use and other toxic residues from soil additives has led many people to question the value of commercially grown vegetables and fruit, especially in terms of cancer protection.

Any adverse effects imposed by farm chemicals must be weighed against probable benefits of consuming vegetables and fruit. Pesticide residue on plants is variable. A 1995 report by the Environmental Working Group ranked forty-two vegetables and fruits according to seven different measures of pesticide contamination. They concluded that more than half the risk of pesticide exposure comes from twelve vegetables and fruit (see box below). Choosing organic varieties of these foods, or limiting intake by substituting nutritionally comparable alternatives, could reduce pesticide consumption substantially.

★ ENVIRONMENTAL WORKING GROUP'S PRIZE FIVE AND DIRTY DOZEN* ★

Crops lowest in pesticides: avocados, sweet corn, bulb onions, cauliflower, asparagus.

Crops with the most pesticide residue, ranked in order starting at the top: strawberries, bell peppers and spinach (tied for second place), cherries (domestic), peaches, cantaloupe (Mexican), celery, apples, apricots, green beans, grapes (Chilean), cucumbers.

*Based on 15,000 food samples tested by the U.S. Food and Drug Administration during 1992 and 1993.

How Vegetables (and Fruit) Influence Your Health

Cancer

Evidence to date indicates that a diet high in vegetables and fruit may reduce the risk of several types of cancer. This is most firmly established for cancers of the lung, stomach, esophagus, pharynx, and larynx. Less persuasive but highly credible data support a decreased risk for cancers of the mouth, colon, rectum, cervix, pancreas, and bladder. Evidence is weaker but still favorable for hormone-related cancers, such as breast, endometrial, and prostate.

More than two hundred studies, looking at people all over the world and using a variety of assessment methods, designs, and analytical approaches, have yielded convincing findings in relation to vegetables and fruit. Regina Ziegler, M.D., with the National Cancer Institute, believes "this is the most consistently supported of all the diet-and-cancer relationships, including those pertaining to fat and calories."* She estimates cancer risk doubles for those eating the least as compared to those eating the most fruit and vegetables in a typical population. In the United States, only about one-fourth of the population is at the level that the National Cancer Institute sees as optimal. If lack of vegetables and fruit turns out to be causative, 10 to 30 percent of potential cancers could be prevented if everyone's intake rose to the recommended level of five to nine servings of vegetables and fruit a day.

The produce that most often shows up as protective is raw vegetables in general, followed by allium vegetables (garlic, onions, and their relatives, discussed in Chapter 3), carrots, green vegetables, cruciferous vegetables (notably broccoli, brussels sprouts, cabbage, cauliflower, and dark leafy greens), tomatoes, and citrus (in that order). This doesn't mean other varieties aren't of equal importance; they may not have shown up in studies simply because fewer people eat them on a consistent basis.

Overall, vegetables appear to be more protective than fruit. Fruit exerts its strongest influence on cancers of the upper digestive and respiratory tracts (mouth, pharynx, larynx, and esophagus). Some benefit from fruit is conceivable for cancers of the pancreas, liver, bladder, and cervix. The farther along tumors are in the digestive system, the less power fruit appears to wield. Most studies of lung cancer haven't looked closely at the role of fruit; however, a few studies examining lung cancer patients indicate a preventative role for fresh fruit, especially those rich in vitamin C. Some investigators even contend that this vitamin is more favorable than beta-carotene, on which most researchers have pinned their hopes (see the discussion of lung cancer that follows).

For hormone-dependent cancers such as breast, ovary, endometrial, and prostate, which are correlated with other dietary factors, there is no convincing evidence from population studies that overall fruit intake plays any protective part. On the other hand, breast cancer suppression is attributed to specific phytochemicals in citrus fruits, while lycopene (found in pink grapefruit, dried apricots, and tomatoes) has been shown to inhibit the growth of prostate and mammary tumors.

At least twenty-two studies of mice, rats, or hamsters have measured the effects of specific vegetables and fruits (primarily cruciferous vegetables, allium extracts, and citrus components) on experimentally induced cancers (using chemical carcinogens or irradiation). The majority unequivocally found that the animals

*From her presentation "Carotenoids and Human Cancer," at the meeting of The Olestra Project on Potential Effects of Reducing Carotenoid Levels on Human Health, held at the Harvard School of Public Health, January 17, 1996.

given the vegetables or fruit experienced either fewer tumors, smaller tumors, less metastases, less DNA damage, high levels of enzymes involved in the detoxification of carcinogens, or other outcomes indicative of lower cancer risk. Of course, the extrapolation of results of animal studies to human beings isn't conclusive, given species differences and the manner in which these experiments are designed.

We don't know what it is in many of these foods that deserves the credit. Initially, attention focused on the vitamins beta-carotene and C. Then people started to think about fiber, vitamin E, selenium, and folate. Certain phytochemicals are now being considered. In fact, an assortment of compounds have the potential to be effective, and a number of factors may be operating independently or in unison. What we currently know is so new that it certainly can't be considered definitive.

There is no reason why we have to wait for this puzzle to be solved. It's enough to recognize that vegetables and (perhaps to a lesser extent) fruit can protect our health, without deciphering exactly why.

Lung Cancer

Lung cancer risk goes down as vegetable consumption rises. Smoking remains the major risk factor, but even among smokers, vegetables—particularly dark green and yellow-orange ones—have a protective effect. (Because cigarette smoking is so detrimental, even with the best diet possible a smoker is still believed to have a much greater risk of lung cancer than a nonsmoker. Diet can modestly diminish the harmful effect of smoking, but it can't abolish it!)

Prospective studies—where a chosen group is followed for a set period of time during which diet, illness, and deaths are tracked—lend support to the link between lung cancer and vegetables and fruit. Of eight such studies, all show a protective effect. In eighteen out of twenty retrospective studies—in which data on individuals with a particular disease are compared to nonafflicted controls—lung cancer incidence decreased as reported vegetable and fruit intake increased.

Attempts have been made by researchers to qualify which elements in particular deserve the credit. As many as forty studies indicate that high blood levels of beta-carotene and increased intake of foods containing carotenoids (discussed earlier in Chemoprotection and Phytochemicals) decrease lung cancer risk. Various conclusions have been drawn regarding what to attribute this to. Since until recently relatively little was known about possible benefits of carotenoids other than beta-carotene, it was presumed that this was the effective agent. Knowledge accumulated within the last decade points to other health-promoting carotenoids.

It is in the area of lung cancer that we have been provided with one of the strongest arguments for food over supplements. Many population studies suggest that diets high in beta-carotene parallel a lower incidence of lung cancer. This gave scientists great hope for substantiating the relationship in clinical trials using beta-carotene supplements. To their great surprise, in the widely publicized

Beta-Carotene and Retinol Efficacy Trial (CARET), smokers taking the vitamin A and beta-carotene supplements developed lung cancer at significantly higher rates than those taking a placebo.

There have been many attempts to explain the outcome of the CARET study. It has been argued that the supplement was chemically synthesized rather than derived from food sources; that high concentrations of beta-carotene inhibited absorption of other protective nutrients; that beta-carotene in excess could be a pro- rather than antioxidant; that beta-carotene alone isn't effective, but in combination with some other substance or substances it affords protection; that alpha-carotene should have been considered rather than beta-carotene; that results using high-risk smokers as subjects can't be applied to the nonsmoking population; and that the apparent benefits of diets high in beta-carotene may have nothing at all to do with this vitamin, but actually reflect another constituent that is present in the same foods.

All these excuses represent different paths to the same conclusion: Food is more than a simple collection of isolated nutrients; when eaten in the whole form, what you get is what is intended to be there.

Gastrointestinal Cancers

There is strong evidence that increased consumption of raw vegetables of all types, as well as green vegetables (cooked and raw), reduces the risk of both stomach and colon cancers.

A large retrospective study of stomach cancer conducted in Italy, which pointed to a protective role for raw fruit as well, was among the first to recognize that the influence of vegetables and fruit couldn't simply be accounted for by vitamin C, as most people would have presumed a few years earlier. As discussed in Chapter 3, vegetables in the allium family such as onions, garlic, chives, scallions, leeks, and shallots (none of which offers notable amounts of vitamin C) have been isolated as particularly beneficial, possibly due to their ability to induce cancer-fighting enzymes, as well as their inhibition of cancer-causing nitrites.

Although attempts to prove a protective role for the fiber in grain and legumes have been inconsistent with regard to colon cancer, vegetables do appear to be beneficial. It's conceivable that fiber is just part of the protective mechanism. Folate, which is found in many plant foods and is particularly plentiful in artichokes, asparagus, avocado, bean sprouts and dried beans, beets, broccoli, brussels sprouts, leafy greens, and okra is associated with a reduction in both precancerous colon polyps and colon cancer itself.

399

Mentor

Breast, Prostate, and Other Hormonally Influenced Cancers

Studies indicate that higher consumption of vegetables and fruit may be connected to a modest reduction of breast cancer, in the area of 20 percent. Vegetables are consistently viewed as more influential than fruit, and green vegetables and carrots have both been singled out in some studies. As with other cancer studies, attempts to isolate particular food constituents haven't been productive. (However, as you will see from the table on pages 381ff., breast cancer suppression has been accomplished in animal experiments using several specific phytochemicals.)

The argument for the advantage of food over supplements is well summarized in a study of premenopausal women in upstate New York, where reduced cancer risk associated with increased vegetable intake was independent of such separate factors as vitamin C, vitamin E, folate, and fiber, and only mildly explained by certain phytochemicals. The conclusion drawn was "no single dietary factor explains the effect. Evaluated components found together in vegetables may have a synergistic effect on breast cancer risk; alternatively other unmeasured factors in these foods may also influence risk."

Development of abnormal cells in the cervix has been associated with marginal consumption of folate and vitamin A. If this is a causal relationship, dark green and leafy vegetables could reduce the risk for cervical cancer.

For prostate cancer, total vegetable and fruit intake shows no correlation. However, men whose diets include lots of tomatoes appear to have a reduced risk. This has been attributed to the specific carotenoid lycopene, which is plentiful in tomatoes and has potent antioxidant activity. Analysis of prostate tissue indicates the presence of lycopene in biologically active amounts, supporting this link. Processed forms of tomato (especially tomato sauce and tomato paste) appear to have a stronger influence than fresh tomatoes; one determinant may be that absorption or potency of lycopene is enhanced by heat or the simultaneous consumption of either oil or some form of fat. (Note that raw tomatoes are considered protective in other forms of cancer, particularly in sites along the digestive tract.)

Other Cancers

For bladder cancer, too, evidence of protective effects of green vegetables and carrots is particularly consistent.

Both vegetable and fruit consumption show some relationship to lowering pancreatic cancer risk. Frequent consumption of dried fruit among Seventh Day Adventists was rated as especially significant here.

Heart Disease

The classic Seven Countries Study, initiated in 1958 to follow 12,400 men from seven different countries, was the prototype for establishing a relationship between dietary fat, cholesterol, and heart disease (see Chapter 2). At the twenty-five-year follow-up, the research team declared that "from a public health perspective it is not enough to focus solely on serum cholesterol levels to decrease the burden of CHD [coronary heart disease] in populations. It appears that reductions in total serum cholesterol levels are not likely to bring cultures with a high CHD risk, such as the United States and Northern Europe, back to a CHD mortality level characteristic for the Mediterranean and Japanese cultures unless other factors are also changed." Those other factors are largely connected to vegetable and fruit consumption.

The quest to discover how vegetables and fruit protect against heart disease is ongoing. The antioxidant effect of vitamins C, E, and beta-carotene have been proposed, but researchers have been repeatedly disappointed by trials using supplements to substantiate this. One of the most highly regarded of these is the Physicians' Health Study, which followed more than 22,000 doctors in the United States who were given either a beta-carotene supplement or placebo for an average of twelve years. There was no sign of even a slight reduction in mortality from cardiovascular disease as a result of supplementation. This doesn't necessarily mean that antioxidant nutrients don't account for any of the beneficial effects of diet, but it might be that isolated from the original food source, their potential may not be fulfilled.

The relationship between some nutrients and heart disease may be subtle. For example, low blood levels of vitamin C are associated with a higher risk of heart attack and are also related to greater infection rates. A perceptive connection is proposed for these two circumstances: The production of infection-fighting prostaglandins raises plasma levels of the blood clotting factor fibrinogen, and thus susceptibility to infection could raise the risk of heart attack and stroke. The study illuminating this maintains that the pivotal determinant of vitamin C status is food, not supplements. Subjects deficient in vitamin C only needed the equivalent of about one orange to adequately boost vitamin C and reduce fibrinogen levels to a point associated with a 10 percent decline in coronary risk. This is in keeping with data from population studies demonstrating that where fruit and vegetable intake is marginal, adding two to three daily servings can lower stroke risk by 20 to 40 percent, and overall heart disease by about 25 percent.

Another interesting experiment was inspired by the observation that after an acute heart attack, blood levels of vitamin C tend to be low. To test the value of dietary intervention, a hospital in India provided a group of patients with a vegetable- and fruit-enriched diet as part of an overall fat-restricted menu during the first week following their heart attacks. The diet included 400 grams of vegetable/fruit each day—consistent with the amounts proposed in How Much Vegetables (and Fruit) Is Enough? Blood levels of all cardiac risk factors improved on this regimen compared with a control group given a diet with only half as much of these foods. In fact, the blood tests of participants who consumed extra vegetables and fruit (as much as 680 grams per day) exhibited even greater improvement. Short-term follow-up reported a decreased rate of repeat incidence, and a year later there were fewer deaths from all causes in the initial intervention patients.

Blood levels of various carotenoids have been tied in to heart disease: As the former goes up, coronary risk declines. When diets are matched against heart disease incidence the same pattern is witnessed. In the Health Professionals Follow-up Study, when beta-carotene consumption was calculated from food diaries, among the 40,000 men involved there was about a 30 percent reduction in risk for those in the highest fifth compared with those in the lowest fifth. The effect was attributed solely to food. Moreover, when the smokers in each of these sectors were compared, the spread was even greater, suggesting an enhanced benefit for men who smoke. Similar results were observed in the smaller but more focused Lipid Research Clinics Coronary Primary Prevention Trial and Follow-up Study (LRC-CCPT) of 1,899 men aged forty to fifty-nine with elevated blood cholesterol and triglycerides, but no preexisting heart disease or other major illnesses. Blood carotenoid levels (which are considered an accurate marker for dietary intake) were compared with coronary heart disease over a thirteen-year period. Among the nonsmokers, those in the top quarter had 60 percent fewer coronary events than those in the lowest quarter. Mortality rates declined to a similar degree. Smokers also fared better as their carotene levels improved, but this time to a lesser degree than nonsmokers.

Because most of the long-term studies of heart disease focus on men, there is some question as to whether women are similarly protected. The Nurses' Health Study, initiated in 1976, follows more than 87,000 female nurses without prior history of cardiovascular problems. When food intake was charted against eventual health outcomes, the risk of stroke was more than 50 percent higher for women in the lowest fifth of vegetable and fruit intake versus the highest fifth. Spinach and carrots showed the most correlation. In a high-risk female population (women with previous coronary incidents) diet emerges as even more determinative.

Among the countries taking part in the Seven Countries Study referred to at the beginning of this section, the Dutch researchers added another piece to the puzzle by investigating the foods most commonly eaten by the men with the lowest risk of coronary heart disease mortality in the study they conducted. Among the common denominators were apples, onions, and tea (discussed in Chapter 8). In other words, the men routinely consuming the most apples and onions (and tea) had the most favorable outcomes. A similar trend was seen in Finland. Analysis of these foods gives credit to the phytochemicals making up the category known as flavonoids. In a review of sixteen populations that were part of the Seven Countries Study, flavonoid intake explained about 25 percent of the variation in deaths from heart disease when viewed in conjunction with other risk factors, and on its own accounted for 8 percent of the risk reduction.

When risk reduction is associated with specific foods, as in the studies cited above, it's important to recognize that the vegetables and fruit routinely eaten by people living in the region being investigated are likely to be the ones that show up as protective. Other less common selections with similarly active nutritional components—kale instead of spinach, pumpkin in place of carrots, mangoes rather than apples—are presumed to be equally beneficial. The listing of foods containing specific nutrients that are cited throughout this chapter and in the table, Phytochemicals: Which, What, and Where, on pages 381ff., illustrate many more such examples.

Elevated levels of a compound known as homocysteine in the blood were discussed as a coronary risk factor in Chapter 3. The B vitamin folate, which helps control homocysteine accumulation, is easily provided by a diet ample in vegetables (see list of sources in Gastrointestinal Cancers, on page 399). But because of their food choices, as much as 40 percent of the U.S. population may be lacking this important nutrient.

Vitamin C and potassium, widely available in vegetables and fruit (with the most notable sources listed below), may reduce strokes as a result of their capacity to normalize blood pressure. Moreover, blood pressure levels don't appear to be adversely affected by salt intake when adults follow diets with adequate potassium, calcium (discussed in Chapter 7), and magnesium (introduced in Chapter 3). Furthermore, animal studies indicate that dietary potassium decreases the risk of stroke independent of its effects on blood pressure.

★ THE VITAMIN C TOP TWELVE ★

red and green bell peppers, guavas, citrus fruits, kiwis, broccoli, brussels sprouts, papayas, red and green cabbage, strawberries, kohlrabi, cauliflower, snow peas

---

A benefit from calcium is uncertain and may be limited to a subset population, just as salt affects blood pressure in only some individuals with hypertension and has little effect on people in the normal range.

The role of fiber in relation to heart disease was covered in Chapter 1. As noted there, it's often difficult to isolate the effect of fiber in food from other protective constituents. Nonetheless, as part of the total package, vegetable and fruit fibers are believed to positively influence outcomes as a result of their impact on cholesterol, insulin sensitivity, and blood clotting. Fiber, and fruit fiber in particular, also emerges as having a beneficial influence on blood pressure (although once again the concurrent presence of some other protective factor in fruit can't be ruled out).

Although fruit can furnish many of the same nutrients and phytochemicals as vegetables, a compounding factor may make it less useful in reducing coronary heart disease. As noted in earlier chapters, elevated triglyceride levels are associated

---

★ POTASSIUM PREFERENCES ★

Three to six servings per day of the following vegetables and fruit will add up to a reasonable 1,875 mg potassium: artichokes, arugula, avocado, bananas, beets, bok choy (Chinese cabbage), broccoli, brussels sprouts, cantaloupes, carrots, cauliflower, fennel, dried fruit, cooked greens, green soybeans, Jerusalem artichoke, kiwi, kohlrabi, fresh lima beans, mushrooms, okra, oranges, plantains, radicchio, rutabagas, soy sprouts, sweet potatoes, tomato puree, watercress, white potatoes, winter squash, yams, yucca (cassava).

To preserve potassium, use only a modest amount of liquid during cooking and consume this as well.

with lipoprotein profiles that are considered to be artery clogging (atherogenic). Diets high in carbohydrate, and sucrose and fructose in particular, elevate triglyceride levels. Thus, while modest fruit intake may be advantageous, too much fruit could tip the scales in the wrong direction.

Diverticulosis

Diverticular disease—outpouching and muscular weakness along the walls of the colon—is one of the most common disorders of the colon among older people in Western societies. In North America, an estimated one-third of the population over forty-five years of age, and two-thirds of those over eighty-five are affected, although only between 10 and 25 percent develop significant symptoms, which include abdominal pain, loose stools, and intermittent bouts of constipation and diarrhea.

What is particularly interesting about this disease is that, prior to the early part of the twentieth century, it was considered to be extremely rare. Due to this, and the fact that the condition remains uncommon in most developing countries, it has been dubbed "a twentieth-century problem" or "a disease of Western civilization." The popular interpretation lies in the parallel with fiber consumption between countries with high and low incidence.

Attempting to clarify this phenomenon, the Health Professionals Follow-up Study, initiated in 1986 to track heart disease and cancer in more than 51,000 U.S. males aged forty to seventy-five, matched diverticular disease against a variety of dietary factors. The results indicated grain fibers weren't of relevance; however, vegetable and fruit fibers were. The presence of more fermentable fiber in the vegetables and fruit has been offered as an explanation of their protective effect.

Diabetes

We've already discussed the protective role fiber can play in diabetes in Chapter 1. Again, the fiber in vegetables makes an enormous contribution. In experimental diets exhibiting significant improvement in insulin use, the fiber in starchy vegetables (including peas, corn, and legumes), combined with other vegetables, generally accounts for the largest benefits, followed by grains and then fruit.

Cataracts and Macular Degeneration

Vegetables and fruit are the only foods whose consumption hints at protection against degenerative eye conditions, including cataracts and macular degeneration.

Cataracts occur in about 4 percent of people age fifty-five to sixty-four years, 18 percent of those sixty-five to seventy-four years, and 50 percent of people seventy-five years and older. Studies analyzing the nutritional composition of diets and comparing them to cataract frequency suggest benefits from vitamin C and the carotenoids lutein and alpha-carotene. When blood carotenoids were assessed at the USDA Human Nutrition Research Center at Tufts, individuals with low levels showed a nearly sixfold increase in cataract risk relative to individuals with high levels. (Foods containing these phytochemicals are listed in the table Phytochemicals: Which, What, and Where, on page 381ff; for the Vitamin C Top Twelve, see page 403.)

Age-related macular degeneration (AMD) is caused by changes in the small central part of the retina of the eye called the macula. The macula is the part you use when you read, drive a car, and recognize faces. Damage to the macula can result in blurred vision, distortion, and, in many cases, blindness. In the United States, AMD affects about 10 percent of people who are sixty-five to seventy-four years old, and about 30 percent of those seventy-five and over. It is the leading cause of irreversible blindness among U.S. adults over age sixty-five, and there is no effective treatment. Although AMD usually doesn't manifest until the later years, it originates much earlier and evolves over decades.

People who routinely eat such vegetables as kale, spinach, and other dark leafy greens have a notably lower incidence of AMD. There's also a beneficial correlation with sweet potatoes and winter squash. It just so happens that these foods are abundant in lutein and zeaxanthin—the two carotenoids concentrated in the macula. These carotenoids help filter out blue light rays, to which this area of the eye is especially susceptible.

Since the body doesn't synthesize these carotenoids, lutein and zeaxanthin must be supplied by our diet. It should also be noted that they were only discovered in 1985, and even then few scientists guessed at their nutritional significance.

Less weighty evidence intimates that foods rich in vitamin C, vitamin E, and zinc may play a small protective role in visual health. Dietary vitamins C and E seem to be more influential in nonsmokers, who start out six times less likely to have AMD than smokers. (Note that trials using A, E, and C supplements report that they are of no help.)

Osteoporosis

In our Historic Perspective, we talked about the relatively recent attention paid to vitamin K and its presence in three proteins that influence calcium levels. Blood levels of vitamin K are generally low in hip fracture patients. Utilization of the bone protein osteocalcin is improved when vitamin K is introduced, and urine calcium loss, as well as other urine indicators of osteoporosis, diminishes.

Phylloquinone is the form of vitamin K found in plant foods, which are the primary dietary source of this vitamin. As discussed in Chapter 2, vegetable oils are potential contributors, particularly canola, soy, and olive oils, with lesser amounts in almond, safflower, sesame, sunflower, and walnut oils. Vegetables are the other principal source. In general, the greener the vegetable, the higher the vitamin K content. Moreover, higher concentrations are generally found in outer leaves. The vitamin K found in other vegetables and fruit resides primarily in the peel, compared with the fleshy portions. Vitamin K isn't well stored in the body, signifying the need for a continuous dietary supply.

Phylloquinone-rich foods include:

Dark leafy greens (beet greens, collards, endive, escarole, kale, mustard
    greens, spinach, Swiss chard, turnip greens, watercress)
Broccoli
Brussels sprouts
Cabbage
Looseleaf lettuce, especially romaine
Parsley

More modest contributions come from:

Artichokes
Asparagus
Avocado
Carrots
Cauliflower
Celery
Green beans
Green peas
Kiwi fruit
Okra
Pumpkin

The need to protect the vitamin K in oils from light was mentioned in Chapter 2. When it comes to maximizing levels obtained from vegetables, note that cooking has minimal impact, but providing some fat at the time of ingestion is important for vitamin K to be absorbed.

Another nutrient that has received minor attention is the mineral boron. For a long time considered insignificant, in the late 1980s studies at the U.S. Human Nutrition Research Center in Grand Forks, North Dakota, found that boron may be a key to preventing osteoporosis. After years of animal studies indicating that boron plays a role in regulating the nutrients and hormones involved in bone building, a six-month study began using twelve postmenopausal women. After switching from a low boron intake to an ample intake, urine analysis showed the women lost 40 percent less calcium and one-third less magnesium. More significantly, their blood levels of estrogen doubled, matching those of women on estrogen replacement. Measures of testosterone, which the body converts to estrogen, more than doubled.

Boron is found primarily in the plant kingdom and is highest in foods (and beverages) made with apples, grapes, cherries, pears, and broccoli (especially the florets). Other fruits, vegetables, herbs, and legumes offer some boron. There is very little in grains and almost none in animal products.

Calcium is the mineral most people associate with bones. In Chapter 7, the relationship between calcium, bone strength, and osteoporosis is covered quite extensively. What many people aren't aware of is the contribution vegetables can make to calcium intake.

NIKKI'S DIALOGUE BOX

Calcium from Vegetables

"People are usually stunned when I tell them they can eat foods other than dairy products in order to get calcium. In the fresh vegetable and fruit kingdom, for example, spinach, bok choy, beet greens, mustard greens, Swiss chard, kale, arugula, broccoli, okra, yucca, various seaweeds such as kelp, arame, hijiki, and wakame, and dried figs are all good sources. This is yet another example of the importance of diversity in the diet."

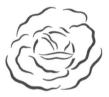

CHAPTER 5

In Praise of Soybeans

It's remarkable that with all we know about the benefits of soy foods, and the fact that approximately half of the world's soybean harvest is grown in the United States, we don't reap more of their benefits. It's time to acknowledge that with such a large soybean crop, soybean farming is as American as cattle ranching.

Even though the direct consumption of soybeans and the numerous foods that are made from them is quite limited in Western diets compared to those of the Pacific Rim, the growth of soy foods on the North American table has been phenomenal. In 1996, the Soy Foods Association of America reported that in the previous decade, sales of soy foods in the United States rose 350 percent.

Soy's Special Assets

What makes us so ardent about soybeans? Soy's special assets include:

• A variety of phytochemicals with both antioxidant and direct cancer-fighting capabilities.

• Natural estrogenlike compounds that may block hormone-induced cancers, such as those of the breast and prostate, help maintain bone strength, and reduce side effects of menopause.

• An ample supply of protein that compares favorably with beef, but without the high levels of saturated fat found in most animal foods. In fact, soy protein has been identified as heart-protective.

• A good source of fiber, which may be one way soybeans help stabilize blood sugar, reduce cancer risk, and lower blood cholesterol levels.

• Phytosterols that help reduce cholesterol levels and thus may offer additional protection against heart disease. (For a discussion of plant sterols, turn to page 340.)

• The essential linoleic and linolenic fatty acids that make up the roster of healthy fats (see Chapter 2).

• Lecithin, choline, and biotin, vital elements discussed in Chapter 3 that, among other roles, assist the body's use of fats and support the production of neurotransmitters and other messenger molecules responsible for sending messages to the brain and central nervous system.

Soybeans are also kinder to the environment than animal protein foods and help share resources more equitably. They conserve land use by providing fifteen times more protein and using 200 percent less water than an acre of land devoted to beef, according to the trade publication *Natural Food Merchandiser*. Moreover, soybeans enrich the soil by adding nitrogen.

The Phytochemical Furor

The excitement about phytochemicals has given a huge boost to the reputation of soybeans. Among the various phytochemicals found in soy, the most notable are the polyphenol isoflavones genistein and daidzein, lignans, and the terpenes known as soyasaponins. Soybeans are the most commonly eaten food that contains appreciable amounts of these phytochemicals.

Isoflavones appear to inhibit the activity of enzymes that participate in the conversion of normal cells into cancerous cells. They block estrogen from entering cells, possibly reducing the risk of breast, ovarian, uterine, endometrial, and prostate cancers. They may also inhibit lung and colon tumors. In postmenopausal women with low estrogen, isoflavones have an estrogenic effect, so perhaps their true value is an ability to properly balance estrogen activity. An isoflavone derivative known as ipriflavone protects bone mass in studies investigating osteoporosis.

The isoflavone known as genistein, which is especially abundant in soy, has the additional attribute of being an especially strong inhibitor of angiogenesis. This means it stifles new blood vessel formation and may thereby prevent tumor growth and metastasis, as well as other diseases dependent on angiogenesis such as rheumatoid arthritis and diabetic retinopathy. Interestingly, data clearly show that genistein specifically targets overactive, proliferating cells. This means that it's unlikely to disturb the desirable formation of new blood vessels for reproductive function, normal growth, and wound healing.

There are also indications that genistein protects the cells lining the blood vessels, deterring the buildup of fatty deposits that cause arteries to become constricted and susceptible to life-threatening blood clots. Genistein may even help prevent blood clots from forming.

Isoflavones such as genistein and daidzein are found in just a few botanical families and make only a small appearance in the modern American diet. Their presence has been confirmed in soybeans, soy sprouts, soy nuts, soy flour, and such derivatives as soy milk, tofu, tempeh, and miso. Levels in low-fat soy milk and low-fat tofu are less certain, however. Some studies claim that products such as tempeh and miso, which rely on fermentation, show higher availability.

(Although the addition of nonsoy ingredients such as rice, barley, or other grains to some varieties of tempeh and miso dilutes their isoflavone concentration, they remain noteworthy sources.) Fermentation also changes the nature of these isoflavones. The implications of this aren't clear, but some researchers feel these altered forms are more easily absorbed by the body and exhibit increased antioxidant strength.

Isoflavones in soy sauce and soy cheese appear to be minor. Soy protein concentrates and soy protein isolates manufactured using alcohol extraction also display minimal amounts of isoflavones. As a result, textured vegetable protein (TVP), meat analogs, infant formulas, and other supplemental soy formulas made from these soy proteins will likewise be insignificant. (The water-extraction method of preparing soy proteins preserves isoflavones, but there's currently no way to determine how products on the market have been prepared; the soy industry has proposed standardized levels of isoflavones for some isolated soy protein products.) Analysis of frozen desserts such as Tofutti, which is made from soy protein isolates, shows insignificant amounts of isoflavones; in brands prepared using the whole beans, such as Ice Bean, isoflavone content rises.

The typical Asian diet includes 25 to 100 mg of isoflavones daily, which is considered a good model. This is the amount found in from 4 to 12 ounces of a variety of soy products.

The lignans in soybeans also have estrogen-balancing activity, are antiangiogenic, act as potent antioxidants, and in animal studies regulate cholesterol metabolism.

Soyasaponins, found in soybeans as well as other legumes, interfere with DNA replication in tumor cells, preventing cancer cells from multiplying. They also may block the entry of estrogen, thereby inhibiting breast, cervical, uterine, and other estrogen-related cancers. Another way in which soyasaponins work is to bind with bile acids and cholesterol in the colon, decreasing levels of lipids in the blood and conferring a possible protective effect against colon cancer. They're particularly strong combatants against free radicals, and even show inhibitory activity against HIV and Epstein-Barr virus infections. Note that the alcohol-extraction of soy proteins removes saponins.

Other phytochemicals found in soy include anthocyanins, the flavone apigenin, which inhibits conversion of androgens (male hormones) to estrogens, caffeic acid, and ferulic acid (see Phytochemicals: Which, What, and Where, on pages 381ff. for more information).

Protein Plus

In Chapter 6, we discuss the body's need for dietary protein. To be considered a reliable source of protein a food must provide two components: (1) The amino acids—or building blocks of protein—that are nutritionally indispensable; these amino acids must be supplied by food in order for the body to effectively carry out its protein-dependent activities. (2) Nonspecific nitrogen needed for the synthesis of additional amino acids and other physiologically important nitrogen-containing compounds. It is the availability of specific indispensable (or essential) amino acids that accounts for the difference in caliber of various food sources of protein.

The protein value of foods—alternately referred to as their biological value, protein efficiency ratio, or net protein utilization—is based on their assortment of amino acids, as explained in the discussion of eggs on page 361. Our bodies need a certain amount of each amino acid in order to build protein. If one is lacking, this process slows down or ceases altogether. While these amino acids can be combined from many different sources, individual foods that have the right proportion of the essential amino acids have the highest biological value. Because the essential amino acids in eggs come closest to matching the ideal usable pattern, egg protein is considered the model for rating all other foods.

According to numerous methods of analysis, soybeans contain all the amino acids required to meet both childhood and adult needs. Thus they would suffice even if they were the only dietary source of protein, which is unlikely for most people. Their biological value is comparable to that of beef or milk.

Since soybeans have an abundance of the essential amino acid tryptophan, they're a more reliable source of protein than most other beans, which lack this amino acid. Their protein is also more concentrated, so that soybeans have about twice the protein content of other legumes, such as chickpeas, kidney beans, or lentils.

The protein in soy has been commended for its heart-protective effect. Studies investigating soy's ability to reduce blood cholesterol focus on about 40 grams of soy protein, but indicate that benefits arise from daily soy protein intake of as little as 17 to 25 grams. Protein levels of various soy products are shown in Mixing and Matching Soy Protein, on page 412, and can be used to meet the suggested goal of 25 grams a day or more.

Soy Fiber

Dietary fiber is believed to have physiological functions, such as assisting the passage of waste matter through the intestinal tract, as well as health-protective potential. All of this is covered in Chapter 1. Recommendations for fiber intake vary, but by all accounts the average North American diet is lacking. A suggested range for adults is 25 to 50 grams a day. Soy foods can help by furnishing:

- 11 grams fiber per cup of cooked dried soybeans
- 7.5 grams fiber per cup of cooked green soybeans
- 7 grams fiber per 1/2 cup of dry roasted soybeans (known as soy nuts)
- 7 grams fiber per 4-ounce serving of tempeh
- 3.5 grams fiber per 1/4 cup soy flour

Soybeans contain both soluble and insoluble fibers. Soluble fibers are generally credited with a cholesterol-lowering and blood sugar–stabilizing effect, and indeed studies indicate that soy has both of these capabilities. (Note that because

★ MIXING AND MATCHING SOY PROTEIN ★

Food	Amount	Protein (grams)*
Soybeans		
fresh green	1 cup	22
dried, cooked	1 cup	28
roasted (soy nuts)	1/2 cup	32
Soy sprouts	1 cup	8
Soy flour		
full-fat	1/2 cup	15
defatted	1/2 cup	20
Tofu		
extra firm	4 ounces	14 to 16
firm	4 ounces	11
regular	4 ounces	9
soft	4 ounces	9
silken	4 ounces	6
Tempeh		
all-soy	4 ounces	24
soy + grain	4 ounces	12 to 21
Soy milk		
full-fat	8 ounces	6 to 10
low-fat	8 ounces	4
fat-free	8 ounces	3
Miso		
all-soy	1/4 cup	8

*Compiled from manufacturers' data and The Food Processor® Nutrition Analysis Software, ESHA Research, Salem, OR. Values may vary by brand.

current methods of determining fiber composition are still crude, it could be that soy fiber is considerably different than reported.)

Vitamins and Minerals

With all the talk about such recently recognized food constituents as phytochemicals, phytosterols, and fiber, the old standards tend to fade into the background. This doesn't lessen their importance. Soybeans are a powerhouse of many long-prized vitamins and minerals, and some of them are receiving renewed interest.

The vitamin E content of soy is of particular interest because the majority of its tocopherol content isn't as alpha-tocopherol, long believed to be the only active form, but as gamma- and delta-tocopherols. As discussed in Chapter 2, noted cancer researcher Bruce Ames and his colleagues have determined that gamma-tocopherol is actually more protective against certain mutagenic compounds than alpha-tocopherol. They believe it may play a role in fighting cancer, heart disease, and other degenerative diseases. Moreover, it could be that various forms of tocopherol complement each other, making their mutual presence most advantageous.

Other nutrients for which soybeans are renowned include biotin, lecithin, and choline. The B vitamins thiamin, riboflavin, niacin, and folate are all found in the soybean, as are the minerals calcium, iron, zinc, potassium, phosphorous, and magnesium. Not all of these nutrients remain in every one of the products formulated from the bean, however. Whereas soy tempeh, soy nuts, and soy flour all furnish notable amounts of calcium, the calcium contribution of soy milk and soy cheese is minimal. (Many soy milks are now fortified with calcium to come closer to the nutritional profile of cows' milk.) The calcium value of tofu varies, depending on whether the coagulant used in the manufacturing process is a calcium or a magnesium salt. Iron, zinc, and folate levels in soy milk are much lower than in other traditional soy foods, and soy sauce doesn't add any recognized nutrients other than sodium.

Soy Concerns

Despite soybeans' numerous attributes, they aren't perfect.

One consideration is the presence of compounds known as protease inhibitors. Protease inhibitors bind to digestive enzymes and reduce the body's ability to digest and utilize the beans' inherent protein. (Although protease inhibitors interfere with the action of many enzymes, they are often generically referred to as trypsin inhibitors.)

Protease inhibitors are dramatically reduced by heat or fermentation. It's unlikely that anyone would choose to eat soybeans raw. In the case of most soy-based products, protease inhibitors are diminished during manufacture. Thus, the soy food most likely to pose a problem is the sprouted bean, which should always be cooked before eating.

Although some soy bashers make a big deal out of the ability of protease inhibitors to interfere with protein digestion, raw potato contains twice the amount as raw soy flour, and raw eggs are comparable. Furthermore, cooked potatoes and hard-boiled eggs contain relatively higher levels of protease inhibitors than toasted soy flour does. (If soy products make up a substantial part of the diet, one way to allay any concerns you might have is to take supplemental enzymes to assist digestion.)

Protease inhibitors may also have some positive effects. For example, they're thought to suppress enzyme production in cancer cells, thereby slowing tumor growth. This may be one way in which soy protects against cancers of the breast, prostate, and colon.

There is also a concern that despite the beans' attractive nutritional profile, their minerals may not be readily available to us. In fact, minerals from many plant foods are poorly absorbed by humans. Because certain crucial minerals aren't widely consumed in the typical U.S. diet, this issue merits attention.

Published reports based on animal studies point to poor zinc availability from soy. What has been shown, however, is that the processing employed to prepare soy products greatly influences the body's use of the minerals they contain. The presence of phytic acid in soybeans is the main culprit, and the way in which soy foods are manufactured affects phytic acid content. For example, fermentation of the bean to make such products as tempeh and miso breaks down almost all of the phytic acid and enhances mineral availability. Cooking also reduces phytic acid. Ultimately, inhibition of minerals appears to be most problematic in the least traditional, high-tech soy products such as soy protein concentrate and isolated soy protein. These are the fabricated forms used by industry as filler and often in processed products like soy cheese and meat analogs. In addition, while the availability of zinc in soy may be reduced by phytic acid, there's no indication that zinc provided by other foods is obstructed by the presence of soy.

A similar situation exists with calcium. When phytic acid is present, calcium absorption can be reduced by about 25 percent. The impact of this is mainly on those who rely exclusively on soy as a source of calcium, such as infants on soy formula or adults taking soy formula as supplemental feeding. As you will read below in the discussion of cancer in Soy for Health, phytic acid may play a helpful role as well.

Iron is another mineral that is poorly absorbed from all legumes, including soy. Once again this doesn't seem to extend to iron from other sources. The fact that soy products are relatively high in iron partially makes up for its low availability. Moreover, the iron uptake from soy—as with all legumes—can be greatly assisted by the simultaneous presence of vitamin C. Therefore, coupling soy foods on the menu with tomatoes, peppers, cooked greens, potatoes, citrus, and similar C-rich foods improves their nutritional worth.

Because isoflavones influence hormones, concern has been expressed about the suitability of soy for children, and the effects it might have on both female and male fertility. In Asian populations that eat soy on a regular basis, and have done so for centuries, no such problems have been seen. (However, soy is a relatively new food in Western diets.) In our opinion, as with any food, soy is meant to be a part of a varied diet, and not the sole or necessarily even the principal protein. Traditional foods that are made from the whole bean provide nutrients in the balance intended by nature. These foods are the ones worth noting.

Soy Food Selection

Does eating more soy mean we're recommending an Asian diet laden with tofu? Not that long ago this might have been the case, but anyone who has visited a natural food store recently knows things have changed when it comes to the choice of soybean-based products. Yes, tofu is there (and in many supermarkets); in fact, now there are even several types of tofu to choose from.

What's so exciting for all those who want to take advantage of soy's enormous potential is that the legume is now available in a myriad of forms, so that it wouldn't be far-fetched to say that it is virtually a convenience food. Thanks to centuries of Asian culinary ingenuity and modern technology, the benefits of soy can be enjoyed without ever eating it in the shape of the bean (although a dish of soybeans can indeed be delicious).

In addition to traditional soy products (discussed below), food manufacturers now make soy foods with Western taste buds in mind—everything from soy cheese to soy-based imitation meat to soy ice cream. As noted earlier, when concentrated soy protein or soy protein isolate is the starting point, these items may lack the native constituents of the whole bean. The addition of fats, sugars, and various food additives may further compromise their value. Because most of the evidence of soy's beneficial effects is based on foods that have been popular in the Pacific Rim for generations—tofu, tempeh, soy beverages, and miso, for example—they should be given priority, along with products made from them.

As you can see from our recipes, dishes using soy foods appeal to a broad range of tastes and time constraints.

Stick with Traditional Soy Foods

The soy foods described here are available in natural food outlets and Asian markets, and are becoming more common in supermarkets as well. Directions for storing soy foods can be found in "The Golden Pantry."

Tofu

Tofu, also known as soybean curd, is a soft cheeselike substance. To make tofu, soybeans are soaked overnight, ground, cooked, and then filtered. The result is a milk that looks a lot like cows' milk. Next a coagulant is added and the soy milk separates into curds and whey. The selected coagulant, noted on the ingredients list, determines the calcium content of the finished product. When calcium sulfate or calcium chloride is used as a coagulant, a 4-ounce serving of firm tofu contributes about 160 to 230 mg calcium; if only a magnesium coagulant (or nigari) is listed, the calcium level drops appreciably, to around 50 mg. (Within these parameters, the firmer the tofu, the higher the calcium. Thus, soft and regular varieties made with a calcium coagulant would have relatively less calcium, and extra firm tofu, more.)

After the curds form they're pressed to remove a portion of the residual moisture. The degree of pressing determines the type. Tofu varieties include:

- Extra firm and firm, which are dense and solid
- Soft, which has less water pressed out, resulting in a delicate texture
- Silken (sometimes referred to as Japanese), manufactured in a different way to produce a more creamy product

The firmer the tofu is, the more concentrated its nutrients. Low-fat varieties of tofu, manufactured from specially processed beans, may not measure up to full-fat tofu. For example, analysis for protective isoflavones reveal that low-fat tofu is lacking.

Today, most of the tofu on the market comes in sealed plastic packages. They should be dated with last date of recommended sale. Some markets offer "bucket tofu," where blocks of tofu are displayed in an open container. This is the traditional marketing format, but hygiene is difficult to control. Japanese-style silken tofu is sold in shelf-stable packages that don't need refrigeration until they're opened. Several preseasoned varieties are available as well.

Tofu is quite bland and easily absorbs the flavors of other ingredients it's cooked with.

Tempeh

Tempeh is the traditional form of soybean consumption in Indonesia. Its dense chewy texture has been compared to that of tender chicken cutlets, while its taste has been described as smoky, nutty, and mushroomlike. When prepared from a combination of soybeans and grains, the flavor becomes rather mild.

The manufacture of tempeh knows no parallel in Western cuisine; the closest process is perhaps the making of blue cheese. To make a slab of tempeh, prepared soybeans are incubated with a mold known as *Rhizopus oligosporous*. After about twenty-four hours, a cottony matrix of fine threads (called mycelium) bind the soybeans into firm cakes. (The harmless mycelium may appear as white or gray areas on the surface.) Sometimes the beans are mixed with a grain such as rice, millet, or quinoa.

The fermentation involved in tempeh production increases the digestibility of the protein and reduces the flatulence that some people experience when they eat beans. As noted earlier, it also modifies the structure of the isoflavones, which human studies show enhances their availability. Other positive changes include an increase in the B vitamins riboflavin, niacin and nicotinic acid, pantothenic acid, folate, and biotin, and a decrease in fat content.

Tempeh made with soy alone has the highest protein content. When grains are added the protein content, although still quite high, is reduced (see Mixing and Matching Soy Protein on page 412).

Tempeh is sold in refrigerated slabs and, while capable of many culinary incarnations, makes particularly great burgers (see recipe page 39). Note that unlike tofu, tempeh must be cooked before eating.

Soy Milk

Soy milk is the rich creamy milk of whole soybeans. The preparation of soy as a beverage has been practiced for a long time in Asia. The standard Asian soy drink is quite beany in taste. New processing techniques that have been applied since the 1980s have greatly improved the flavor, and the shelf-stable (aseptic) box it's typically packaged in makes it long-lasting and convenient. A limited amount of fresh soy milk is sold from the dairy case (sometimes referred to as soy dairy milk). Soy milk is also available powdered, in which case it must be mixed with water. Because powdered soy milk is usually made from a concentrated soy protein rather than the whole bean, its protein and fat content may differ from traditional soy milk's, and it may not be a reliable source of isoflavones.

A growing number of people are using soy milk instead of cows' milk. According to research conducted by Spence Information Services, 44 percent of soy products sold in 1996 were in the beverage category.

Different brands of soy milk vary considerably in both nutrition and flavor, so you may want to compare and taste several to see what you prefer. In cooking, it's difficult to discern much difference between dairy and nondairy milks. In comparison to whole cows' milk, soy milk has less fat, a different proportion of fatty acids (mostly unsaturated, with both omega-3s and omega-6s), and no cholesterol. Many soy milks are fortified with calcium, vitamin D, and vitamin B_{12} to improve their nutritional profile. Unlike cows' milk, soy milk made from the bean also contains isoflavones and soysaponins. Some other aspects of the nutritional issue are presented in Nikki's Dialogue Box, below.

Soy Nuts

Soy nuts are prepared from whole dried soybeans that have been soaked in water and roasted. They have the nutritional value of the whole bean and make an excellent snack food.

NIKKI'S DIALOGUE BOX

Just Because They Call It "Milk": Nondairy vs. Dairy

"Soy milk, dairy milk, and all the other nondairy milk alternatives work equally well in recipes and most other applications. However, using them to replace one another has significant nutritional implications. Some of these you will be able to detect from the nutritional panel on the label. Other less obvious effects include how they alter fatty acid balance, blood sugar levels, insulin release, steroid and regulatory hormones, and other influential elements that derive from these factors.

"Soy, rice, oats, and almonds are all used in the production of retail dairy milk substitutes. The nutritional content shown on their labels reveals that fat, protein, and carbohydrate composition of these products can be quite dissimilar. They even vary from brand to brand. How meaningful this is depends on your overall diet. Considerations might include whether or not you rely on these beverages for protein or calcium, and the effect their increased carbohydrate might have on blood sugar and insulin levels. Note that the G-Force of soy and other nondairy milks hasn't been measured.

"Among the popular brands of soy milk on the market, the amount of protein for full-fat products ranges from 6 to 10 grams per 8-ounce serving, and the carbohydrate content ranges from 13 to 18 grams, of which 7 to 12 are in the form of sugars. Low-fat soy beverages contain only 4 grams of protein and 14 to 15 grams of carbohydrate, of which sugar is 4 to 9 grams. Fat-free soy beverages generally contain even less protein and a little more carbohydrate. (What doesn't show on the label is the loss of important isoflavones in fat-reduced soy milks.)

"Other nondairy 'milks,' such as rice milk, oat milk, and almond milk, are much lower in protein than soy and dairy milks (only 1 to 4 grams in 8 ounces) and can have anywhere from the same to twice the amount of carbohydrate."

Mentor

Whole Soybeans

Soybeans, which grow in a pod like peas and other legumes, can be harvested when the bean is still green and cooked fresh. The Japanese call these "sweet beans" or "edamame." They're available in Asian markets both fresh in season and frozen, as are canned shelled green soybeans, which are sold in natural food stores as well.

As soybeans mature in the pod they ripen into hard, dry beans. Most dried soybeans are yellow; however, there are brown and black varieties. Dried soybeans can be cooked like any other dried beans.

Soy Sprouts

Whole dried soybeans can be sprouted like any other bean to produce a nutritious vegetable. Sprouting increases the isoflavone level and generates notable amounts of vitamin C. Soy sprouts should be cooked prior to eating to deactivate the protease inhibitor contained in raw soybeans.

Soy Flour

Soy flour is made by grinding roasted soybeans into a fine powder. There are four kinds of soy flour available: Full-fat soy flour contains the natural oils found in the soybean; defatted soy flour has the oils removed during processing. In between are high-fat soy flour, made by adding soy oil back to defatted soy flour at a level slightly less than the full-fat variety, and low-fat soy flour, with about one-third the fat of full-fat soy flour. All give a protein boost to recipes.

Soy Grits

Soy grits are similar to soy flour, but here the roasted soybeans are milled into coarse pieces rather than a fine powder. Soy grits can be cooked as cereal alone or along with grains for added protein.

Soy Sauce

Soy sauce is one of the few soy foods familiar in North America. Unfortunately, soy sauce has few of the attributes of the bean it derives from. Nonetheless, traditionally made soy sauce warrants a place in the kitchen as a flavorful seasoning agent (see "The Golden Pantry").

Miso

In Japan, the fermented soybean paste known as miso is the characteristic flavoring in many foods, including the famous miso soup. This rich, salty condiment is prepared by inoculating rice with a bacteria, mixing this with soybeans (and often a grain such as rice or barley), plus salt and water, and then aging the mixture in cedar vats for one to three years. The bacterial strain used in the

The Question of Salt

"The effect of sodium on blood pressure, and in turn the risk of heart attacks and strokes, has always been controversial. There are sound studies supporting a relationship, and equally convincing reports discounting one. Maintaining a moderate sodium intake is undoubtedly good advice. This is judged to be in the range of 2,500 to 3,000 mg sodium per day. Salt (regardless of whether it is land or sea salt) is the principal contributor, with 2,100 mg sodium per teaspoon.

"The food industry makes a greater impact on most people's sodium intake than the salt shaker. By following a diet consisting largely of unprocessed foods this can be minimized. Taking note of the sodium content listed on the nutrition panel of food labels is another way to reduce the impact.

"Some popular soy foods are high in sodium. Most soy-based meat analogs would be tasteless without the addition of high-sodium seasonings. Moreover, some basic soy condiments such as soy sauce and miso add a heavy dose. (One teaspoon of soy sauce contributes from 270 to 345 mg sodium; one teaspoon of miso adds around 210 mg sodium.)

"Despite its high sodium levels, miso may actually have blood pressure–lowering capability. This is accomplished by the presence of short chains of amino acids (known as peptides) that inhibit the action of an enzyme that promotes hypertension. Substances that act in this way are known as ACE inhibitors. A particularly potent ACE inhibitor is formed during the fermentation process used to make miso."

process is *Aspergillus oryzae*, and it produces a product with particularly high antioxidant activity.

The flavor of miso varies according to how long it's aged and the variety. Lighter misos with added grains are milder and sweeter than the robust, dark, all-soy products.

Okara

Okara is the pulp that remains after soy milk manufacture. It has a high fiber content and less protein than the whole soybean; however, the protein remaining is of high quality. Okara is used in some commercial meatless sausages, burgers, and similar products. It also has the potential to be added as fiber to granola, cookies, and other baked goods (where it tastes similar to coconut).

Natto

This rather exotic soybean product is made of fermented, cooked whole soybeans. It has a sticky, viscous coating with a cheesy texture. In Asian countries natto traditionally is served as a topping for rice, in miso soups, and is used with vegetables. It can be found in Asian food stores. Although regarded as a premier soy food, natto is quite foreign to the Western palate and, we admit, not to our liking because of its unusual consistency.

Soy for Health

Soybeans are documented in the Asian diet as early as 3,000 B.C., and have been grown commercially in the United States since World War I. Nevertheless, most of the research looking into their potential health benefits didn't begin until the early 1980s.

As is apparent from this chapter, we are very impressed with the health potential of soy foods. However, finding out which of the elements in soybeans have positive health benefits, and in what amounts, is a monumental and complex task. As research continues, progress is being made and will go on. It must be noted, though, that current enthusiasm in the media sometimes surpasses the data.

Cancer

Breast, Prostate, and Other Hormonally Influenced Cancers

In countries where people eat substantial amounts of soy foods, such as Japan, China, and Korea, breast cancer rates are much lower than in the West and death from prostate cancer is minimal. (In the United States, these are the second most lethal cancers in women and men, respectively.)

The link between breast, ovarian, uterine, cervical, endometrial, and prostate cancers, and possibly colon cancer as well, is that they all appear to be sensitive to sex hormones. Scientists suspect that diet can similarly influence them all.

Because the isoflavones in soybeans closely resemble human estrogen, the potential for soybeans to mimic its negative effects has been questioned. Specifically, if these phytochemicals behave so much like the natural hormone, couldn't they raise a woman's risk of breast and ovarian cancer? In fact, they're touted for doing just the opposite.

Explaining how this happens isn't simple, since it seems to contradict much of what we know about estrogen's relationship to certain cancers. For example, inside breast tissues, estrogen can encourage cancerous tumors to develop. But in order to do so, the estrogen must enter the tissues, a feat accomplished with the aid of estrogen receptors within breast cells that facilitate its uptake.

The explanation most researchers give as to how phytoestrogens work is that the potency of phytoestrogens is just a fraction of that of human estrogen. While they're close enough in structure to fit into the estrogen receptors, they're too weak to stimulate them. By acting in a competitive manner, they block the entry of the more potent, cancer-promoting hormone. Direct studies on human breast cancer cells in the laboratory, some dating back to 1978, confirm the ability of isoflavones to act in this manner. This argument makes sense to cancer researchers because the anticancer drug tamoxifen is thought to work in the same way.

Another hypothesis is that the lengthening effect phytoestrogens have on a woman's menstrual cycle decreases her lifetime exposure to estrogen. At the onset of each cycle until ovulation women experience a surge of estrogen. From ovulation to menstruation, which is known as the luteal phase, estrogen diminishes.

Therefore, the longer the luteal phase and thus the longer the time between periods, the fewer the number of estrogen surges during the reproductive years. This reduced exposure to estrogen may lessen the occurrence of estrogen-related cancers.

Of course, it's possible that other dietary, lifestyle, or genetic factors make Asian women less prone to breast cancer. For example, the fact that Asian girls begin menstruating later than American peers, and thus are exposed to estrogen for fewer years, could be due to overall calorie intake. That is, American girls take in more calories and lay down fat stores earlier, a prerequisite for ovulation to occur. The possibility that breast cancer is genetically determined is less likely, since descendants of Asian immigrants living in the United States have much higher breast cancer rates than their ancestors. Even within their native environment, Chinese women with breast cancer have been shown to eat less soy than comparable Chinese women who are cancer free.

Additional support for a dietary explanation comes from comparing blood hormone levels of vegetarian women, omnivores, and women with breast cancer. The hormonal pattern evidenced in women with breast cancer resembles that seen in meat-eating women whose diets are low in fiber and high in animal fat, whereas vegetarian women with diets rich in plant foods exhibit a distinctively different range of values. Their profile is similar to that of Japanese men and women consuming a traditional diet emphasizing soy, rice, vegetables, seaweeds, and fish. Most significant is the variance in levels of the hormone called sex-hormone-binding globulin (SHBG), which influences the clearing rate for sex hormones. High levels of SHBG, seen in the women consuming vegetarian diets and in the Japanese study, are associated with lower sex hormone activity.

Just as phytoestrogens limit breast cancer in women, they may also reduce prostate cancer in men. The hormone testosterone is responsible for the development of numerous male characteristics. But once a man develops prostate cancer, testosterone can hasten its progression. If phytoestrogens can harness testosterone, the path of prostate cancer can be altered.

The likelihood of this is reflected by the fact that in Asia, where phytoestrogen-rich soy foods are popular, the ratio of deaths from prostate cancer is dramatically less than that in the United States. It isn't that Asian men aren't afflicted with this cancer. In fact, autopsies indicate similar incidence in both populations. But their tumors grow so slowly that the Asian men tend to die from other causes long before the tumors become lethal. (Moreover, the average life expectancy for Japanese men is about four years longer than for American men, so their rate of survival may be even greater.)

There are a few theories as to how phytoestrogens might accomplish this. One is that estrogen slows down production of the male hormone testosterone, a factor that has led to the use of female hormones to treat prostate cancer. If phytoestrogens act like estrogen they can perhaps have the same effect. The ability of phytoestrogens to stimulate liver synthesis of SHBG, and thereby decrease the biological activity of male hormones, could also contribute to this protective effect. In addition, there is good experimental evidence that isoflavones inhibit an enzyme that converts testosterone to a more proliferative form within the prostate itself. Men might be comforted to know that although phytoestrogens may alter testosterone's activity, unlike hormone therapy, they do so without compromising masculinity.

Another way in which isoflavones might arrest prostate cancer is by obstructing the growth of blood vessels that normally form around prostate tumors and nourish them. It was noted earlier, in The Phytochemical Furor, that genistein and to a lesser degree lignan, which are both abundant in soy, exhibit this antiangiogenic ability.

An important aspect of this account is that the bacteria present in the gastrointestinal tract play an important role in the body's ability to make maximum use of isoflavones. Intestinal bacteria are activated by fiber—and particularly resistant starches, which were discussed in Chapter 1. Soybeans are a good source of resistant starch. (For other foods containing resistant starch, see page 293.) Foods that are fermented or cultured with bacteria, such as tempeh, miso, and yogurt, also make a contribution. (Antibiotics, on the other hand, can wipe out these helpful bacteria.)

Other Cancers

Most of the attention to soy's cancer-protective action focuses on its hormone-inhibiting capabilities; however, the ability to act against other forms of cancer is likely. For instance, the isoflavone genistein inhibits the action of the Phase 2 enzymes, including tyrosine kinases, discussed in Chapter 4. These enzymes promote tumor growth in a wide range of cancers; consequently, the power of genistein may be widespread.

Studies of mice show that dietary intake of genistein stimulates the activity of antioxidant enzymes in the skin and small intestine. In a skin cancer study, genistein significantly lengthened the period in which tumors remained dormant and stifled tumor growth. The researchers at the University of Alabama who conducted these studies noted that the high level of genistein in soybeans makes them a "promising candidate" for the prevention of human cancers.

Genistein's antiangiogenic ability, which prevents the formation of new blood vessels, is an additional powerful mechanism by which tumor growth and the spread of cancer to other sites is halted.

Soyasaponins are another of the presumed anticarcinogens in soybeans. Studies in which human cancer cells were directly exposed to soyasaponins showed an inhibitory influence on growth and proliferation.

Ironically, animal studies also show that the protease inhibitors, which for years detracted from the soybean's image, may now be one of its selling points. Protease inhibitors were one of the first compounds identified in foods to inhibit the promotion of experimentally induced cancer. In a variety of experiments, protease inhibitors derived from soy have suppressed the activity of carcinogens in different animal species and at different sites, including the colon, liver, lung, esophagus, and mouth. While consuming raw soybeans as a cancer-prevention measure certainly isn't advisable due to the potentially negative actions of protease inhibitors, the fact that not all protease inhibitors are destroyed by cooking or various processing procedures may add to the cancer-fighting capability of soy.

While some nutritionists criticize soybeans because of their phytic acid content, researchers at the University of Maryland applaud the soybean for just this reason. In their laboratory studies on rats, phytic acid halted the growth of experimentally induced cancer tumors in the colon.

Heart Disease

Early animal studies, followed by human trials, have led to a general consensus that dietary soy protein is cardioprotective compared with a variety of animal proteins.

In the late 1970s, a team of Italian scientists from the University of Milan began to investigate the use of soy protein to reduce cholesterol. What they found was that when patients with elevated cholesterol levels were switched from a standard low-fat diet to a similar diet containing soy protein in place of all animal protein, most of them displayed a striking reduction in cholesterol. This occurred mainly in the undesirable low-density lipoprotein (LDL) fraction, with no significant reduction in high-density lipoprotein (HDL). They were able to dupli-

423

Mentor

cate this effect in people with familial hypercholesterolemia, a genetic form of elevated cholesterol that doesn't respond to conventional intervention, such as low-fat diets, and therefore is usually treated with cholesterol-lowering drugs.

Soybean farmers have a lot to gain if North Americans can be enticed to eat more soy foods. To help them realize this dream, the University of Illinois, located in a major soy-growing state, has commenced research to provide the incentive. Since most prior studies focused on men, they looked at reducing cholesterol levels in a group of women volunteers. For six months, the women agreed to add soy protein at every meal, adding up to 40 grams daily. The school provided them with baked goods containing isolated soy protein and soy protein powder for drinks. After six months, LDL cholesterol had gone down about 8 percent, and HDL was elevated by about 4.5 percent.

A scientific analysis of thirty-eight studies designed to test the effect of soy protein on cholesterol levels revealed positive outcomes in thirty-four of them. The most marked changes typically occur in people who start out with the most unfavorable cholesterol profiles. On average, those with extremely high levels (over 300 mg/dl) show decreases of as much as 24 percent. Even subjects with normal initial levels are able to lower them by around 7.7 percent. Unlike many other dietary intervention models, where preferred HDL levels often go down along with LDL, soy maintains HDL and may even produce a small increase. Triglyceride levels also respond favorably when soy foods are added to the diet.

The medical community maintains that every 1 percent reduction in cholesterol decreases heart attack risk by 2 to 3 percent. If so, based on the thirty-eight-study review, people in the highest risk population could possibly reduce their chances of a heart attack by as much as 48 to 72 percent just by eating about 50 grams of soy protein daily. Even if these figures are exaggerated, a mere 8 percent decrease in cholesterol levels would translate to 16 to 24 percent less risk. While the more soy protein consumed, the greater the effect, researchers conclude that as little as 17 to 25 grams of soy protein per day can be meaningful.

The mechanism by which soy wields its cholesterol-reducing powers is probably multidimensional. Most researchers give credit to the protein faction, but can't explain exactly why.

One interpretation of the cholesterol-lowering effect is the proportion of specific amino acids in soybeans. Soy protein has a relatively high ratio of arginine to lysine compared with animal proteins. Animal studies show that arginine induces changes in blood levels of the thyroid hormone thyroxine, along with other related hormones. Likewise, feeding soy to laboratory animals consistently elevates plasma thyroxine levels. Furthermore, this change in thyroxine precedes changes in cholesterol concentrations. In humans, high plasma thyroxine is generally accompanied by satisfactory total and LDL cholesterol.

An additional argument in favor of the arginine-lysine balance is the role arginine plays in a factor in the blood called endothelium-derived relaxing factor (EDRF). EDRF (discussed on page 329) relaxes arteries and also decreases blood platelet stickiness. EDRF is the compound nitric oxide, for which arginine is a

Twenty-five grams of soy protein a day?

"Several times this chapter has targeted 25 grams of soy protein per day as a protective amount. I recognize that this may seem unreachable if you aren't accustomed to eating soy foods. The key is to find places within your diet to easily integrate soybeans, tofu, tempeh, soy milk, soy flour, and miso. While it isn't very difficult to accomplish this, the process may be different for everyone. Some will pour soy milk on cereal or drink it in shakes; some will eat tempeh burgers and scrambled tofu; adding soy flour to baked foods will add to other people's intake; and for everyone, snacking on soy nuts can help fill in. In addition to the numerous recipes found in 'In Nikki's Kitchen,' here are some simple ways to go about adding more soy foods to your daily diet:

"Snack on roasted soy nuts alone, or turn into a trail mix with nuts, whole-grain ready-to-eat cereal, and dried fruit. Or try this Japanese snack: Boil fresh unshelled soybeans in salted water until tender and eat out of the pod as a treat. (Snacking on soy not only supports Golden Guideline #5, but also the goal of eating more than just three times a day.)

"Purchase preseasoned tofu and tempeh in the natural food store for quick sandwich fillings; add tofu cubes to soups during the last 10 to 20 minutes of cooking; top salads with chunks of plain or seasoned tofu or (cooked) tempeh; prepare chili with crumbled tofu or tempeh and use to fill tacos or burritos; add strips of tofu or tempeh when stir-frying vegetables; marinate tofu and tempeh in your favorite barbecuing sauce and cook on the grill. You can also dice tofu or tempeh into bite-size pieces and simmer in marinara sauce for 10 minutes to serve over pasta.

"Try soy milk as a beverage on its own, cold or hot. (If taste is an issue, try mixing it with dairy milk and decreasing the proportion over time.) Create shakes by blending with fruit and ice; pour on cereal; use to lighten coffee and tea; use in place of dairy milk in baking, sauces, and other favorite recipes.

"If you bake, replace up to one-fourth of the flour in muffins, pancakes, cookies, and quick breads with soy flour. (As soy flour has a tendency to brown quickly, lower the cooking temperature by 25 degrees or check for doneness ahead of schedule to prevent overbaking.) When making yeast breads, substitute 1 to 2 tablespoons soy flour for this amount in each cup of wheat flour called for. (Because soy flour lacks gluten, which gives structure to yeast breads, it must be used in lesser amounts than in baking powder–leavened products.)

"You can also use soy flour instead of eggs to bind ingredients; for each egg omitted, use 2 tablespoons soy flour mixed into a paste with an equal volume of cold water. In addition, soy flour can be used as a thickener for gravies, sauces, and soups. (Use about twice the amount of wheat flour called for.)

"To add more miso, try this when you make soup or stew: Before turning off the heat, stir 1 to 2 tablespoons of miso into each quart or every four servings. Cover, remove from the heat, and let sit a few minutes for the flavors to meld. (A good approach is to mix a little of the hot soup or stew with the miso in a separate bowl to make a smooth, loose paste. Then add it back to the hot pot. Miso is more nourishing if it isn't subjected to high temperatures, which is why this technique is preferred.) You can also use miso as a flavoring in salad dressings. (It's a good substitute for anchovies in Caesar salad.) For some tasty dips and spreads, mix miso with nut butters, yogurt cheese, mashed tofu, or pureed beans."

precursor. People with high cholesterol levels have reduced concentrations of EDRF in their arteries, indicating a relationship between the two.

Another proposition is that diets high in soy protein affect cholesterol generation by altering bile production and loss. However, this theory has fallen out of favor with a number of researchers, who propose that soy may have a more direct impact on liver production of cholesterol.

Some researchers admit that perhaps another constituent may be influential. For example, the fiber in soybeans, like other forms of fiber discussed in Chapter 1, may be beneficial to people with elevated cholesterol levels. Or perhaps the phytic acid or minerals play an important part.

The potential estrogenic activity of soy isoflavones suggests a heart-protective role based on the well-established evidence that natural estrogen protects premenopausal women from heart disease relative to men of the same age. Studies on monkeys point to the isoflavones in soy as a central mechanism, independent of any cholesterol lowering. They appear to be a deterrent to LDL cholesterol oxidation, which many researchers believe damages arterial walls, initiating the accumulation of artery-clogging plaque. It has also been proposed that isoflavones act by keeping blood platelets from clumping and forming clots that can plug blood vessels. Blood-thinning drugs (including aspirin) are a common therapeutic approach to coronary artery disease. That isoflavones can act similarly has been demonstrated in the laboratory but awaits confirmation in live species.

Diabetes

People with diabetes respond quite differently to foods than normal people as far as blood sugar levels are concerned. Repeated experiments indicate that soybeans, like other legumes, are particularly useful in modulating blood sugar responses. The fiber content is one explanation, apparently delaying the release of glucose and fatty acids into the bloodstream. This has the effect of modifying the rise in blood sugar, as well as decreasing blood triglyceride synthesis. Moreover, unlike that of most other legumes, the overall carbohydrate content of soybeans is low. Thus they are a good choice for anyone concerned about glucose tolerance.

A further benefit from soy foods is envisioned due to their isoflavone content. In the earlier discussion of soy's role in cancer prevention, its ability to inhibit the activity of tyrosine kinase enzymes was mentioned. Although there isn't uniform agreement on this subject, data indicate that tyrosine kinases take part in a negative feedback system that depresses insulin release, resulting in high blood sugar levels. Administration of genistein in a laboratory setting blocks this action, increasing insulin release appropriate to rising glucose levels. This may enable some diabetics to control blood sugar more effectively.

Osteoporosis

There is a lot of enthusiasm about the part phytoestrogens might play in preventing postmenopausal bone loss and osteoporosis.

The lumbar region of the spine, a key area used to assess osteoporosis, has many estrogenlike receptor sites. Based on animal studies, scientists think that the isoflavones in soy may bear a strong enough resemblance to the natural hormone to fill in when a woman's own estrogen levels start to decline. In a study of rats whose ovaries were removed, administering the isoflavone genistein reduced rates of bone loss, corroborating this hypothesis.

Population studies show that vegetarian women who eat a lot of soy products have lower rates of osteoporosis than meat-eating women. Moreover, even though the bone density of Japanese women is low, their rate of hip fractures is only half that of American women.

To help illuminate this, while conducting their cholesterol-lowering studies, researchers at the University of Illinois looked at bone activity as well. By comparing before-and-after bone scans, they found that daily intake of 40 grams of soy protein (with quantified amounts of isoflavones) over a period of six months had a positive influence on bone maintenance, particularly in the lumbar spine. It should be noted that this is a relatively short-term study for evaluating changes in bone structure.

Whether soy can increase bone mass as well is unclear. An Australian trial in which the diets of fifty-two postmenopausal women were supplemented with soy grits for twelve weeks did demonstrate improved bone mineral content with increased soy intake. However, this isn't a large enough sample on which to draw conclusions, since other studies support a protective effect, but not a role in reversing bone mineral loss.

Further evidence of a bone-protective effect of the isoflavone genistein is the use of ipriflavone, a structurally similar isoflavone derivative, to treat postmenopausal women. Ipriflavone preserves bone mass by slowing down bone resorption, a naturally occurring, continuous process of bone breakdown.

Some soy foods even make a notable contribution to calcium intake:

1 cup cooked green soybeans = 260 mg calcium
1 cup cooked dried soybeans = 175 mg calcium
1/2 cup dry roasted soybeans = 230 mg calcium
4 ounces firm tofu (calcium coagulant) = 160 to 230 mg calcium
4 ounces regular tofu (calcium coagulant) = 119 mg calcium
4 ounces tempeh = 105 mg calcium
8 ounces fortified soy milk = 200 to 300 mg calcium

Women and Soy

The performance of soy may become most evident in women as they age and become more susceptible to such hormone-mediated events as breast cancer, heart disease, and osteoporosis. All of these conditions are shared by men, and are explored above. But one is unique to women—menopause.

Several phytochemicals mimic the natural hormone estrogen and have thus been dubbed phytoestrogens. Because of their estrogenlike activity, their effect on women could be substantial. More than three hundred plants exhibiting estrogen potential have been identified, including many common foods. The most potent seems to be the soybean. One of the ways this has been documented is by assessing the effect of daily soy consumption on women's menstrual cycles.

It has been observed that Japanese women eating a traditional diet rich in soy have blood levels of phytoestrogens fifteen to twenty times those of American women. Moreover, the interval between periods for Asian women is typically two to three days longer. Experimental diets measuring the impact of various isoflavone-containing soy foods on young women confirm its influence on the hormones that regulate menstruation.

It's often pointed out that in Japanese there's no word for "hot flash," suggesting that this isn't a common condition of menopause. Indeed, in a cross-cultural study, only 12.6 percent of Japanese women going through menopause acknowledged an incidence of hot flashes in the preceding two weeks, and just 3.6 percent reported night sweats; by contrast, among perimenopausal Canadian women, 47 percent professed to hot flashes during the previous two weeks, and 19.8 percent suffered night sweats. It's possible that Asian women are raised to complain less or to be more reserved when it comes to talking about health issues, which might explain why they report less discomfort. On the other hand, researchers are inclined to believe that their diet has a lot to do with actually reducing side effects.

A British study of a small sampling of women showed a reduction in reported frequency of hot flashes during the span of two months in which they consumed a soy protein drink daily. When matched against control subjects who drank a placebo beverage, blood analysis showed significant changes in hormone levels.

Soy also holds promise in alleviating another common side effect of menopause—thinning of the vaginal lining. Human research substantiating this theory comes from Australian researchers. Using soy and flaxseed, another food high in phytoestrogens, they were able to strengthen cell growth in the vaginal walls, leading them to conclude that these foods were indeed estrogenic and might reduce the thinning of vaginal tissues associated with menopause.

One reason phytoestrogens may have a more pronounced effect as women age is the natural decline of estrogen. In premenopausal women, who have high concentrations of circulating estrogen, the estrogen receptors (special sites on cells located in various parts of the body that bind to estrogen and escort it into the tissues) are occupied. The isoflavones in food must compete with natural estrogen for a place on these receptors, but due to their lower binding activity have only a mild influence. As women age and their natural supply of estrogen declines, there's less competition for estrogen sites and phytoestrogens become more functional.

If enough research can eventually validate a positive role for soy during menopause, a soy-enhanced diet could become the routine prescription rather than estrogen-replacement therapy.

Infant Feeding

Questions have been raised as to whether soy-based formulas are a proper source of nutrition for infants. Unlike mother's milk, they lack cholesterol—but so do commercial formulas based on cows' milk. Studies show that exposure to cholesterol in infancy reduces the rate at which the body intrinsically manufactures its own cholesterol. Compared to infants raised on (cholesterol-rich) breast milk, babies fed (cholesterol-free) dairy-based formula have elevated rates of cholesterol synthesis, and this rises even more with soy formula. Presumably, this is an adaptive mechanism, providing the cholesterol needed during this period of rapid growth. How this might affect blood cholesterol levels later on, when "challenged" with rising dietary intake, is unknown.

An additional concern is related to phytoestrogens. Between the area of risk of disorders due to estrogen excess and risk of disorders due to estrogen deficiency lies a zone of optimal estrogen activity. It has been proposed that this optimal zone is smallest prior to puberty. If this is true, the introduction of estrogenlike substances early in life could more easily interfere with such narrow bounds.

Depending on the manufacturing process, soy formulas made from isolated soy protein have varying concentrations of phytoestrogens. Scientists in New Zealand estimate that the quantity of formula consumed by an infant each day could provide an isoflavone intake that, based on relative body weight, is three to five times higher than amounts that disrupt the menstrual cycle in young women. A study of soy infant formulas in the United States concludes that exposure of infants to isoflavones is six- to eleven-fold higher on a body-weight basis than levels that exhibit hormonal effects in adults eating soy foods. Adequate estrogen is necessary during infancy for the development of many physiological and behavioral characteristics. While specific research hasn't looked at how phytoestrogens might interfere with this by competing with estrogen, it has been confirmed that phytoestrogens are absorbed by infants. The repercussions of this warrant investigation.

Because phytoestrogens exhibit both pro- and antiestrogen capability, scientists worry not only that they may decrease estrogen availability, but also that phytoestrogens may elevate estrogen-related activity. Their fear in either case is that sexual development, which is patterned beginning in infancy, could be affected. While no such evidence of genital idiosyncrasy is seen in populations who traditionally consume large quantities of phytoestrogen-rich plant foods, infants in these areas have customarily been breast-fed.

Also worth considering is that more and more infants are being weaned from formula or breast onto soy milk, a practice that has been sanctioned after the age of one year. Soy milk contains measurable amounts of phytoestrogens. Since there is little history to look back on, long-term effects of soy-dependent diets early in life are unpredictable. Consequently, parents may want to be more cautious regarding the routine use of soy-based formulas and soy milk for infants and young children.

CHAPTER 6

The Beauty of Beans

❧❧❧

Beans may be unattractive to some people; perhaps this is because they've never taken a really good look at them. In fact, beans are quite a feast for both the palate and the eye. Beans are suited to every course in the meal, as shown by their international popularity in soups, dips, stews, casseroles, salads, and even sweet bean desserts. "Proof of the plate" is found in cultures throughout the world and reflected in our recipes.

One of the easiest ways to eat beans is out of hand, warm or cold, as a snack or hors d'oeuvre. (In Spain, a bowl of room-temperature chickpeas liberally spiced with fresh ground pepper is as common at the cocktail hour as peanuts and pretzels in the American barroom.) Cooked beans can be tossed into salads or marinated in dressing for a salad in themselves. Stuff this salad into a whole wheat pita pocket and you have a substantial lunch.

Seasoned in a variety of ways, beans provide a sauce for grains (for example, Indian dahl), a filling for tortillas, or a side dish to round out the meal (as in Mexican refritos). Then there are soups, stews, and bean-based casseroles. Among the most familiar are minestrone soup, split pea soup, Cuban black bean soup, chili, and baked beans.

In addition to serving them whole, beans can be pureed to make wonderful dips (such as the garlic-laden chickpea puree called hummus), mashed into pâtés, or ground to chopped meat consistency and used in the same way to make bean balls and burgers. Beans can even be turned into fresh vegetables by sprouting them.

And, if you haven't done so before, take a look at their natural beauty, which can be as intricate and surprising as that of any flower. Beans come in deep pink, dusky purple, inky black, creamy white, pale green and yellow, mottled brown, with startling "eyes," and speckled and splotched with some surprising colors.

Seeds of Life

Dried beans are the mature seeds of plants that have a characteristic pod—or legume—that protects these seeds while they're forming and ripening. If you take a single bean and plant it, more will grow. This is because except for water, all the elements needed to generate life are concentrated in each tiny seed. Different varieties provide us not only with food, but also medicines, oils, chemicals, dyes, and ornamental plants. The USDA's Agricultural Research Service has set up a special legume collection, with more than four thousand varieties that their scientists describe as an "unopened medicine chest."

Lentils are thought to be one of the earliest plant foods to be domesticated by humans. Soybeans, so extraordinary that they merit their own Golden Guideline, have been eaten by populations for about five thousand years. And in spite of its name, the peanut (or in some cultures groundnut) is a legume rather than a nut. Not every kind of bean is grown on a commercial scale, but a good assortment is easily found. (For details see "The Golden Pantry.")

All beans, with the exception of soybeans and peanuts, are similar in nutritional content. They're rich in protein, carbohydrate, and fiber, and low in fat. (Soybeans and peanuts, while also excellent sources of protein and fiber, have a low carbohydrate content and rather generous amounts of fat.) Beans supply several B vitamins, including folate, B_6, niacin, thiamin, and pantothenic acid. They're an excellent source of the minerals potassium, iron, copper, and magnesium, and provide modest amounts of calcium and zinc. Sodium is minimal in all but canned varieties, which get their salt (and sometimes sugar) at the processing plant.

Protein

The *American Cancer Society 1996 Dietary Guidelines* advise: "Choose beans as an alternative to meat." While the benefits of beans have been known for a long time, this is the most emphatic recognition that beans are a preferred source of protein.

In First Place

The importance of protein can't be overemphasized. Every cell in every living organism—from the tiniest microbe to the biggest animal—is dependent on protein.

What makes proteins essential is their constituent amino acids, which the body must have to build its internal structure and manufacture other nitrogen-containing substances that make life possible. There are twenty recognized amino acids that can be configured into precise patterns according to use. If the right materials are available, the liver can manufacture most of the amino acids the body needs. But in order to complete the job, nine to eleven specific amino acids must be supplied. These are referred to as "essential" or "indispensable."

The body's demand for protein is divided among several functions:

1. *Structural:* To build and repair tissues and muscles (including every major organ such as heart, kidneys, liver, intestines) and create the fibrous proteins found in connective tissue, skin, bone, hair, and nails.

2. *Regulatory:* As components of enzymes that direct most body processes (discussed in Chapter 3); in hormones such as insulin, glucagon, parathyroid hormone, adrenocorticotropic hormone (ACTH), somatotropin (growth hormone), and vasopressin, which indirectly control many body functions by regulating the synthesis or activity of numerous enzymes; as precursors for a variety of neurotransmitters that modulate brain and nerve function, such as serotonin, dopamine, epinephrine, and norepinephrine; for the creation of other brain chemicals, such as endorphins and enkephalins, which have structures similar to chemical opiates and a wide range of jobs, including tempering pain sensations, blood pressure regulation, control of body temperature, hormone secretions, and influencing movement and learning ability; as antibodies, which defend the body against disease and foreign substances.

3. *Transport:* Found in the bloodstream as hemoglobin, albumin, ceruloplasmin, transferrin, retinol-binding protein, and more, where they act as a transport system for many vital substances, including vitamins and minerals that must be carried to diverse sites.

4. *Energy source:* In conditions of calorie deprivation or when more protein is consumed than the body needs for its primary jobs, protein is converted into glucose and absorbed into the bloodstream, where it functions like carbohydrates. Protein is converted to glucose more slowly and more gradually than carbohydrate, peaking in about three hours. Thus it has a very low G-Force.

Inside the body, proteins are constantly being assembled and disassembled. This synthesis and degradation are independent—sometimes they occur at the same pace, but for a variety of reasons (growth, exercise, illness), the rate of either one can surpass the other. This "protein turnover rate" is strongly intertwined with the available pool of amino acids, which is composed of amino acids that are released after digestion and absorption of dietary proteins, plus amino acids unleashed by the breakdown of tissue protein. While the entire process is directly controlled by steroid hormones that govern specific messenger RNA, food wields an effect by altering hormone balance, which is particularly sensitive to changes in the amino acid concentration of the blood.

If the body doesn't have enough dietary protein to meet its needs, it compensates by slowing down certain protein-requiring processes or by breaking down muscle tissue to release amino acids. Likewise, if the body doesn't receive sufficient calories from food and has depleted all its energy reserves of glycogen and adipose tissue, it will tap into protein stored in its tissues. (This is a highly undesirable situation and a strategy of last resort that is generally seen only under conditions of severe malnutrition. However, it can also be triggered by certain disease states, and chronic, long-term dieters who take in minimal amounts of food run a similar risk.)

Even in this rich country with ample protein sources, deficits do occur as a result of poor food choices. But when the population is viewed as a whole, most Americans can be said to eat too much protein. What this means in terms of actual amount is that the general adult requirement of 45 to 65 grams a day is frequently exceeded, often as much as twofold.

Too Much of a Good Thing

Many people, especially athletes, believe that if protein is good for you, then a lot must be better. This is untrue. Consuming protein above recommended levels serves no useful purpose. Moreover, it can be harmful if it results in excessive consumption of fats (which accompany many protein foods) or insufficient carbohydrates (which can be crowded out by high-protein diets).

A more direct outcome of an overabundance of protein is that it can speed up the rate of protein turnover. This, in turn, increases the chances for "programming errors" to occur, leading to uncontrolled cell division and tissue growth. This is a description of what happens during tumor growth. There are other problems associated with overconsumption of protein, such as added work for the kidneys and an inclination toward osteoporosis.

★ CALCULATING YOUR PROTEIN PROFILE ★

There are a variety of recommendations by different official sources as to how much protein a day is needed by people in various age groups. The most widely used formula for calculating a reasonable intake is to multiply your body weight in pounds by .36. This is considered to be a good estimate of how many grams of protein someone in good health should be eating each day. There is some indication, however, that this may be too little to meet everyone's needs. For example, studies of elderly individuals, who were once thought to need less protein, suggest a daily protein intake of .45 to .54 grams per pound of body weight is more protective, and that marginal amounts of protein can compromise the immune system and recovery from illness or surgery. Stress, illness, pregnancy, and heavy weight training all boost protein requirements. Here's how to predict how much protein you should aim for each day:

If you are an adult in good health and sedentary to moderately active:

Daily protein target in grams = body weight × .36

If you are an adult in good health and regularly engage in heavy physical pursuits, or a child between the ages of five and eighteen:

Daily protein target in grams = body weight × .45

If you are pregnant or nursing, a competitive athlete, under great emotional or physical stress, recovering from illness or surgery, or a child under five years old (you can also use this formula if you don't feel alert, energetic, and content at the suggested lower amounts):

Daily protein target in grams = body weight × .54

Because beans are extremely low in fat, get about 70 percent of their calories from fiber-rich carbohydrate, and have a distinctive amino acid balance, the ill effects of excess protein are unlikely when beans are the primary contributor (see Beans Boost Health, on page 436).

More Than a Match for Meat

Beans are the healthiest and most economical source of protein. Meat eaters who try to convince people otherwise might be startled by the following comparisons:

• One cup of chickpeas and 2 ounces of broiled extra lean ground beef both furnish the same amount of protein (about 14 grams). However, the chickpeas (which are considerably higher in fat than most beans) contribute just 4 grams of (unsaturated) fat, while the ground beef is accompanied by 9 grams of (mostly saturated) fat.

• One cup of lentils furnishes 17 grams of protein and .75 grams of fat. Two ounces of trimmed sirloin steak (one of the leanest cuts of beef) deliver an equal quantity of protein, but six times as much fat.

As you can see, fat, and saturated fat in particular, which makes meat a concern, isn't an issue when it comes to beans. An argument that is used to discredit bean protein, however, is that with the exception of soybeans, legumes have a shortage of the essential sulfur-containing amino acids (methionine/cystine) and tryptophan. This would only be a concern if the availability of other foods were quite limited. Because methionine/cystine and tryptophan are plentiful in grains, beans and grains are often touted as ideal companions. In fact, a variety of foods can fill in the missing amino acids, including nuts, dairy products, eggs, and even some vegetables. Most nutrition authorities concur that the protein in beans is likely to be ample in a varied diet that meets overall caloric needs.

NOTE: The nutritional profile of soybeans is different from that of other beans, with about twice as much protein and half the carbohydrate. (For comprehensive information, see Chapter 5.)

Bean Fiber

Of considerable importance is that beans contain ample amounts of both insoluble and soluble fiber. The former aids the passage of foods through the digestive tract and is believed to confer protection against colon cancer; the latter is the kind that studies show helps lower blood cholesterol and regulate blood sugar.

A cup of cooked beans averages between 12 and 15 grams of fiber, slightly less if canned. This makes a substantial contribution to the daily suggested intake of 25 grams or more. (A slice of whole-grain bread offers only 2 grams; an apple, skin included, contributes 4 grams; even a cup of cooked oat bran provides just 6 grams of fiber. Foods of animal origin have no fiber at all.)

Beans also contain the fiber-associated lignan precursors (introduced in Chapter 1) that appear to inhibit hormonally induced cancers, such as breast, ovarian, prostate, and colon, and reduce some symptoms of menopause in women. Lentils are a particularly good source, while lesser but still significant amounts are reported in kidney beans, navy beans, fava beans, yellow split peas, and pinto beans. As not all beans have been included in the published data, others may have equal or greater lignan-generating capability.

Beans and Bloating

Some people complain of flatulence from eating beans. This is a reflection of the resistant carbohydrates (both starches and sugars) they contain. Basically, resistant starch (and sugar) is the undigestible matter that remains in the small intestine after eating certain carbohydrates. What the body can't break down with digestive enzymes, bacteria attack by fermentation. In the process they produce gas—which the body then expels.

It may be embarrassing or uncomfortable, but it also may be reassuring to know that this is one way beans exert their anticancer and heart-protective properties. (The potential benefits of resistant starch are explored in Chapter 1.)

Here are some ways to modulate flatulence:

• Those who are bothered by excessive gas may find canned and mashed beans less troublesome. (Resistant starch is reduced somewhat by these procedures.)

• Another way to minimize this problem is to eat beans often, but in small quantities at each sitting. This helps your body adapt.

• The manner of cooking makes a difference. Begin preparation by boiling beans in water for three minutes, turning off the heat, and letting them soak for a few hours. The boiling softens the plant cell walls and releases as much as 85 percent of the indigestible carbohydrates into the water. After soaking, discard the water and replace with fresh water for cooking. (Unfortunately, some water-soluble vitamins and minerals are lost with this technique, but if it enables you to enjoy beans, the trade-off is in your favor.)

• Cook beans with herbs and spices that are reputed to reduce their flatulence. Among these are fennel, dill, caraway seed, coriander, ginger, and the seaweed kombu. In Mexico and India, the herb epazote is used in bean dishes to improve their digestibility.

• Select some of the least reactive varieties such as adzuki, anasazi (a specialty bean that was originally cultivated by Native Americans), and mung beans. Split peas and lentils are also thought to be gentler on the digestive system. (If you can't find the beans you want locally, check "Resources" for mail-order sources.)

• Try pressure-cooking beans, as some people report this helps reduce gas.

• Discard the cooking liquid, if the recipe allows. (If you aren't plagued by gas, however, this liquid provides a flavorful and nourishing cooking medium that we often recommend in our recipes. It keeps foods moist during cooking, enabling preparation without adding fat.)

- Rinse canned beans to remove residual cooking liquid.
- Avoid eating beans with other gas-producing vegetables such as broccoli, cabbage, cauliflower, and brussels sprouts.
- Try one of the over-the-counter digestive enzyme preparations made expressly for this purpose.

Beans Boost Health

Beans and Blood Sugar

Beans are slowly digested, causing a gradual and sustained release of glucose into the bloodstream. As a result, they're especially useful in curbing hunger. But most significant is that their moderate effect on blood sugar levels makes them ideally suited to people who experience overproduction of insulin or persistent peaks in blood sugar in response to other carbohydrate-containing foods. This includes anyone with mild carbohydrate intolerance, as well as those with diagnosed diabetes.

The G-Force of Beans

The lower the G-Force, the less upsetting a food is to blood sugar levels and insulin production. Keeping these two blood factors within normal range has numerous health benefits, as discussed in Chapter 1. The G-Force for those beans that have been tested is shown in The Low-Force Bean, on page 437. A G-Force below 69 is rated as having only a modest impact; the lower you go, the more stable blood sugar levels are likely to remain.

Home-cooked beans have a lower (and thus preferable) G-Force compared with canned varieties. This is because canning is more disruptive of bean fiber. Correspondingly, beans in the whole state have a lower G-Force than when mashed or pureed. Likewise, the G-Force is less favorable in beans that are commercially processed to reduce cooking time, as in soups that reconstitute within five minutes of adding hot water and bean dips that only need rehydration.

Carbohydrate Loading: Beans Are a Winner

"Carbohydrate loading" for several days before an athletic event to increase endurance is practiced by many competitors. But while consuming carbohydrates during exercise has been shown to delay fatigue, whether carbohydrates should be eaten shortly before starting out is uncertain. According to a study comparing the endurance time of eight trained cyclists, beans may offer the most rewarding profile for athletic performance.

★ THE LOW-FORCE BEAN ★

In general, beans have a low G-Force. (The lower the G-Force the better in terms of stabilizing blood sugar.) Note the differences between conventionally prepared dried beans (as in home cooking) and canned beans, as well as the particularly low G-Force of soybeans.

Legume	G-Force Rating
Black beans	43
Black-eyed peas (cowpeas)	59
Chickpeas (garbanzos)	47
canned	60
Fava beans	109
Green peas, dried	32
Kidney beans	49
canned	74
Lentils, green	42
Lentils, red	36
Lima beans	50
Navy (white)	54
Pinto beans	55
canned	64
Soybeans	25
canned	20
Split peas, yellow	45

About an hour before the test subjects began an exhausting workout, they ate equal quantities of carbohydrate from either lentils, potatoes, or glucose. Endurance time was twenty minutes longer after the lentil meal than after the potato meal. (Comparative endurance figures weren't reported for the glucose trial; however, blood levels of all markers put glucose in last place.) The researchers concluded that the winning formula was a result of beans' ability to sustain blood sugar and produce relatively low concentrations of insulin and lactate compared with potatoes and glucose. Beans were especially good at conserving blood sugar and fatty acids for use during the later stages of exercise.

Taking Beans to Heart

A daily intake of relatively large quantities of oat bran significantly lowers blood cholesterol. This fact has received widespread publicity. What hasn't been promoted is the finding that a more practical amount of beans is of equal benefit. In a study assessing the potential cholesterol- and triglyceride-lowering effects of oat bran and beans, eating 1½ cups cooked dried beans each day elicited similar reductions to consuming a cup of oat bran (prior to cooking). Moreover, by combining these two foods on the daily menu, there was an equally successful outcome using lower, more realistic amounts of oat bran (about ⅓ cup dry weight).

437

Mentor

Even the daily inclusion of only about ½ cup canned beans made a significant difference in cholesterol and triglyceride levels.

Their cholesterol-reducing capacity isn't the only way beans are heart-healthy. Some researchers believe that as many as 30 to 40 percent of heart attacks and strokes suffered by men in the United States each year are related to inadequate folate intake. High blood levels of a protein known as homocysteine are associated with increased heart attacks and strokes (see page 352). Since skimping on the B vitamin folate raises homocysteine, and clinical trials demonstrate a profound ability to reverse this with a folate-rich diet, foods with a high folate content are considered protective. Legumes are among the best source of this vitamin; many varieties of cooked beans offer about 200 mcg folate in just one cup. Lentils and black-eyed peas (also known as cowpeas) have almost double this amount, which is extremely desirable since, in light of folate's importance, the government guidelines were doubled in 1998, and a daily intake of 400 mcg is now recommended for everyone over the age of fourteen.

Other important cardioprotective nutrients supplied by beans include copper and magnesium.

Beans for Pregnant Women (and Those Who May Be)

Boosting folate consumption, mentioned above as an important B vitamin for cardioprotection, is even more strategic for pregnant women. Folate is required during fetal growth for brain and spinal cord development. Insufficient levels of folate during pregnancy are linked to spina bifida and other neural tube defects in infants. Legumes are about the richest source of folate in the grocery store.

The tricky part is that these problems can occur in an embryo in the early stages, before many women even realize they're pregnant. A target for women prior to conception is 400 mcg folate daily, and double this amount during pregnancy. Eating beans regularly can provide this insurance. Lentils, black-eyed peas, and cranberry beans contain the highest amounts, with about 355 mcg per cup. Many other legumes deliver more than 200 mcg per cup. Split peas are among the lowest, with about 130 mcg, which still surpasses most other foods that are touted as a good source of this vitamin.

Copper is required for infant brain development, which begins in utero. Without adequate copper, nerve cells in the part of the brain that governs learning and memory can't fully develop. Magnesium is another mineral linked with brain function. Animals deprived of magnesium turn in circles obsessively, mimicking behavior symptoms often ascribed to people who are characterized as "obsessive." Beans are a good source of both copper and magnesium.

Beans and Cancer

Beans contain estrogen-related compounds that appear to boost estrogen levels when called for, yet also protect against the harmful estrogen-activated mechanisms that promote hormone-related cancers. This phenomenon is discussed in Chapter 5.

While soybeans are particularly rich in the phytoestrogens that form the category known as isoflavonoids, other members of the legume family make some contribution as well. Researchers believe that this may account for why Mexican American women, who have a bean-rich diet, have lower rates of breast cancer than non-Hispanic American women, even though they tend to have higher body weights (another risk factor associated with breast cancer).

One reason that beans are often neglected in reports recommending foods with significant amounts of protective isoflavonoids is that direct scientific measurements sometimes miss meaningful subtleties. In the case of legumes, what gets overlooked is that they're equipped with precursors of the critical isoflavonoids. Once ingested, the body turns these precursors into the desirable phytoestrogens. Moreover, accurate assessment of food phytoestrogens is still in development. Preliminary testing indicates estrogen potential in lima beans, chickpeas, kidney beans, pintos, pink peas, great northern beans, black turtle beans, green and yellow split peas, red lentils, adzuki beans, fava beans, mung beans, and black-eyed peas. Sprouting the beans increases isoflavonoid levels.

Another estrogen-related category of phytochemicals found in legumes is saponins. Saponins appear to block estrogen from entering sensitive tissues, thereby inhibiting breast, cervical, uterine, and other estrogen-related cancers. They have been identified in many different beans, including chickpeas, kidney beans, black-eyed peas, mung beans, and soybeans. They are presumed to exist in most other legumes as well.

Saponins are reputed to have several cancer-protective actions. Studies indicate they interfere with DNA replication in tumor cells, preventing cancer cells from multiplying. They also may work by binding with bile acids and cholesterol in the colon, conferring a protective effect against colon cancer. In addition, saponins are especially good at reducing free radicals, and saponins isolated from some beans have shown an ability to suppress HIV and Epstein-Barr viruses.

Beans and Bones

One of the problems with the high-protein diet common in Western nations is the deleterious effect protein can have on calcium retention. It has long been noted that protein causes urinary levels of calcium to rise, a sign that this mineral is being poorly conserved. This situation calls for more calcium to be ingested. What has been discovered, however, is that the source of protein makes a big difference in maintaining what is called "calcium balance."

When diets contain modest amounts of protein—for example, 45 to 50 grams daily for women, which is in line with the U.S. Recommended Daily Allowance (RDA)—even when calcium consumption is as little as 500 mg, calcium balance is maintained. Despite a recommended intake for calcium of as much as 1,200 mg, at this reasonable protein intake adding more calcium is of no advantage. But when daily protein climbs to around 90 grams, calcium loss occurs at the 500 mg level and at least 800 mg of calcium are needed daily to prevent it. When protein rises higher, it's difficult to preserve calcium even at 1,400 mg, which exceeds the RDA and the more recent Dietary Reference Intake (DRI). What this means is that women who take in large quantities of protein could be at greater risk for osteoporosis.

But when beans are the principal source of protein this isn't the case. Even with as much as 90 grams of bean protein daily, calcium balance can be achieved with as little as 500 mg. One explanation for this is the proportion of the sulfur-containing amino acids methionine and cystine in various protein sources. Animal proteins contain a surfeit of these amino acids, while bean protein is somewhat meager. The presence of excess sulfur in the bloodstream creates an acidic environment. In order to return the blood to an appropriate acid-base equilibrium, calcium is drawn from bones.

This helps clear up why osteoporosis isn't common in many cultures where calcium intake is quite modest. The traditional diets of people in these places is lower in overall protein, and beans, not animal foods, take first place among their protein sources.

Beans and Blood Pressure

It is well known that sodium promotes urinary calcium loss. Conversely, calcium causes sodium to be excreted. This intricate interconnection appears to be responsible, in part, for the blood pressure–lowering effect attributed to calcium in salt-sensitive individuals.

What does this have to do with beans? It appears that a third factor—protein—is involved in this equation. Raising the level of dietary protein from about 50 grams to more than 100 grams, without altering sodium, increases urinary calcium loss and inhibits sodium excretion. This protein-induced retention of sodium

NIKKI'S DIALOGUE BOX

Is calcium really the solution?

"When I work with people at risk for osteoporosis the first thing I ask about is their protein intake—not how much calcium they consume. Where diets are high in animal protein, making a transition to more beans instead is an important step."

appears to have an additional link to animal protein. In one study, adding about half a pound of beef to the daily diet of strict vegetarians caused a significant increase in systolic blood pressure (which is the first and higher reading compared to diastolic blood pressure). Furthermore, studies show that consuming vegetarian diets of equal protein and sodium content to omnivorous diets results in blood pressure normalization of both systolic and diastolic readings. The difference in amino acid proportions (see page 440) is credited with this outcome.

Beans and Kidney Stones

Considerable evidence points to an increased risk of kidney stone formation when the diet is rich in animal protein of any kind. This has been confirmed in a number of studies connecting diet to calcium oxalate stone formation.

A particularly creative research design compared diets identical in total protein, fat, carbohydrate, calcium, phosphorus, and sodium, but with different foods supplying the protein. What the researchers discovered was that as the diet increased in sulfate content (which is low in beans and high in animal foods) urinary profiles coincided with increased risk factors for stone formation. During the phase in which subjects totally avoided animal protein, urinary chemistry was most favorable; adding eggs made things moderately worse, while shifting to a predominantly animal protein diet was even more undesirable, with nearly three-fold higher levels of urinary markers. Unlike earlier studies that dwelt primarily on calcium oxalate stones, this one implicated animal protein in the creation of uric acid stones. Yet another example of the beauty of beans.

CHAPTER 7

Yogurt: Beyond Milk

Yogurt is made by culturing milk with specific bacteria that convert some of the milk sugar (lactose) into lactic acid, causing the formation of the curds that give it its custardlike consistency. All the nutrients in the original milk are carried over and then some.

The most significant contributions milk makes to the diet are protein, calcium, and the B vitamins riboflavin and B_{12}. Because most low-fat and nonfat yogurts are fortified with dry milk solids, they generally provide considerably more of all these nutrients. Moreover, nonfat yogurt cheese, introduced in Golden Guideline #7 and featured in "In Nikki's Kitchen," not only supplies 55 percent more protein than milk, but also offers 35 percent more than yogurt itself.

Friendly Flora

Where yogurt and milk really differ is a result of the culturing process that brings about the growth of certain strains of bacteria. These bacteria make the milk (now yogurt) more acidic by changing some of the milk sugar into lactic acid. This has several advantages:

1. Since the natural milk sugar content is reduced during the creation of yogurt, people who suffer from gastric distress caused by lactose intolerance are generally able to eat yogurt with little or no difficulty.

Ordinarily, after it enters the gastrointestinal tract the milk sugar lactose is broken down by the enzyme lactase. In people who are lactose intolerant, this enzyme is deficient and as a result the milk sugar molecules pass undigested into the intestines, where they're acted upon by bacteria. The gases produced during this bacterial fermentation can cause cramps, bloating, flatulence, and diarrhea. Certain ethnic groups are more predisposed to this condition, which is attributed to the fact that historically milk wasn't a large part of their diets. Consequently,

★ SKIM MILK, YOGURT, AND YOGURT CHEESE COMPARED* ★
(100 grams)

Protein
  skim milk = 3.42 grams
  nonfat yogurt = 5.74 grams
  nonfat yogurt cheese = 7.80 grams
Calcium
  skim milk = 123 mg
  nonfat yogurt = 199 mg
  nonfat yogurt cheese = 199 mg
Riboflavin
  skim milk = .14 mg
  nonfat yogurt = .23 mg
  nonfat yogurt cheese = .23 mg
B_{12}
  skim milk = .38 mcg
  nonfat yogurt = .61 mg
  nonfat yogurt cheese = .61 mg

*Based on a composite of nutrient databases and scientific sources, published in The Food Processor® Nutrition Analysis Software from ESHA Research, Salem, OR. Depending on their formulation, yogurts (and the yogurt cheese made from them) will vary somewhat in nutritional content.

those of Hispanic, African, Asian, Native American, and Eastern European ancestry are often less tolerant of lactose than other peoples.

The active cultures in yogurt produce an enzyme capable of splitting a portion of the lactose molecule into its simple sugars before it's ingested. Numerous studies report improved digestion and fewer symptoms in both children and adults when yogurt is consumed.

For people who count on dairy products as their main source of calcium, better tolerance improves their calcium status.

2. The bacteria in yogurt is associated with several health-protective changes.

During the fermentation stage of yogurt production, some of the protein is partially broken down or predigested. As a result, allergenic proteins in milk that cause reactions in some people are decreased, allowing yogurt to be tolerated when other dairy foods aren't.

In a small study of women prone to vaginal yeast infections, daily consumption of 8 ounces of yogurt reduced recurrence from a mean of 2.5 infections over a six-month period to less than one episode.

Subjects eating twice this amount for four months had higher levels of gamma interferon, a protein in white blood cells that boosts the immune response. Immune system stimulation by lactic acid bacteria, indicated by levels of various antibodies and other markers, corroborate this effect.

Children with chronic diarrhea are helped by yogurt. Likewise, regular consumption of yogurt reduces common "travelers' diarrhea." Animal studies confirm yogurt's ability to fight intestinal infections.

Mentor

Antibiotic therapy alters the microflora balance in the intestines and often causes gastrointestinal side effects. Yogurt consumption has been shown to eliminate common secondary gastrointestinal infections, presumably by recolonizing the intestine with competing, healthy microflora.

When yogurt is eaten on a continuous basis, human intestinal microflora activity is altered, resulting in the suppression of enzymes associated with the conversion of procarcinogens (substances that have cancer-causing potential) into carcinogens.

Cells tested with extracts of live yogurt culture exhibit enhanced resistance to chemicals known to induce cancers.

3. Foods that are fermented or cultured with bacteria (such as yogurt) promote the body's use of the protective phytochemicals known as isoflavones, most abundant in soybeans.

In addition to the benefits enumerated above, there is a long list of supposed cures that are derived from the friendly flora that yogurt brings to the digestive tract. Some of these claims seem exaggerated; even so, there are enough good reasons to support yogurt and none to discredit it. Note, however, that all of the activities associated with its microbial action are dependent on the presence of *live* bacterial strains. This is of supreme importance. Not all commercial offerings meet this criteria. If yogurt is pasteurized after manufacture it will no longer contain viable cultures.

NIKKI'S DIALOGUE BOX

Things to Do with Yogurt Cheese

"Yogurt cheese can be used to replace mayonnaise, sour cream, and cream cheese in many dishes. It doesn't take much trouble to find ways to use it. Here are some of our favorite quick applications:

"Serve on baked potatoes (a few chopped chives make this especially nice); use in dips in place of sour cream or mayonnaise; for a healthy 'cream cheese and jelly' sandwich, spread on whole-grain bread along with some all-fruit preserves; use in place of butter or mayonnaise to moisten the bread for sandwiches; spread on hot toast or muffins and let it melt in like butter; spoon a generous dollop on chili, tacos, burritos, and bean stews; stir into pasta sauces just before serving to make them creamy; spread a thin layer on top of casseroles before baking; serve soups and vegetable stews with a spoonful of yogurt cheese in the center.

"In addition, spread on crackers or toasted squares of whole-grain bread and top with cucumber slices, diced sun-dried tomatoes, thin wedges of artichoke hearts, a few capers, olive paste, or something similar for instant hors d'oeuvres.

"To end a meal, sweeten yogurt cheese lightly with pure maple syrup and a few drops of vanilla extract and use on top of berries, baked apples, or other fruit desserts as you would whipped cream."

The Healthiest Diet in the World

Animal Fat Gets a (Slight) Reprieve

As described in Chapter 6, protein is essential to every living cell. In the human body, protein is concentrated in muscles, organs, hair, nails, and blood. Numerous regulatory substances, including enzymes, hormones, and genes, are also composed of various proteins. And in order for many vital nutrients to get to where they're needed, proteins provide the transport system.

Animal products are generally an excellent source of protein—but they come packaged with saturated fats that can undermine health. Yogurt and yogurt cheese offer the best of both worlds.

Prime Protein

Consuming ½ cup of yogurt cheese or 1 cup of yogurt provides about 9 grams of protein, or 12 to 20 percent of the U.S. Recommended Daily Allowance (RDA) and Canadian Recommended Nutrient Intakes (RNI) for healthy males and females over the age of eleven years (44 to 73 grams per day). For younger children, ages two through ten, these foods satisfy 32 to 64 percent of the daily protein need (14 to 28 grams).*

If yogurt cheese is prepared with nonfat yogurt, the resulting product is fat free. This compares quite favorably to ½ cup cream cheese, with 9 grams protein and 40 grams of fat; an ounce of hard cheese (a 1-inch cube or modest slice), averaging about 7 grams protein and 7 to 9 grams fat; ½ cup sour cream, supplying 3.5 grams protein and 24 grams fat; or the same quantity of mayonnaise, which is not a source of protein and contributes a whopping 88 grams of fat. Obviously, using nonfat yogurt or yogurt cheese in their place is quite an asset to anyone trying to lower fat intake.

Make Way for CLA (Conjugated Linoleic Acid)

When yogurt cheese is made with low-fat or whole-milk yogurt, its fat content rises. Despite the problems attributed to animal fats, there may be something here to pursue: an unusual polyunsaturated fatty acid called conjugated linoleic acid (CLA).

CLA occurs primarily in animal fat, although it's related to linoleic acid (LA), the essential fatty acid found in vegetable oils that was discussed extensively in Chapter 2. CLA is highest in foods derived from both the flesh and the milk of ruminant animals (cows, sheep, goats). The CLA content of the meat and dairy from these animals varies with the animal's diet. CLA appears to be enhanced by heat, and as a result, cheeses and yogurt, which are heated prior to culturing, have higher levels than milk. The addition of whey (a milk component that is added to many brands of yogurt) may also increase CLA levels. Overall, the

---

*Regarding protein, the U.S. RDA and Canadian RNI differ a little in several age categories. The figures here reflect the lowest and highest recommendations within the given age spreads.

amount of CLA per gram of fat in yogurt and cheese is generally more than the amount per gram of fat in beef.

CLA has the ability to inhibit chemically induced skin and stomach tumors in mice and mammary tumors in rats. This fatty acid has also been found to suppress human melanoma cells in laboratory cultures, as well as lung, colorectal, and breast cancers. A protective effect during the initiation phase of cancer progression has received the majority of attention, although several studies suggest CLA may be suppressive during the promotion stage as well. Since many tumors take years to develop following exposure, lifelong intake of yogurt and yogurt cheese seems like a wise strategy.

In addition to its cancer-inhibiting activity, CLA reduces serum cholesterol and triglyceride levels and the severity of induced atherosclerosis in rabbits. David Kritchevsky, a researcher with the Wistar Institute in Philadelphia who has conducted several CLA studies, makes this interesting observation: "It is ingenious of nature to provide a fatty acid, linoleic acid, which is essential for tumor growth and also to find ways to convert it to a protective modification." (This modification being CLA.)

Of additional note is the theory that nonruminants also have the capacity to produce CLA with the aid of intestinal microflora. Synthesis of CLA in humans hasn't yet been determined. If people do have this capability, yogurt, which increases the number of friendly bacteria in the colon, should boost CLA potential.

NIKKI'S DIALOGUE BOX

What Are the Lessons of CLA?

"The discovery of possible health-protective factors in animal fats doesn't mean we should now view fat as a 'health food.' What these studies underscore is what we've been saying for years: It's best to eat a wide variety of wholefoods. Moreover, we have to be wary of food companies or supplement manufacturers who start seeking ways to use CLA as an additive, or process it into pill form, since other health-enhancing compounds in yogurt and other dairy foods are likely to be missed. This holds true for most of the nutrients, phytochemicals, and other coincidental food constituents, known and yet to be discovered."

Benefits to Bones

Calcium is indispensable to the body's skeletal structure. The U.S. Daily Recommended Intake (DRI) for calcium ranges from 800 mg for children between the ages of four and eight, to 1,300 mg thereafter until age eighteen. The recommended intake then decreases to 1,000 mg, until age fifty-one, when it rises to 1,200 mg. These standards, revised in 1997, are above previously set goals.

As we explained in Chapters 3 and 6, in a diet that isn't overwhelmed by phosphorus and animal protein, the need for such high levels of calcium is doubtful. Nonetheless, good sources of this mineral are imperative at all ages, and government surveys indicate that many people aren't measuring up (see Osteoporosis, on page 448).

Nonfat yogurt and yogurt cheese can make an ample contribution to calcium intake, supplying 245 mg per ½ cup. The same volume of milk, a food widely promoted for its calcium value, provides only three-fifths of this amount (150 mg). Cream cheese, which is easily replaced as a spread by yogurt cheese, offers a mere 93 mg calcium per ½ cup. Likewise, sour cream, which is rendered unnecessary in dips, hot dishes, and even baking when yogurt and yogurt cheese are on hand, provides just 133 mg. And mayonnaise, which also becomes obsolete in some applications, offers a negligible 20 mg.

The Biology of Bone

Bones are made up of a network of collagen tissue permeated by calcium phosphate salts. Bone growth takes place by a complex process that is directed by specialized cells called osteoblasts. At the same time bone construction is going on, an opposing process called resorption is continuously taking place. Even fully mature bone is constantly undergoing this transformation, which is known as "remodeling."

Bones are classified into two general types—trabecular (or cancellous) bone, which composes the spongy interior of many bones, and the more dense cortical bone that makes up the exterior. Certain bones, such as the spinal column, hip bones, and the end portion of long bones (knees, elbows), are primarily trabecular bones; the skull, shin bones, and shaft portion of long bones are cortical by nature. In adults, approximately 25 percent of trabecular bone is renewed annually, while cortical bone has a yearly turnover rate of only about 3 percent.

Bred in the Bone

Bone conformation, as animal breeders have known for a long time, is the result of the interaction between genetic endowment and environment. Population studies confirm this effect in humans by tracking height against diet changes. Observations have consistently shown that where calcium intake is limited, people are shorter. As calcium consumption rises, so does height. This particular outcome isn't necessarily of any use, unless, of course, you want to be a professional jockey or play basketball. Of more genuine interest, however, calcium also helps determine the strength of bones, an issue of considerable concern.

More than 99 percent of the calcium in the human body is deposited in the skeleton. During the first two decades of life, skeletal growth and calcium accumulation in bones tend to rise in tandem. But by the end of the third decade, when skeletal growth has been over for a decade or so, the relationship between the storage of calcium in bones and its removal starts to go in reverse. As a result, the reservoir of bone calcium tends to decrease. This process is usually quite gradual; in fact, it is almost imperceptible until the age of about fifty, when it generally starts to accelerate.

During menopause, the onset of bone calcium loss in women tends to be sudden and continues at a rapid pace until about the seventh decade of life. On average, during the first ten years following menopause about 13 percent of bone mineral mass is lost, largely affecting trabecular bone, although cortical thinning is also significant, particularly in women diagnosed with osteoporosis. This explains why the spine and hips are common trouble spots. In men, this decline is in a more gradual, linear fashion, with a rate of less than half a percent a year from age thirty on. Eventually, the rate of loss for women becomes much slower, on par with that of men. Of course, not every person follows this pattern—some women lose bone mass more slowly, and some men lose bone mass at a faster than average pace.

The conditions that lead to optimum bone density in childhood, and optimum bone retention for adults, are diverse. As mentioned, genetics plays its part, but so does nutrition, which has a large share in whether or not people reach their maximum genetic potential. Calcium, as the preceding description of bone development makes clear, is a critical nutrient in the accumulation of bone mass. This helps the body defend against later losses. If calcium loss can't be curtailed and is too extensive, bones become fragile, causing the all-too-well-known condition osteoporosis.

The progression of osteoporosis and the potential role of calcium are discussed next. Keep in mind, however, that calcium isn't the only crucial element in this equation. In other chapters we discuss the possible effects of the following dietary factors on osteoporosis:

- Improper fat ratios (see Fat and Osteoporosis, on page 336)
- The presence of zinc and copper (see Bring on the Metal, on page 354)
- The availability of vitamin K and boron (see The "Koagulations" Vitamin, on page 373, and Osteoporosis, on page 405)
- The potential role of phytoestrogens (see Osteoporosis, on page 426)
- Mineral depletion from excess animal protein and sodium (see Beans and Bones, on page 439)
- What you drink (see Chapter 8)

Nondietary factors such as heredity, exercise, and vitamin D also play critical roles.

Osteoporosis

Osteoporosis, the thinning of bone structure that makes bones susceptible to fracture, affects more than 20 million people in the United States. The lifetime risk of hip fracture for a woman is as high as 15 percent, approximately twice that of a man. After menopause, a woman's risk doubles with every seven years of age. This is more than a mere inconvenience; 15 to 30 percent of those affected die because of this disease.

The causes of this disorder are puzzling. There is general agreement that calcium intake during the time of initial bone growth—the first twenty years of life—greatly influences bone integrity. But once bone is fully formed, the impact of calcium is still somewhat obscure.

Absorption of calcium is regulated by vitamin D. Although classified as a vitamin, vitamin D is considered to actually be a hormone whose production depends not on diet, but on the exposure of skin to sunlight.* Its principal action is to stimulate calcium transport in the intestine and kidneys, increasing the amount of dietary calcium that gets absorbed by the body and decreasing the amount that's lost in urine. Vitamin D also stimulates production of osteoblasts, the specialized cells mentioned above that produce proteins required to build and harden the network of collagen and calcium salts that compose bone.

With the help of vitamin D, the body can adapt to varying levels of calcium availability during the growth period. When less calcium is present, absorption and retention becomes more efficient. Once the skeleton is fully developed, however, the primary path by which calcium is absorbed changes. When this happens, the body's internal regulating system becomes less dependable and the actual amount of calcium ingested may have greater influence over how much is assimilated. This means more calcium (along with adequate vitamin D) is needed to keep calcium in a favorable balance.

At the same time that calcium absorption becomes more dependent on diet, the loss of calcium in urine starts to accelerate. While children are able to retain the most calcium, the reverse is true in postmenopausal women.

It has been postulated that too much phosphorous in the diet limits calcium absorption, and high protein intake from animal foods causes increased excretion. Thus an individual's personal calcium needs are determined to some extent by how much of these other nutrients is present in the diet. The availability of hormonelike food factors (phytoestrogens)—with soy foods being a principal source—may also influence needs by improving calcium retention.

Nonetheless, consuming enough calcium remains extremely important for everyone, and government studies reveal that this nutrient is lacking in many people's diets, particularly those of young girls and women. Results from the USDA's 1995 Continuing Survey of Food Intakes by Individuals (CSFII) indicate that in the survey group of women age thirty and older, only 25 percent reached the 1989 RDA of 800 mg, with a mean intake ranging from 615 to 670 mg. Moreover, although the adolescent females and young adult women polled averaged an additional 100 mg calcium daily, fewer than 15 percent met the RDA at the time of 1,200 mg for this age group, at a stage of life when optimizing intake is called for.

*Most foods don't contain vitamin D, and fortified foods aren't viewed as a reliable source. Exposure to sunlight provides most humans with their vitamin D requirement. Inhibiting this with sunscreens can dramatically affect the skin's production of vitamin D. This isn't an excuse to overexpose skin to harmful ultraviolet rays, but if bone strength is to be maintained, spending time outdoors in good sunlight with some skin fully exposed for fifteen to thirty minutes a day is suggested.

The ability of yogurt and yogurt cheese to furnish generous amounts of calcium was presented at the beginning of this section. As with other animal proteins, the excess of calcium-draining sulfur-containing amino acids in yogurt could cut into this generous supply. However, the fact that yogurt and yogurt cheese start out with so much calcium sets them above all other dairy foods. In addition, it has been speculated that the calcium in yogurt is better absorbed as a result of bacterial fermentation. Animal flesh foods, with their scant amounts of calcium, are no match for yogurt and yogurt cheese. And those who might think supplements are the best choice of all should think again. Nature doesn't provide a single food that contains just calcium, or even one where it is as concentrated as it is in a supplement. With such an onslaught of calcium, the absorption of two other essential minerals, zinc and magnesium, can be hindered.

Yogurt's Extended Reach

Even though 99 percent of the calcium in the body is found in the skeleton, the remaining 1 percent has an important job to do in regulating nerve transmissions, muscle contractions, blood clotting, and blood pressure. Once again, yogurt can contribute to this and more.

Yogurt and Heart Disease

Many investigators have reported that yogurt has a cholesterol-lowering ability in man and animals. Due to numerous variabilities in studies purporting this effect, as well as no conclusive explanation of how this occurs, the hypothesis cannot be definitively confirmed or disproved.

In an attempt to answer the question "Is there a hypocholesterolemic factor in milk and milk products?" research that looked at a number of studies came to the conclusion that the key may be an interplay between many factors, and that the "complex food" itself, rather than any individual constituent, is responsible for whatever influence yogurt has on blood lipid levels.

A variety of mechanisms have been proposed regarding the impact of yogurt on blood lipids. The influence of specific bacteria has been suggested, along with the ability of some component in yogurt or milk itself to inhibit cholesterol synthesis. One plausible connection for yogurt is decreased levels of a substance called orotic acid as compared with milk, which is supported by the fact that orotic acid causes fatty livers in rats. However, this effect could be species specific, as the relationship between orotic acid and lipids in the human liver is still undetermined. Another theory is that calcium binds with bile acids, increasing their excretion and thereby preventing cholesterol from being reabsorbed. Since calcium absorption is possibly improved as a result of bacterial fermentation, this could account for yogurt being more active than milk in lowering cholesterol.

According to studies on monkeys conducted by David Kritchevsky, Ph.D., the milk sugar lactose may shed some light. What Kritchevsky discovered was that some sugars influence the rate of triglyceride synthesis and the deposition of fat on artery walls (or atherogenesis) more profoundly than others. It was already noted in Chapters 1 and 4 that fructose is thought to elevate triglyceride levels more than sucrose, and substantially more than glucose.

The effect of lactose, the sugar found in milk, is especially intriguing. Kritchevsky found that lactose, when ingested in a fat-free milieu, had little impact on blood fats; however, when ingested in the presence of dietary cholesterol, it increased the level of fat in arterial tissue more than any other sugar. This implies that the form and context in which milk is ingested can have quite different coronary outcomes. Because yogurt is low in lactose, it would be expected to have much less negative impact, even if the yogurt isn't fat (and thus cholesterol) free.

Calcium and Hypertension

Hypertension, another way of saying high blood pressure, is brought on by an increase in vascular resistance due to a decrease in diameter inside the arteries. What causes this is a shortening (or contraction) of the smooth muscle tissue.

Hypertension is viewed primarily as an adult problem, since it appears mainly in older individuals. But now that blood pressure measurements are a routine part of pediatric care, there is evidence that its roots extend back into childhood, and elevated measurements in some children are an early warning sign. Addressing this at the onset could prevent serious repercussions later.

A relationship between calcium and hypertension was first recognized in the early 1970s when researchers noticed lower death rates from cardiovascular disease in communities with hard water (that is, a high mineral content, including calcium). Since then more than two dozen population studies, as well as laboratory work and clinical trials, have supported an association between blood pressure and calcium. One particularly indicative dietary intervention study involving men and women, Caucasians and African Americans, found that when a diet high in vegetables and fruit was administered there was a significant lowering of systolic pressure (the higher of the two numbers); when modest amounts of low-fat dairy products were added on top of this, both systolic and diastolic pressures improved. In fact, this "combination" diet—consisting of eight to ten servings of vegetables and fruits and two to three servings of dairy—was twice as effective in reducing blood pressure in all subjects; moreover, in those who were classified as hypertensive at the start, reductions were comparable to what is accomplished with antihypertensive drug therapy.

Various attempts have been made to explain how low levels of dietary calcium are implicated in the problem. As with many conditions that have a nutritional component, calcium most likely interacts with other nutrients (in this case phosphorus, sodium, and magnesium). Understanding this mechanism would enable more specific dietary intervention. Regardless, what has been observed is that low dietary calcium consumption is identified with increasing arterial pressure, rather than high intakes of calcium being responsible for decreasing blood pressure. This means intake of calcium-rich foods to a reasonable level by people whose diets fall short is expected to have the most impact. Increasing calcium beyond normal needs is ineffectual.

As with sodium, not all people with hypertension are responsive to calcium, but most often the same population reacts to both; that is, where blood pressure is aggravated by sodium, it's helped by eating more calcium-containing foods.

In addition to furnishing calcium, yogurt may have an enhanced role in reducing hypertension. Certain protein compounds formed during the fermentation of milk are able to inhibit the enzyme that transforms a compound known as angiotensin I into angiotensin II, a potent artery constrictor. In fact, drugs known as ACE inhibitors work according to the same premise. This could explain how some "sour" milk products exert a distinctive blood pressure–reducing capacity.

Calcium, Yogurt, and Cancer

Deaths from colorectal cancers rank number three in the United States for both men and women. Diets high in calcium are associated with lower risk of colorectal cancer, but whether or not this is a causal relationship hasn't been proven.

Noted cancer researcher Edward Giovannucci believes that striking increases in colon cancer rates in populations migrating from low- to high-incidence areas implicate an environmental factor, probably related to diet. Abundant data corroborate this, although specific dietary elements have yet to be elucidated. Among the list of suspects is a protective role for calcium, with a possible heightened advantage from fermented dairy products such as yogurt. The likely means is via the binding of calcium to bile acids, which are key factors in the promotion and development of tumors, to render them inert and reduce cell proliferation.

The relationship between calcium and stomach cancer reported in a study investigating dietary risk factors in China is of great interest, since this association isn't often made. Animal studies hint that calcium might exert its effect by reducing salt-induced damage to the stomach lining.

While increasing calcium-rich foods in the diet is a good idea, overdosing on calcium may not be. In examining a possible connection between calcium and cancer, there are some indications that this mineral may have a role in both enhancing and inhibiting tumors. Excessive amounts can stimulate cell division (which could be tumor promoting). But calcium is also essential for cell maturation, and certain cancers arise as a result of a block in normal cell maturation. It is difficult to get too much calcium when food is the only source.

Calcium seems to encourage healthy differentiation and inhibit unhealthy proliferation of a number of epithelial cell types, such as the colon. On the other hand, some cancer cells appear to be adversely sensitive to calcium, such as breast, lung, and specific brain tumor cells. These cells secrete calcium-inducing factors to assist their own growth. Researchers believe that the negative effects of high calcium may be buffered by vitamin D, which acts as an antagonist, but nonetheless suggest using caution regarding long-term prophylactic, high-dose calcium supplements. Here again is an indication that nutrients within food and supplements aren't interchangeable.

Another nutrient that has been correlated with reduced cancer risk in animal models and human studies is riboflavin. Riboflavin is an essential cofactor for a number of enzymes, including some involved in disarming certain carcinogens. Yogurt and yogurt cheese are excellent sources of this nutrient.

In addition to calcium, riboflavin, and CLA (discussed on page 446), yogurt may have another cancer-suppressing mechanism that derives from its bacterial fermentation. Comparative laboratory tests on cells to determine activity against colon cancers show that something other than CLA makes yogurt two and a half times more potent than either unfermented milk with added lactic acid or yogurt with low bacterial growth. This phenomenon is believed to come from a suppressing action on enzymes that activate potential carcinogens. Milk containing *Lactobacillus acidophilus* at levels consistent with commercial products decreases the activity of at least three such fecal enzymes by two- to fourfold. When consumed daily in a controlled study, the impact was most pronounced after four weeks; that is, enzyme levels exhibited the least activity. But even after only ten days, some reduction in enzyme activity occurred. Moreover, when the lactobacillus-containing food was removed from the diet, significant effects persisted for at least ten days, although there was a progressive increase in activity, which after thirty days returned to prestudy measures. This suggests that continued, regular consumption of bacterial cultures is most protective.

Because the bacterial strains used to culture yogurts vary, and this can influence their ability to alter intestinal microflora, more research into individual effects is needed before medical conclusions can be drawn. Based on what has been shown in the laboratory and reflected by yogurt-eating populations, many of these organisms could have similar health-enhancing properties.

Calcium and Kidney Stones

The majority of kidney stones are classified as "calcium oxalate" stones, with calcium being one of the main constituents; therefore, many people think that calcium contributes to kidney stone formation. In fact, the influence it has is in the opposite direction; that is, consuming calcium-rich foods can reduce kidney stone formation. This is explained by the ability of calcium to bind with oxalates in food as well as with oxalates produced spontaneously by the body (the predominant source). This keeps the level of urinary oxalates from rising. High urinary oxalate levels are used as a marker for pinpointing people who are likely to develop kidney stones.

Studies show that when eaten in combination with calcium-containing foods, high-oxalate foods, including spinach, nuts, tea, chocolate, beets, rhubarb, strawberries, and wheat bran, have a much smaller impact on urinary oxalate levels.

While consuming calcium along with these foods is a good idea, research also supports the value of incorporating small portions of high-calcium foods into each meal of the day as a means of reducing kidney stone production.

The ease of using yogurt and yogurt cheese as a complement to many high-oxalate foods, as well as at other times of the day, makes them a valuable resource for decreasing the likelihood of painful kidney stones. In the Health Professionals study that has been referenced in many of the chapters, dietary intake of about 600 mg per day of calcium (largely from dairy) was associated with significantly reduced risk of kidney stones. In this report, only foods, not supplements, were protective. The renowned Nurses' Health Study (of women) found calcium from food to be similarly protective. Moreover, for the women taking calcium supplements the reverse was shown; that is, they were at the highest risk for kidney stones. Note, too, that while the credit was given to calcium, it was proposed in these studies that perhaps some other aspect of the dairy foods that furnished the calcium was involved; if so, yogurt and yogurt cheese would still be effective.

Get the Best (Not BST)

BST stands for Bovine Somatotropin, a naturally occurring hormone that increases milk production in cows. The possible economic advantages to dairy farmers of greater yields prompted development of genetically engineered BST (rBST or rBGH). This synthesized BST was approved for use by U.S. milk producers in the fall of 1993. Since then there has been a vocal movement to reverse this decision.

Some of the problems associated with BST are described below. One of the biggest challenges concerned consumers face is the fact that use of this hormone isn't indicated anywhere on food labels; indeed, efforts in some states to permit dairy products to claim that the cows' milk they contain is free of BST have been prohibited. Many manufacturers also claim that because milk is generally pooled from several sources, it's impossible for them to substantiate a BST-free claim.

"Don't Worry"

The injection of rBGH into dairy herds increases the concentration of an insulinlike growth factor (IGF), designated IGF-1, in their milk. This is agreed upon. The consequence to humans of ingesting more IGF, however, is hotly debated. There is an extensive bibliography of articles attesting to the safety of BST and the appearance of IGF-1 in milk, and an equally heavy body of scientific papers repudiating it. Despite the U.S. FDA's "Don't Worry" attitude, these concerns merit attention:

1. Human IGF-1 is identical to bovine IGF-1. In humans, IGF-1 intercedes in the activity of pituitary growth hormone, thereby controlling cell growth, division, and differentiation, among other things.

2. Milk from cows receiving the hormone injections show a four- to twenty-fold increase in IGF-1 levels.
3. Pasteurization increases IGF-1 activity.
4. Although some scientists and the FDA insist that ingesting IGF-1 isn't dangerous, a study by Monsanto, the manufacturer of rBGH, indicates that mature rats fed modest doses of IGF-1 for just two weeks exhibited significant changes, including increased body weight, liver weight, heart weight, and bone length, and a decrease in bone cartilage width. Moreover, most of the company's study designs have been criticized as being of too-short duration, using mature rather than young animals (the latter probably being more vulnerable), and not directly employing IGF-1 taken from milk samples of rBGH-treated cows.
5. IGF-1 in milk survives digestion and passes across the intestinal wall. It may be absorbed most efficiently by infants.
6. IGF-1 may promote the growth of invasive breast and colon cancer cells. Animal studies show that recombinant forms of growth hormone induce mammary development beyond internal controls. In addition, the U.S. National Institutes of Health Expert Committee noted a need to determine possible "acute and chronic actions" of IGF-1 in the upper gastrointestinal tract, including the esophagus, stomach, and intestines. In his comprehensive review of the considerations due rBGH, Samuel Epstein, of the University of Illinois School of Public Health, summarizes several mechanisms by which these forms of cancer could accelerate.
7. Since infants are most affected by IGF-1, babies and young children drinking milk from BST-injected cows may be especially vulnerable. A twenty-two-pound baby drinking just over a quart of milk a day would be subjected to a dose of IGF-1 12.5 times the recommended minimum needed to display biological activity.

There hasn't been enough time to confirm adverse outcomes in humans. Treated cows show higher concentrations of IGF-1 in their udders, and increased rates of an udder infection known as mastitis. Mastitis requires the use of antibiotics. Fertility rates in cows are also altered, and this too is often addressed by the use of drugs. Increased medications in these animals could have a secondary effect on humans from consuming milk with residual traces.

There have been numerous criticisms of the FDA's acceptance of rBGH, along with claims of inconsistencies between scientific studies and interpretations of the findings. Not everyone agrees that these concerns are valid. The Institute of Food Science & Technology issued a Position Statement on March 27, 1996, in which they state: "Objective scientific assessment of the use of bovine somatotropin (BST) to improve milk yield in cows indicates that it carries no harmful effects to humans, to the treated animals or to the environment; the resulting milk and meat is not significantly different from milk and meat from untreated cows, in composition or quality; and in consequence there is no basis for requiring special labeling of milk or meat from BST treated cows." They back this up by rebutting the previously reported concerns.

While we don't have the answer, we aren't willing to complacently accept its approval by the FDA. We support Dr. Epstein's statement that "the entire nation is currently being subjected to an experiment involving large-scale adulteration of an age-old dietary staple by a poorly characterized and unlabeled biotechnology product."

"Be Happy"

One recourse consumers have is to query companies that manufacture yogurt, notify them you won't purchase their products if they don't satisfy your request for a BST-free product, and support dairies that are trying to keep BST out of the food supply. There are several brands that conform; products labeled "organic" are among them.

CHAPTER 8

Drink Up

The modest-size supermarket in the small rural community where we live devotes sixteen aisles to foodstuffs. When you add up the space allocated to things to drink—shelf-stable bottles, cans, and boxes; tea, coffee, powders and concentrates to reconstitute; and the juices and milk found in the dairy case—four of these aisles are taken up by beverages. Our local natural food store, which is rather ample, allots more space to drinkables than any other comestible. We have also seen that although the number of dedicated fruit and vegetable stores and private bakeries have decreased over the years, stores devoted to beer and nonalcoholic beverages have flourished.

Do we really need all these options? From a health standpoint, it hardly seems justified. So rather than waste time talking about every possible item, we'll use the final chapter to clarify some of the publicity that has boosted the sales of such popular drinks as water, tea, and alcohol. Are claims about their benefits true and should they be more widely promoted? The answers, as you will soon see, depend on such factors as what your health goals are, your age and gender, and even where you live.

Water: The Worldwide Paradox

One of the only things you could get every human being to agree on is that water is indispensable to human existence. Despite this, throughout the ages water has been the cause of massive health problems. This is a remarkable paradox: Water can be deadly, as evidenced in many locales that lack adequate sanitation equipment. And even in places that have sophisticated purification facilities, pollution of drinking water is still a health concern.

Water All Around Us

Although popular in Europe for decades, bottled water has become such a phenomenon in North America that it's now the primary source of drinking water for one in six inhabitants. Today, toting a personal water bottle is chic. This confirms that people are willing to embrace health-enhancing activities, particularly when they can be made stylish. But this attention also makes us prey to sometimes unfounded and ofttimes persuasive messages about the (assumed poor) quality of our water supply and the (assumed better) value of the water we can buy. Indeed, there are problems; but they aren't always remedied by the widely publicized solutions.

A vast quantity of the world's beverages besides drinking water—from reconstituted juices to soft drinks—rely on water as an ingredient. This brings the concern beyond our immediate faucets to the water used by beverage makers. We make this point primarily to alert people who, fearing the quality of drinking water, turn to bottled and canned juices and soft drinks as alternates. Moreover, even where the quality of the added water used in these items is assured, the importance of water itself to health isn't always fulfilled by other water-containing drinks. In addition to H_2O, they may contain sugars, artificial sweeteners, caffeine, sodium, phosphates, colorants, and other additives that aren't among the body's preferences.

What's Good About Water

People rarely identify water as an "essential nutrient." However, considering that our bodies are composed of nearly two-thirds water, one would expect it to be an essential part of the diet. The brain, for example, is about 75 percent water, and even moderate dehydration can cause dizziness and headaches. Water also makes up 92 percent of blood, 75 percent of muscle, and 22 percent of bone.

Water plays a vital role in digestion and gastrointestinal function. It helps the body convert food into energy, absorb and transport nutrients and oxygen to all cells, and maintain the proper balance of internal fluids. Water aids in the removal of excess minerals, vitamins, waste matter, and other unwanted elements from the body via the kidneys and digestive tract. In addition, the body uses water to regulate internal temperature, thereby avoiding hypo- and hyperthermia. This is why water is particularly important during physical activity, where rapid loss through sweat can lead to dehydration. Water loss due to illness (such as fever, diarrhea, and vomiting) poses a similar threat.

Individual thirst is one indicator of how much fluid a person should drink each day. But unfortunately, we aren't all equally adept at noticing the signs our bodies give us. Moreover, in some people—and this is a common occurrence with aging—the thirst sensation is diminished. Even for those who claim they rarely "feel" thirsty, this doesn't mean body fluids don't need to be replenished. Therefore, having a clinical guideline is useful. A variety of parameters have been proposed (see How Much Water Should You Drink? on page 460).

Water needs vary with exertion, climate, and body size. Some people aim for a routine six to eight 8-ounce glasses, or 1½ to 2 quarts per day. This is within reason, but it doesn't necessarily match individual circumstances, as the formulas on the next page indicate.

Keep in mind that not all of this liquid has to come from a glass; the water in vegetables, fruit, and what is absorbed by cooked grains and legumes also counts. On the other hand, beverages high in added sweeteners, caffeine, and/or alcohol may be counterproductive due to their water-depleting (diuretic) effect. Another drawback to satisfying your need for water with such beverages is the number of calories involved—on average, 100 to 150 per 8-ounce glass for juices and soft drinks—which for most people is apt to cause weight gain.

- Vegetables range from seventy percent water for dense varieties like potatoes, to more than ninety percent for such juicy items as tomatoes, cucumbers, and cooked greens. On average, with each cup of vegetables you consume you take in 4 to 5 ounces of water.
- Seventy-five to ninety percent of fruit is water. A cup of fruit or medium-size apple, pear, or orange furnishes about 4 ounces. Smaller specimens such as plums, kiwis, and peaches add 2 to 3 ounces. Even a dense fruit like a banana offers 3 ounces water in an average-size 4-ounce piece.
- Cooked rice, kasha, millet, and cracked wheat (bulgur) contribute 5 to 6 ounces water per cup. Wild rice, barley, and whole wheat berries are slightly drier, with just 4 ounces, while cooked cereals (oatmeal, cornmeal, Cream of Rye, Wheatena) are as high as 7 ounces water per cup. Even a cup of pasta offers 3 ounces of water.
- On average, with a cup of cooked dried beans you receive 3.5 to 4.5 ounces water.

What's Wrong with Water

What's wrong with water is primarily a matter of its purity. Water is subject to contamination by microbes and environmental chemicals, including heavy metals from automotive and industrial emissions, corroding copper and lead from ancient plumbing systems, pesticides and herbicides from agricultural applications, and some or all of these from direct animal contact and feedlot runoff. Efforts to clean it up lead to the use of other chemicals that are suspect, such as chlorine. There's also a concern about the addition of fluoride to some municipal water systems. (Fluoride is a natural element found in varying amounts in all drinking water and soil. It's present in trace amounts in the body and is a beneficial nutrient; however, above certain levels it may pose health risks.)

★ HOW MUCH WATER SHOULD YOU DRINK? ★

Following are three formulas health professionals use to calculate adequate fluid intake. Use the one that suits you best.

Formula #1: One of the simplest equations used to target fluid intake is 30 ml (1 ounce) per kilogram (2.2 pounds) of body weight. This should be calculated using a reasonable body weight for your height, which could differ from actual weight if you're particularly heavy or thin. This is an important caveat, especially for people with low body weight who might otherwise underestimate their fluid need. For heavier people, who have a lower percentage of water content due to increased fat mass, fluid needs may be less than estimated using true body weight; however, over-consumption of water isn't harmful.

Using this preceding formula, for someone weighing 150 pounds, the calculation comes to 68 ounces, or 8$\frac{1}{2}$ 8-ounce glasses (a little over 2 quarts) of water daily. (150 lbs ÷ 2.2 kg/lb = 68 kg × 1 oz/kg = 68 oz)

Hot weather and heavy physical exertion increase fluid loss; to compensate under these conditions the water multiple can be increased to 35 ml (1.17 ounces). Using the same illustration, a 150-pound person would strive for 80 ounces of water a day, or 10 8-ounce glasses. (150 lbs ÷ 2.2 kg/lb = 68 kg × 1.17 oz/kg = 80 oz)

Formula #2: The U.S. Recommended Daily Allowances proposes a figure linked to energy expenditure of 1 ml per calorie. In other words, if your body burns 2,000 calories in a day you would need to take in 2,000 ml or about 68 ounces fluid (30 ml = 1 ounce). This can be modified to 1.5 ml per calorie to cover activity, sweating, climate, and such, which in this example brings suggested intake up to 3,000 ml or 12.5 cups. Since most people don't have an accurate way of measuring how many calories they use up daily, this gauge isn't very practical for individual use. If calculated based on the caloric value of the diet, which is an approach nutritionists often use, a low-calorie regimen could easily underestimate actual need. However, viewed along with the other two methods, you can see what the range is, and how this might differ from the conventional notion of 6 to 8 cups of water per day.

Formula #3: A third approach, which compensates for extremes in body weight, is based on a three-phase formula. Accordingly, allow 100 ml per kilogram (kg) for the first 10 kg body weight; 50 ml per kg for the next 10 kg; and 15 ml per kg for each remaining kg. Using this rule, for a 150-pound person the goal would be 9$\frac{1}{4}$ cups. (1,000 ml/10 kg + 500 ml/10 kg + 720 mg/48 kg = 2,220 ml ÷ 30 ml/oz = 74 oz, which is 9$\frac{1}{4}$ cups)

Entire books have been written on the subject of water. People have adopted many different approaches to ease their worries. Some buy bottled water. Others invest in home filtering systems.

In order to secure a safe water supply, you need to have information about both the water that comes out of your faucet and the water you can buy. For information about well or municipal water, you should contact a local authority. If you're suspicious about the quality of your home water and don't know where to have it tested, contact your health department to find a sanctioned private laboratory to provide an analysis. Experts recommend that private wells be tested every six months to one year.

Navigating the Water Ways

If you think that the water coming out of your tap isn't of optimum drinking (or cooking) quality, you may be able to correct this with a filter. Filters must be matched to the specific problem that needs solving, as not all systems have the same capacity.

When it comes to purchasing bottled water, whether for purity or simply for taste, there are some things that apply universally. Health standards for bottled drinking water are enforced in the United States by the Food and Drug Administration (FDA). They require all bottled water, whether domestic or imported, to meet the purity requirements mandated for potable tap water by the EPA. This means it must be below a certain microbial count and residual contaminants, including arsenic, lead, mercury, cadmium, copper, and volatile organic chemicals (benzene, carbon tetrachloride, PCBs, herbicides, pesticides, radioactive substances, and the like) mustn't exceed levels deemed acceptable by the EPA. The amount of fluoride present in bottled water is also regulated by federal standards; the maximum allowed is 1.3 to 2 mg per liter, compared to 4 mg per liter in tap water.

If you aren't satisfied with the EPA water standards due to concern about some of these allowed substances, the water you buy may not be preferable. On the other hand, most bottled water (about 75 percent) comes from a protected source, such as an underground aquifer or spring, while tap water generally originates in rivers and lakes, which are more susceptible to environmental and industrial contamination. In addition, about 85 percent of companies selling bottled water in the United States conform to the somewhat stricter guidelines set forth by the International Bottled Water Association, so your chances of getting a better product are greater.

The current standards for bottled drinking water specify what certain keywords on labels mean. Bottled waters, by definition, contain no sweeteners or chemical additives, with the exception of minimal amounts of flavor extracts or essences. Beverages such as seltzer water, soda water or club soda, and tonic water aren't included in these categories.

Spring water is obtained from an "underground formation from which water flows naturally to the surface of the earth." The location of the spring must be identified.

Artesian water is tapped from a confined underground source, such as a spring or a well, in which the water level rises above the top of the source.

Well water comes from a hole drilled or bored into the ground that taps into an aquifer.

Mineral water contains naturally occurring minerals and trace elements such as potassium, calcium, magnesium, sodium, bicarbonates, and chlorides that are picked up as it flows through geological formations to the source. When the minerals dissolve in water they form a measurable solution called "total dissolved solids." The FDA specifies that mineral water must contain between 250 and

461

1,500 mg total dissolved solids per liter, but the particular content of individual minerals isn't dictated. Thus, levels of calcium, magnesium, sodium, and such vary from one brand of mineral water to another. (Some companies list mineral content on the label; all will provide this information if you query them directly.)

Purified water is the name for water that has been altered by distillation, deionization, or reverse osmosis to remove all minerals and other impurities. Most purified waters are reprocessed from municipal water supplies. Depending on the method, some volatile chemicals may still be present. *Distilled water* is one form of purified water.

Sparkling water is water tapped from a source with natural carbonation and must contain the same amount of carbon dioxide that was there when it emerged. This isn't necessarily the same carbon dioxide; sometimes carbon dioxide is added to adjust for losses that occur during processing.

Teetotaling Takes on New Meaning

Tea is reported to be the most widely consumed beverage worldwide after water. This refers specifically to what is called leaf tea, as distinct from herbal tea.

All of the more than three thousand different types of tea grown and drunk throughout the world come from the same plant family—*Camellia sinensis*. The differences between the three principal tea categories—green, oolong, and black—result from processing: For green tea, the fresh leaves are prepared and dried as quickly as possible to preserve their composition. Black tea leaves are kept in a moist atmosphere for up to ninety minutes prior to drying in order to activate natural enzymes that oxidize and modify some of the inherent chemical compounds. This oxidation process (often referred to as fermentation) is responsible for changes in structure, as well as flavor and appearance. Oolong tea is prepared in a similar manner to black tea, but oxidized for a shorter time period.

The tea plant contains a variety of phytochemicals classified as polyphenols, or more specifically various catechins (flavanols), flavonols, and phenolic acids (see the table on pages 381ff.). The health-protective effects associated with drinking tea are attributed to these substances.

Tea catechins, including epicatechin (found in green, oolong, and black teas) and epicatechin gallate, epigallocatechin, and gallocatechin (which are altered by fermentation and thus found primarily in green tea) are potent antioxidants, protecting unsaturated fats in particular. Catechins are also antimutagenic, and there are signs that they even inhibit an enzyme required by the HIV virus to initiate AIDS.

The flavanols that predominate in black tea are called theaflavins and thearubigens. They are produced from catechins during manufacture and give the various types of black tea their characteristic flavor and color. (Some people know them by the name "tannins.") They, too, are antioxidants and exhibit HIV virus–suppressing activity. Theaflavins and thearubigens may have a moderate influence on blood sugar levels as a result of their mild suppressive action on the digestive enzymes that break down starches (amylase) and sugars (sucrase). Moreover, these tea phytochemicals influence the sensitivity of taste buds, lowering the response threshold to salt (in other words, making the perception of salt greater) and increasing it toward sugar (requiring more sugar to achieve the same sense of sweetness).

Another mechanism by which black tea could be protective results from its inhibitory effect on iron absorption. Although iron is an essential mineral, it's also a potent oxidant and can accelerate the production of damaging free radicals and other oxidative compounds that have been implicated in cancer, heart disease, and other chronic conditions (see Chapter 3). For those who need to maximize their iron intake (for example, to offset low blood stores as in anemia), there is evidence that when milk is added to tea, the milk protein casein binds with the iron-inhibiting tannins, making the iron more available. This could explain the common custom in some cultures of adding milk to tea. Ascorbic acid also facilitates absorption of iron from tea, which could be why other cultures adopted the habit of drinking tea with lemon.

Flavonoids, an additional group of polyphenols found in tea as well as numerous other plants, are among the most common and active antioxidants within our food supply. Some flavonoids (those in the category flavonols) are more potent in this regard then others. For example, quercetin and myricetin inhibit oxidative changes and are active free-radical scavengers even at very low levels. Both these phytochemicals, along with the flavonols kaempferol and rutin, are found in green, oolong, and black teas.

In general, flavonoids (which are discussed in greater detail in Chapter 4) exhibit anti-inflammatory and antibiotic activity. Even the small quantities found in food have measurable anti-infectious action against both bacteria and viruses.

One substance found in tea that has been criticized is caffeine. Although caffeine levels in tea are modest compared to those in coffee (see Counting Caffeine, on page 468), people differ greatly in their sensitivity. Moderate caffeine consumption is considered to be about 300 mg, yet some people feel its stimulating effects with lower doses. Moreover, several cups of tea in a concentrated time period are sufficient to reduce cerebral artery blood flow, initiate hormone secretion, and arouse sympathetic nervous stimulation of the heart and vascular system. While acute doses of caffeine can elevate high blood pressure in some individuals, studies don't support a similar effect from intake of caffeine over a prolonged period. Caffeine can also increase blood sugar levels and insulin secretion, and people report feeling hypoglycemic after caffeine ingestion, with symptoms such as trembling, headache, and mental impairment, even when their blood sugar levels don't fall below normal. In addition, caffeine may increase the level of free fatty acids in the blood, although no such direct effect has been connected with drinking tea.

A Proper "Cuppa"

With more than 3,000 choices, deciding what tea to drink could be confusing. In fact, the availability of tea varieties is generally quite limited within a geographic area. And while differences in taste can be quite pronounced, many are rather subtle.

Since all teas are derived from the same plant, growing area, cultivation techniques, harvesting, and production methods are what distinguish one from another. Within any one type, the highest-quality tea is made from the top two or three leaves and the growing bud. The farther down the stem the leaves come from, the less highly regarded the tea. In the factory, tea is sorted by sifting through a stack of mesh sieves. Generally the best tea of a particular type is on the top sieve, which catches the biggest pieces. Successively lower grades fall to the sieves below. The "fannings" or "dust" at the bottom are used in tea bags.

Green tea is considered the best choice healthwise. It contains the most catechins, comparable levels of flavonols to black tea, and, when brewed in the preferred manner (see Basic Green Tea, on page 236), the least caffeine. Yet it accounts for only about 20 percent of the worldwide tea production and is consumed mainly in Asian countries. (Black tea accounts for 78 percent of tea manufacture and is the tea most known in Western nations. Oolong, which makes up just 2 percent of tea, is drunk mostly in southeastern China.)

Despite the preference by dedicated tea drinkers for loose leaves over prebagged tea, which is warranted from a taste standpoint, the phytochemical content of lesser grades doesn't appear to suffer. In fact, when steeped for the same length of time, infusions from tea bags (probably owing to their small particle size) show higher levels of some phytochemicals.

Tea and Health

The general mechanisms by which tea gains its health-promoting reputation were described above, along with the potential for caffeine to make it objectionable to those who are particularly sensitive to its stimulating effect. Below we describe how these factors relate to specific conditions.

Tea Tames Cancer

Cancer researchers have shown that tea catechins prevent cell mutation and deactivate certain carcinogens. They have demonstrated potential to inhibit tumor production in the skin, lungs, esophagus, stomach, colon, liver, pancreas, and breast. They also have a protective effect against lymphomas caused by radiation, and protect skin from damage by ultraviolet rays. These claims have been validated in animal models, but no direct studies on humans have been done.

In addition, the flavonoids in tea act by blocking enzymes that produce estrogen. In this way they may reduce the risk of estrogen-induced cancers such as breast, prostate, and colon.

A phenol in tea known as ellagic acid provides another clue to how tea might inhibit cancer. Ellagic acid prevents certain procarcinogens from becoming carcinogenic, inhibits activity of compounds that initiate cancer, and prevents tumor growth. In animal studies, ellagic acid exhibits potent activity against skin, lung, esophageal, small intestine, liver, and pancreatic tumors. It also reduces genetic damage caused by tobacco smoke and air pollution.

Several highly regarded population studies substantiate these hypotheses by making a strong association between tea drinking and reduced cancer incidence. However, this can't be considered proof, especially in light of the fact that an extensive 1993 review of the research up to that time indicates that many investigations failed to show any connection between cancers and tea consumption, while at some sites (stomach, colon, rectum, lung) tea has been implicated as both protective and causative. Supportive studies have surfaced since this review; however, further investigation is warranted, particularly as to how local habits might impact on the results.

In studies pointing to increased esophageal cancer among tea drinkers, tea itself probably isn't the culprit, but the irritant effect of drinking boiling hot (and salty) tea, which is the custom in certain places. Case-controlled studies with normal-temperature tea and high-temperature tea affirm this. Other dietary components may also help interpret the mixed outcome of research findings. For example, tea is likely to protect against stomach cancer when the suspected cause is nitrosamines (formed from nitrates found in processed meats, some vegetables, and in some places in the water supply), but may not be effective in combating stomach cancer precipitated by other carcinogens. Likewise, while tea might reduce esophageal cancer in nonsmokers who avoid alcohol, it may not be powerful enough to overcome the known damaging effects of these two habits.

Tea Helps the Heart

Animal studies demonstrate that tea catechins play a protective role in heart disease. They suppress excessive elevation of blood cholesterol, especially the damaging low-density lipoprotein (LDL), and help prevent a rise in blood triglycerides, presumably by interrupting the absorption of fats. They inhibit the activity of enzymes that cause arteries to contract, and in this way may curb high blood pressure.

The flavonoids in tea also provide a buffer by inhibiting oxidative changes to LDL that can lead to atherosclerosis, by decreasing blood platelet stickiness, and also by lowering blood pressure.

Supporting evidence for the coronary benefits of tea drinking in humans is seen in several reports comparing heart disease incidence and consumption of green tea (in Japanese men) and black tea (in Dutch men). These results are observed when tea is consumed in fairly large quantities—as much as ten cups a day. In green tea studies, even smokers were at a reduced risk.

As noted earlier, although caffeine levels in tea are modest compared to those in coffee, drinking several cups in a short time period can cause blood pressure to climb. This is usually a transient effect, but it can be frightening, especially for people with angina, arrhythmias, or similar heart problems. (In some instances it may also lead to medical misdiagnosis.)

Tea for Teeth

Tea helps protect teeth in two ways. One is that the catechins in tea inhibit growth of bacteria that cause dental plaque and cavities. Second, tea is a source of natural fluoride, the mineral that strengthens tooth enamel. Although fluoride levels vary with the soil the plant is grown in, and green tea generally contains more fluoride than black tea, an average figure is .1 mg per 5- to 6-ounce cup. This is within the range found naturally in water and considerably less than permitted in municipal fluoridated water systems.

Tea and Kidney Stones

Tea contains oxalic acid, which is the precursor of one of the two main constituents in calcium-oxalate kidney stones. Although urinary oxalate levels, which are used to help predict kidney stones, are influenced more by endogenous synthesis than diet, food intake can't be discounted. The potential for tea to promote kidney stone formation may even be enhanced by the diuretic action of its caffeine, which promotes calcium excretion. Based on this equation, urologists may counsel stone formers to avoid tea.

In fact, although some teas do have significant levels of oxalates, it's uncertain whether tea drinking causes kidney stone formation. For people who aren't predisposed toward stones and those with normal absorption rates of oxalates, tea isn't a particular concern. But for "hyper" absorbers, drinking more than a cup or two of tea daily could be problematic.

If kidney stones are a concern, there are some ways for tea drinkers to reduce oxalate impact. For one, when tea is taken with milk urinary oxalates show only negligible increases. Similarly, eating other calcium-rich foods at the same time and simply maintaining adequate overall calcium intake are also protective.

Brewing black tea for just one minute is another way to bring oxalate levels down to as much as half the measure detected after five minutes of steeping. On the other hand, stirring tea vigorously dramatically increases oxalates, so this practice is best avoided.

In addition, because green tea is usually brewed using fewer leaves than black tea, it averages about 3.4 mg oxalates per 4-ounce serving, considerably less than black tea, which when steeped for a traditional five minutes ranges from 6 to 10 mg oxalates per 4-ounce serving.

Common herbal teas have a low oxalate content and thus are an option for those who tend to form calcium oxalate kidney stones.

Tea and Osteoporosis

Because tea contains caffeine, and high caffeine consumption spurs the body to excrete more calcium, there's a potential for tea to promote bone deterioration. A few studies do show an association between caffeine and hip fractures in women; however, the ultimate effect of tea depends on the rest of the diet, including total caffeine intake from all sources and habitual calcium consumption.

Studies of caffeine and bone loss in postmenopausal women indicate that when calcium intake is low, caffeine has a more pronounced negative impact. In one well-designed study, when average daily calcium intake was 745 mg or more, there appeared to be no detrimental effect on bone mineral density for a wide range of caffeine consumption. However, in women ingesting only 440 to 744 mg calcium daily, routine caffeine intake above 450 mg corresponded to a significant loss of bone mineral density. Based on the estimated caffeine content of various beverages (see Counting Caffeine, on page 468) women drinking about four 6-ounce cups of brewed coffee a day or seven 6-ounce cups of instant coffee who don't have a reliable calcium intake are at greater risk. It would take more than 1½ quarts of tea to reach the same caffeine level. Thus, tea drinkers are seemingly vulnerable only if they drink vast quantities or consume tea in addition to coffee.

Other studies corroborate this sparing effect of calcium as far as caffeine is concerned, with estimates that two cups of brewed coffee or four to six cups of tea can decrease bone density and increase hip fracture risk for older women who don't drink at least one glass of milk or consume its calcium equivalent on a daily basis. For the 3,170 subjects followed in the Framingham Study, one of the classic long-term nutrition studies, heavy caffeine use was deemed a risk factor in hip fracture; however, the investigators were careful to note that since caffeine use may be coupled with other behaviors that are themselves risk factors for fracture, the association could be indirect rather than inducing.

In premenopausal women the connection between caffeine and bone integrity is complicated even more by the fact that younger women who tend toward high caffeine intake often follow such compounding lifestyle practices as smoking and drinking alcohol. Most investigations of this population don't show that, on its own, caffeine has any compromising influence. However, a 1990 study examining the effect of 400 mg caffeine on sixteen healthy premenopausal women, although claiming no significant effects on calcium balance, did admit to evidence of altered bone remodeling. A follow-up report in 1995 by the same researchers, analyzing data from 560 calcium balance studies carried out on 190 women, found that every 6-ounce serving of coffee (which is the equivalent of two or three cups of tea) notably increased calcium loss.

According to several reports, the effect of caffeine on bone integrity may not be measurable solely in terms of bone density, but due to some additional interfering factor. Therefore, moderation is once again a good idea, and in women prone to osteoporosis, limiting tea intake (as well as all sources of caffeine) and

★ COUNTING CAFFEINE ★

A moderate daily caffeine intake is considered to be about 300 mg; however, people differ greatly in their sensitivity to caffeine. Note that the caffeine content of beverages isn't consistent, and varies with preparation techniques and plant variety. The values given below for tea correspond to a typical brewing time of three to five minutes, and are calculated using boiling water. The longer tea steeps and the hotter the water, the greater the caffeine extraction. In addition, the more leaves used per cup, the higher the caffeine potential. While equal quantities of black, oolong, and green teas all have the same caffeine capacity, properly prepared green tea is made using water that has cooled to between 165 and 185°F and is steeped for only one to three minutes. Therefore, when made according to these guidelines, green tea imparts less caffeine than noted here for black tea. Oolong tea is generally comparable to imported black tea in caffeine content.

Beverage (6 fluid ounces)	Typical	Range (mg caffeine)
Black tea, major U.S. brands	35	20 to 90
Black tea, imported	60	25 to 110
Tea, instant	30	25 to 50
Coffee, brewed, drip method	110	60 to 180
Coffee, instant	65	30 to 120
Coffee, espresso, brewed	375	—
Coffee, espresso, instant	126	—
Cappuccino	75	

choosing brewing methods that lower caffeine extraction is a wise precaution. Decaffeinated tea is another alternative.

Alcohol: To Drink or Not to Drink

Moderate intake of alcoholic beverages has been shown to decrease the risk of coronary heart disease, at least in middle-aged adults. The American Cancer Society, which warns people to "limit consumption of alcoholic beverages, if you drink at all," amends this by noting that the "cardiovascular benefits may outweigh the risk of cancer in men over age 50 and in women over age 60." While some people choose to interpret this and similar statements as an endorsement for drinking alcohol, any position on alcohol consumption requires a careful look at all sides of the issue. Only then can each person decide what his or her approach should be.

A warning: Whatever you determine after reading the various arguments for and against alcohol, keep in mind that public health officials advise people who do drink to limit their intake to two drinks a day for men, and one drink per day for women (see The Measure of Alcohol, on page 469). Women generally don't tolerate alcohol as well as men, which is why they're counseled to drink less. Fur-

Moderate drinking is regarded as one drink daily for women, and not more than two drinks per day for men.

A drink is defined as:

12 ounces of regular beer
4 ounces of wine at 12.5% alcohol
5 ounces of wine at 10% alcohol
3 ounces of sherry
1.25 ounces of brandy, cognac, cordials, and similar liquors
1.5 ounces of 80-proof distilled spirits

thermore, those at risk for certain cancers, as well as children, adolescents, pregnant women, and people taking certain medications, should abstain from alcohol consumption altogether. We want it to be clear that the upcoming information shouldn't be used in any way to justify alcohol consumption beyond the amounts just indicated.

Alcohol Is Dangerous

This section covers some of the potential benefits and hazards associated with drinking alcohol. Any decision you make regarding alcohol should take into account its numerous harmful effects on nutritional status. One major criticism of alcohol is that it puts people at risk for various illnesses because those who drink heavily are likely to substitute alcohol for nutrient-rich, protective foods. This seems obvious for heavy users, who typically derive 50 percent or more of their daily calories from alcohol, but even for social drinkers it may account for 10 to 15 percent of calories. Therefore, it's crucial that if you do imbibe alcohol, you don't forgo other healthful habits as a result.

Excessive use of alcohol is a critical health issue. Alcohol contributes to morbidity and mortality not only by its influence on specific diseases, overall nutritional status, and possibly by affecting immune competence, but via its role in motor vehicle and other unintentional injuries, homicide, and suicide. It is implicated in an estimated 100,000 deaths each year, and countless people develop other maladies that are alcohol related. Therefore, any message suggesting that alcohol may offer health benefits must be carefully presented to guard against misperceptions, especially among youths. (According to a 1991 survey by the National Institute on Drug Abuse, 30 percent of high school seniors reported having had five or more drinks at one sitting during the previous two weeks. More than 70 percent of eighth graders reported they had already consumed alcohol at some time, and this increased to 88 percent by twelfth grade. Among eighth graders, 27 percent reported being drunk in the past month, and this figure was up to 65 percent for twelfth graders. For this population there is no hint that alcohol is of any health benefit whatsoever.)

469

Mentor

Alcohol permeates every tissue in the body and affects most vital functions. The liver is the organ most severely impacted, in part because unlike fat, protein, and carbohydrate, which are broken down in the stomach and intestines, alcohol is metabolized primarily in the liver. As a result of this unusual energy pathway, the production of energy (or calories) from alcohol precipitates a variety of metabolic disorders. For instance, the breakdown of alcohol leads to increased levels of uric acid in the blood (which can exacerbate gout or lead to goutlike symptoms); it inhibits proper glucose production, causing symptoms of hypoglycemia; and it disrupts fat metabolism, favoring storage of body fat and increased levels of certain blood lipids, suggesting an influence on the absorption or synthesis of fatty acids. Moreover, alcohol promotes cell death by depleting levels of critical enzymes, inducing oxidation reactions, and generating harmful free radicals.

Alcohol also blocks the secretion of proteins, causing liver cells to retain water, protein, and electrolytes, and to become swollen. This "balloon effect" is a hallmark of alcoholic liver disease.

Also unlike fat, carbohydrate, and protein, our bodies can't store any of the energy generated by alcohol, and chronic intake can change the body's "metabolic efficiency"—that is, the way it burns these other nutrients to generate energy. This can lead to the development of many alcohol-related ailments. Deficiencies of zinc, vitamin B_6, and folate are common in alcoholics. These deficiencies aren't necessarily caused by low dietary intake; rather, levels are compromised by alcohol as a result of decreased absorption, impaired utilization, or increased excretion.

Alcohol depletes liver stores of vitamin A, which in turn affects the integrity of epithelial cells. In addition, it may impair absorption of vitamin C, whereas vitamin C itself protects against alcohol-induced toxicity. Since drinkers are more prone to lipid oxidation and free-radical formation, alcohol places an increased demand on vitamin E, which protects fats from oxidation.

Low dietary intake of riboflavin (vitamin B_2) can complicate alcoholism, contributing to tissue damage on skin surfaces and the lining of such organs as the stomach, colon, and esophagus. Increasing riboflavin has displayed some protection against malignant lesions in the esophagus.

Experiments with rats suggest that diets high in choline, methionine, and protein protect the liver from alcohol-induced injury; however, adding more choline to the diet hasn't been sufficient on its own to help people ward off liver damage due to long-term alcohol use.

Finally, great care is needed regarding alcohol when taking any medication. There are at least three good reasons for this:

1. Alcohol increases the level of the cytochrome P-450 enzymes that have an extraordinary capacity to turn many foreign substances into highly toxic elements. This encompasses chemical agents, as well as many medications, including common over-the-counter pain medication such as acetaminophen.

2. While long-term consumption of alcohol makes certain drugs more potent, metabolism of some medications is suppressed in the immediate presence of alcohol. As a result, instead of traveling to targeted sites, these drugs become concentrated in the brain and liver.
3. Certain drugs, including aspirin and antacid medications, increase the toxicity of alcohol by interfering with the body's ability to process it.

A Drink a Day Could Keep the Cardiologist at Bay

Heart disease is the leading cause of death in the United States. Understandably, any avenue of prevention seems worth pursuing. This is where alcohol enjoys its status as a health-protective beverage, although this must be viewed with many qualifications. The American Heart Association estimates that 80,000 deaths from heart disease are prevented each year by moderate drinking. This is an impressive figure; however, it diminishes in stature when juxtaposed against the 100,000 presumed to be killed every year by alcohol, and the multitude who suffer in its wake.

Depending on whose research you read, moderate drinking reduces the risk of coronary heart disease in men and women in a range of 30 to 70 percent. Studies of drinking populations indicate that consumption of alcohol in amounts typical in France, that is 20 to 30 grams a day, confer a 40 percent risk reduction. For women, as little as 10 to 15 grams of alcohol daily is believed to be protective. There is even a study claiming that compared with nondrinkers, women who consume as few as three drinks per week derive some benefit. One drink

---

NIKKI'S DIALOGUE BOX

Are There Better Ways to Drink?

"In addition to moderating quantity, here are two important rules regarding alcohol.

"First, sipping your drink during the course of a meal is a safer strategy than chugging a few drinks during happy hour.

"Alcohol consumed in a fasting state is more detrimental than alcohol consumed along with food. Although the liver is the primary site of alcohol metabolism, the stomach can break down alcohol to some degree and thereby reduce its toxic effect. When alcohol is consumed with food, it remains in the stomach long enough for this activity to occur. (The reason women tend to be less tolerant of alcohol and more vulnerable to its effects is that they generally have lower levels of the enzyme alcohol dehydrogenase necessary to perform this task. Certain ethnic groups also seem to generate less of this enzyme. It is believed to be absent or markedly decreased in 80 percent of Japanese people.)

"Second, don't mix aspirin, antacids, and alcohol.

"Certain drugs, including aspirin and antacids, further suppress stomach levels of alcohol dehydrogenase. As a result, smaller amounts of alcohol have a more profound effect in their company. Ironically, people often take these medications to reduce symptoms that accompany drinking—headaches and indigestion."

(12 ounces beer, 4 to 5 ounces wine, or 1.5 ounces hard liquor) contains 14 to 15 grams of alcohol.

The benefit conferred by alcohol could be a result of its ability to increase the protective HDL cholesterol, or the fact that it decreases blood platelet stickiness. The latter is more likely; however, this influence on blood platelet stickiness could create problems as well, such as increasing the risk of hemorrhagic stroke. Wine (and red wine in particular) may act in an additional manner by reducing the oxidation of damaging LDL cholesterol, although this is disputed in some studies.

In the now famous report that first declared a relationship between reduced heart disease and alcohol, it was dubbed "The French Paradox" because the population under investigation lives in a part of France famous for its foie gras (fatty goose liver pâté). Naturally, accounts of low coronary heart disease (CHD) in this region seem surprising. Equally intriguing is that worldwide reports relating many different foodstuffs to CHD are in agreement on one only—dairy fat. Once again, the French (and Swiss) confound this: Despite an intake of dairy fat in France and Switzerland equal to that in the United Kingdom, Australia, and Germany, mortality from CHD is lower.

The mystery was unraveled when data from seventeen countries uncovered a correlation between wine consumption and reduced mortality from CHD. Among its other actions, wine has been credited with countering the negative effects of saturated dairy products. Not to be forgotten, however, is that in these wine-drinking cultures intake of fruit and vegetables is generally high, people eat smaller portions of meat, less processed food and fewer "snack" foods, obesity is infrequent, and alcohol is customarily consumed with food.

The positive effects of alcohol on heart disease are reversed at high levels, especially in the form of binge or "heavy weekend" drinking. One indication is that heavy drinkers have elevated blood levels of homocysteine, an intermediary product produced by the body during the conversion of the amino acid methionine to cysteine (see Chapter 3). Homocysteine has been linked to vascular disease leading to heart attack and stroke. Alcohol also increases blood triglyceride levels, which is another possible risk factor for CHD; therefore, it should be avoided by anyone with either of these two markers.

Since alcohol is estimated to be involved in as much as 10 percent of the incidence of hypertension, its therapeutic influence may not be realized in people with high blood pressure. Low doses of alcohol (as in one to two drinks) actually relaxes blood vessels and lowers blood pressure in people with normal blood pressure, but when regular drinkers who suffer from hypertension avoid alcohol, their blood pressure usually improves. Furthermore, even those who respond favorably to one or two drinks show adverse effects on blood pressure when they consume three drinks or more. An interesting observation has been made that sympathetic nerve response, which controls communication between the brain, the nerves that run down the spinal column, and the blood vessels in muscles and internal organs, is highest when alcohol is wearing off, rather than during drinking. This suggests that something produced by the body during the metabolism of alcohol may influence the hormones that regulate such functions as muscle contractions, insulin production, and artery constriction and relaxation.

While most people worry about the effects of long-term chronic alcohol consumption, short-term bingeing could cause a stroke because of alcohol's effects on blood pressure and blood platelets.

Women at high risk for heart disease who have few risk factors for other alcohol-related disorders may view moderate alcohol consumption as part of an overall protective strategy. Nonetheless, there are many more prudent steps that can be taken to prevent heart disease, and no one who doesn't already drink should be encouraged to start in anticipation of any benefits.

Red or White?

For those who wish to pursue the potential health benefits of alcohol, reports are mixed as to which beverages serve this purpose best. Red wine is cited most often by researchers, with credit given to the polyphenols (catechins, flavylium compounds, and flavonols, especially quercetin and myricetin), which are potent antioxidants and antiplatelet aggregants (discussed on page 462 in Teetotaling Takes on New Meaning), along with a compound known as resveratrol, which is found in grape skins. Resveratrol, too, has the ability to reduce blood platelet stickiness.

Although less active or at reduced levels in other grape-based beverages, these substances are present in white wine, as well as some nonalcoholic wines and even grape juice. Observational studies lend support to beer and distilled spirits as well, leading public health researchers to conclude that all of these beverages have a role.

Drinking Your Way to Cancer

Alcohol is second only to smoking as a proven cause of cancer. It exerts its harmful influence in several ways. Although alcohol itself may not be a direct carcinogen, at the initiation stage it arouses the liver enzymes that activate potential cancer-causing agents. It also blocks the enzyme that normally repairs damaged DNA. During the promotion stage, alcohol acts as a tumor promoter by fostering fat oxidation and free radical formation, and by increasing blood levels of the free fatty acids involved in tumor growth. Another way it may contribute to cancer is by reducing the body's store of vitamin A. Vitamin A opposes the activation of certain carcinogens. Prophlyactic supplementation has failed to be effective and actually shows signs of making things worse. This is explained by the fact that alcohol makes the liver more susceptible to damage caused by excessive vitamin A; even the toxicity of beta-carotene (which is normally considered benign) is amplified by alcohol.

Alcoholic beverages, along with cigarettes, snuff, and chewing tobacco, are blamed for cancers of the mouth, throat, larynx, and esophagus. While separately these factors are damaging enough, their combined effect is even more pronounced. For instance, alcohol use increases cancer of the esophagus by 18-fold, smokers have a 5-fold higher risk, and the two behaviors combined result in a 44-fold greater chance of esophageal cancer.

Studies also point to an increased breast cancer risk among alcohol drinkers. As little as two drinks a day are associated with a 25 percent risk increase. (A weak relationship exists for women consuming one half to one drink daily.) The reason for this link hasn't been determined. It may be due to a direct effect from alcohol or a breakdown product of alcohol, or to alcohol-induced changes in levels of hormones such as estrogen, or to some other process.

Since exposure of breast tissue to estrogen is considered a risk factor for breast cancer, and the ability of alcohol to increase estrogen in women has been repeatedly documented, a logical assumption is that hormones are involved. In premenopausal women, even moderate alcohol intake increases estrogen levels, especially around the time of ovulation. Over the course of a woman's monthly menstrual cycle, alcohol can raise the hormone from 7 to 32 percent. In postmenopausal women on hormone-replacement therapy (including estrogen and progestin), an experiment in which approximately three alcoholic drinks were consumed daily during the estrogen phase led to a 3-fold increase in blood hormone levels. In a control group not taking estrogen, blood levels of estrogen weren't significantly changed. The researchers concluded that for women who drink and take estrogen, hormone levels could be as much as 300 percent higher than clinical goals. It isn't known whether this short-term effect is consequential, or if estrogen substances other than Estrace, which was the form administered in this study, produce the same results. Because the degree of exposure to estrogen over a lifetime may be critical, the findings of these studies should be factored into every woman's decision about drinking.

Note that researchers are still hesitant regarding the issue of alcohol and breast cancer, and comment that "association does not prove cause." Even though in some studies there appears to be a dose-response—that is, with more alcohol risk increases—which generally supports causality, not all data agree. And since the effect remains modest, cause is difficult to establish. Researchers believe there could be some other factor that results in both a tendency to drink and a tendency to develop breast cancer.

Earlier, we noted that alcohol consumption is associated with high blood levels of homocysteine. This is because alcohol disrupts the process that converts the amino acid methionine into cysteine. Other nutrients involved in this transformation include folate, vitamin B_6, and vitamin B_{12}. Studies show that men who consume more than two alcoholic drinks daily and don't get enough folate and methionine in their diets are more likely to suffer from colon cancer. This is supported by other research indicating that alcohol reduces vitamin B_{12} (especially in men), and although it doesn't depress folate levels, avoidance of alcohol is associated with rising blood folate measures. (To ensure an adequate supply of these nutrients, see Dietary Sources of Nutrient Helpers, on page 356.)

The devastating effect of alcohol on the liver was reviewed earlier. What wasn't stated is that liver injury to women drinkers is more frequent and progresses faster than for men with comparable habits. This may be due to the fact that female hormones such as estrogen, whether produced naturally by the body or from an exogenous source such as oral contraceptives or hormone-replacement therapy, can impair various liver functions. (Hormones may also influence the pathologic response to alcohol in other tissues, which is perhaps why women who drink are more prone to gastric ulcers and possibly breast cancer.) Daily consumption of only 20 grams of ethanol (less than two drinks) significantly increases the incidence of cirrhosis in well-nourished women; for well-nourished men, risk increases at 40 to 60 grams of ethanol. (A drink, as defined on page 469 in The Measure of Alcohol, contains 14 to 15 grams of ethanol.) You just read how women on hormone-replacement therapy who drink may be getting more hormone than they signed on for. If this is the case, their odds of incurring liver disease could go up, too. Regarding liver cancer, the lipid-oxidizing effect of alcohol is an additional contributor.

Resveratrol, a compound derived from grape skins, does show cancer-prevention activity at all three stages of cancer. It is an antioxidant, an antimutagen, and it induces the activity of cancer-blocking (Phase 2) enzymes. A purified form of resveratrol has been shown to block human leukemia cell proliferation in the laboratory and to inhibit tumor growth in mouse skin and mammary cancers. This doesn't prove it's effective in humans, or that wine has similar capabilities. In light of the adverse effect alcohol has been shown to have on cancer, fresh grapes (eaten with the skin, which is where resveratrol is concentrated), nonalcoholic wines, and other grape products would be better paths to pursue if this agent proves to be useful. (Peanuts are an additional source of resveratrol.)

Alcohol and Blood Sugar

Alcohol disrupts the production of energy by interfering with glucose uptake by the cells. This is a form of insulin resistance that is induced directly by alcohol. As we discussed in Chapter 1, the body can sometimes compensate by pumping out more insulin; however, for people with varying degrees of glucose intolerance, this can create a range of complications. Diabetics whose blood sugar isn't well controlled and elderly men and women (who often have mild to moderate undetected insulin resistance) are particularly susceptible.

Alcohol Builds Bones (and May Also Break Them)

Data culled from the Framingham Study (cited above in the discussion of caffeine) suggest a positive role for alcohol consumption in curtailing osteoporosis. Postmenopausal women participants who drank 7 ounces of alcohol or more weekly maintained higher bone densities than nondrinking peers. This could be due to the fact that alcohol raises the body's natural production of estrogen, a fact that has been documented in several studies. The same report indicated that bone density in men drinking 14 ounces of alcohol or more on a weekly basis was also greater, but this wasn't as significant as for the women. It is important to note that subjects were generally well nourished, so that some of the adverse nutritional consequences of alcohol that could undermine bone density probably weren't present. Several other studies have led researchers to conclude that "social drinking" is associated with higher bone mineral density in men and women.

By contrast, a study of more than 84,000 U.S. women aged thirty-four to fifty-nine years who were followed for six years implicated alcohol in both hip and forearm fractures. Compared with nondrinkers, women consuming an average of two alcoholic drinks or more daily fell into a higher risk group. No explanation was offered as to why.

Studies of long-term chronic alcohol users indicate decreased bone formation, which has been attributed to a direct toxic effect of alcohol on osteoblasts, the cells responsible for orchestrating bone formation (see Chapter 7). In addition, alcoholics have been found to have high levels of corticosteroid hormones in their blood. These hormones can induce bone loss. Chronic use of alcohol can also decrease vitamin D levels, resulting in decreased calcium absorption, which may in turn affect the course of osteoporosis.

There is at least one other reason why incorporating alcohol into a plan to reduce osteoporosis may not be a wise strategy: The danger of falling due to even mild intoxication can result in hip and wrist fractures. In older women especially, who are at greatest risk for osteoporosis and often have a lower tolerance for alcohol, such a mishap could outweigh potential gains.

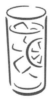

Appendix

The Weight Issue: What (You Eat) vs. Weight

This book isn't about body weight, but as the subject seems to be on virtually everyone's mind, we would be remiss in not discussing it.

We want to state right off that a substantial volume of research validates that *body weight doesn't necessarily parallel health*, although at both the upper and lower ends of the scale it does appear to have an influence. For most people who are "dieting," however, the concern is appearance, not health. The connection between self-worth and weight and the issue of public image and weight are extremely important, but they aren't within the scope of this book, which is about healthy eating, not healthy attitudes. When it comes to health and weight, though, we do have a few things to say.

According to U.S. government statistics, more than one third of adults are considered to be overweight (a figure that has gone up almost 10 percent since the 1970s). Children also appear to be fatter than ever. What has never been adequately determined, however, is what does being "overweight" mean, as well as what are the effects of being "underweight."

While the relationship between weight and health remains unclear, what we know with certainty is that the quality of one's diet is fundamental to good health.

Weighty Questions

Weight isn't just a question of numbers. When evaluating weight-management needs, a knowledgeable health professional considers many factors that individuals trying to lose (or gain) weight should look at as well. But oddly enough, scores of people subject themselves to all kinds of weight-loss schemes without these assessments. Moreover, they resist initiating sensible diet and lifestyle changes that are known to be integral to well-being.

Below are some questions you should examine before making a determination about your weight. They are each addressed in the discussion that follows.

How much extra weight or body fat is too much?

Is the location of fat (for instance, on the abdomen or on the hips and thighs) important?

Does height, which is correlated with weight, play a role?

Is the timing of weight gain or loss a consideration?

Does food matter more than weight?

Are weight and nutritional status connected?

People Are Dying to Weigh Less

Statistics from the mid-1990s indicate that at any given moment in the United States, 40 percent of women and 24 percent of men are trying to lose weight. Whether for reasons of health or appearance, these people average 2.3 diet attempts each year. As many as 16 percent of women age nineteen to thirty-nine consider themselves "perpetual dieters." Many of these dieters aren't actually above recommended weight. Among those who are, more than 90 percent are likely to regain most or more of their lost pounds within five years.

While people view their weight in terms of pounds, a figure known as body mass index (BMI) is the guideline used in health settings. BMI, a number based on a ratio of weight to height, is explained in Finding Your Body Mass Index, on page 482. Within a given range of BMI, people are categorized as being of healthy weight, moderately overweight, or severely overweight. Though there is a big space beneath healthy weight in which people are presumably underweight, much less attention is paid to this segment of the population.

The criteria used to determine weight categories vary and are complicated by socioeconomic issues. Various public health agencies and researchers propose different cutoff points. The life insurance tables that have traditionally been the reference point for weight are widely criticized as being biased in favor of economically stable white men (the population most apt to have health insurance). A legitimate concern of many investigators of weight-health issues is what this means for women and people of different ethnic origins, whose biological programming doesn't appear to parallel that of white males. For example, as a result of this stereotype, older white, non-Hispanic women, and black and Hispanic adult males and females are more apt to be considered overweight. U.S. government figures claim that 50 percent of Mexican American women and 52 percent of non-Hispanic Black American women are overweight! Data on Asian Americans is scant.

Although statistics indicate people are getting heavier, the vision of what people should ideally weigh is simultaneously getting narrower. In 1990, the official USDA weight guidelines raised the cutoff point for healthy weight after age thirty-five (in other words, they added a few extra pounds); in 1995 they withdrew this allowance for healthy weight to increase with age, although evidence confirms a natural trend in this direction and, within limits, improved health outcomes. Currently the USDA considers a BMI of 19 to 25 as optimal for everyone over the age of nineteen years. However, a number of important studies dispute this.

Among the evidence that supports higher ideal weight is an impressive study from Cornell University to the effect that optimal weight for men is about 15 pounds heavier than most recommendations. Consequently, a BMI between 23 to 29 is more suitable for men, with the lowest risk of death related to a BMI of 27. Their conclusion comes from analyzing twenty-two studies correlating weight to all causes of mortality. About one thousand citations were considered to find these studies in order to isolate what the researchers felt was the best controlled and least biased data. A British study published in 1997 (after the Cornell review), which followed more than 7,700 men for almost fifteen years, made a similar determination; mortality from all causes increased only in men with a BMI under 20 or when BMI reached 30.

Figures claiming higher death rates for people with BMIs below the healthy weight range are often discounted due to a belief that smoking or preexisting illness clouds the issue. The Cornell study found this to be a misconception. Contrary to expectations, when smoking and illness were controlled for, mortality rose in almost equal increments both below and above the 23-to-29-point range.

Unfortunately, there is limited information available on weight and mortality in white women, and even less on various ethnic groups, so no conclusions can be drawn regarding these populations.

The Nurses' Health Study, one of the few long-term studies of women's health and the most often cited, affirms that weight gains up to 22 pounds don't increase mortality risks for women. And after age seventy, higher weights are associated with the lowest mortality. Researchers at the National Institutes of Health Obesity Center at St. Luke's–Roosevelt Hospital in New York claim that for older women a BMI of 28 to 32 and for men 26 to 30 is most desirable.

Thus, despite the restrictive nature of the 1995 U.S. Dietary Guidelines, there actually appears to be a rather broad range of weight associated with low mortality. Note, however, that as you stray above and below this realm, what you weigh becomes increasingly risky.

Are You Sick of Your Weight?

In the hundreds of studies that have looked at the link between cancer and obesity, what has been found are mild to moderate associations with rates of prostate and colorectal cancer in men, and gallbladder, breast, cervical, endometrial, uterine, and ovarian cancers in women. Not all studies have found a connection, however, and in none of those that have could weight alone be considered conclusive.

One scientific explanation of how weight might be implicated lies in the fact that fat tissue is capable of converting a major hormone secreted by the adrenal gland into a form of estrogen. This, coupled with the fact that obese women and postmenopausal women exhibit other hormone changes, might account for the increased odds ratio for some of the aforementioned hormone-related cancers.

Another theory as to how extra body weight could affect cancer lies in the hypothesis that fat in the abdomen, which is where men have a tendency to accumulate fat tissue, is more biologically active. A link between this activity and cell development and proliferation may hold a clue as to why heavy men are more likely to get colon cancer.

On the other hand, it's quite conceivable that certain foods and behavior patterns predispose toward both cancer and obesity. For example, colon cancer is consistently associated with increased consumption of red meat and some types of fat, decreased consumption of vegetables, and physical inactivity. Overweight men tend to consume more meat and fat, eat fewer vegetables, and get less exercise than lean men, making it difficult to separate weight from these other potential risk factors.

Although the incidence of heart disease parallels increases in BMI, several studies claim that the association is specifically with fat around the abdomen compared to fat deposited at the hips, thighs, or buttocks. Likewise, higher BMIs, and particularly abdominal body fat, correlate highly with a decline in insulin sensitivity, or the effectiveness of insulin to lower blood sugar levels. When this happens, the body compensates by producing more insulin, resulting in a condition called hyperinsulinemia. Many studies have shown that obese adults have much higher insulin levels in their blood than leaner people. The dangerous health implications of this situation are discussed in detail in Chapter 1.

Even though central girth (that is, belly size) is cited most often in relation to illness, this may not hold true for all ethnic groups. This difference serves as a reminder that the health effects of weight could vary according not only to sex, but also genetic background.

Bigger Bodies

Height and body frame size have also been considered in relation to cancer risk. Taller, larger-framed adults appear to have a somewhat greater risk for both breast and colon cancers (and possibly other sites). Adult stature is a direct consequence of growth and maturation during childhood and adolescence; while this is genetically controlled, nutrition during these years plays a big part in the realization of genetic potential. Again, hormone production could explain this relationship. Taller people have been exposed to more insulinlike growth factors, which play a role in the development of cancerous colon cells and breast tissue development.

Timing

In examining weight changes over time, small gradual weight gain during adulthood generally isn't considered a concern. In fact, there is some indication that health is more compromised by recurrent fluctuations in weight (that is, a pattern of alternating weight gain and weight loss). As mentioned, though, weight gain among adults of more than 10 kg (22 pounds), not weight per se, is associated with greater mortality.

As the preceding section on body frame suggests, obesity during childhood could create an environment that predisposes toward certain genetic inclinations, including insulin resistance. While serious health consequences during childhood are seen only in the severely obese, children who are fat are considered more likely to become fat adults, and thus perhaps more prone to certain outcomes linked to obesity later in life. On the other hand, it's doubtful that coercing children to lose weight and withholding food improve their long-term health.

The BIG Question: Who Needs to Lose Weight?

Obviously, the relationship between weight and disease is extremely complex. Until the genetic determinants of weight can be separated from behavioral causes, predictions about the real effect of weight are speculative. Many heavy people will never develop any of the ailments that are often associated with weight, such as some cancers, heart disease, strokes, diabetes, gallbladder disease, respiratory illness, and osteoarthritis; likewise, lean people are certainly subject to all these conditions as well. However, it appears that in conjunction with other risk factors, including unsound food choices, low activity level, menopausal status, and a genetic predisposition toward insulin resistance, weight places people at higher risk. How much or how little, and how influential this is we don't know.

Every responsible health practitioner would probably agree that the worst way to address weight is to jump from one restrictive diet to another. The reason for this is that getting to the "right" weight doesn't mean your diet is sound, and conversely, as we have said, being over- or underweight doesn't establish that someone is poorly nourished. *What you eat is more important than what you weigh.* A rational approach for children and adults is to maintain a healthy weight by making sensible food choices and keeping the body "busy" through regular activity or exercise. Even if you aren't satisfied with the weight that results, the health-protective effects of proper diet and exercise will prevail.

481

Appendix

★ FINDING YOUR BODY MASS INDEX ★

Body mass index is calculated by dividing your weight in kilograms by your height in meters squared (kg/m²). Since in the United States we use pounds and feet/inches to measure these parameters, this mathematical formula becomes a bit more complicated. If you don't want to take the time to do the conversions (1 pound = 2.2 kg and 39.37 inches = 1 meter), there is an alternative formula of pounds/inches² × 705.

Example:
Based on a weight of 150 pounds and a height of 5 feet 3 inches (63 inches):
$$150 \div 2.2 = 68.18 \text{ kg}$$
$$63 \text{ inches} \div 39.37 = 1.6 \text{ m}^2 \text{ or } 2.56 \text{ m}$$
$$68.18 \div 2.56 = 26.6 \text{ rounded up to a BMI of } 27$$
or
$$150 \div 3{,}969 \ (63 \times 63) = .0378 \times 705 = 26.6$$
The following table allows you to determine BMI with one quick glance.

Body Mass Index (kg/m²)*

Height (in.)	19	20	21	22	23	24	25	26	27	28	29	30	35	40
						Body Weight (lb.)								
58	91	96	100	105	110	115	119	124	129	134	138	143	167	191
59	94	99	104	109	114	119	124	128	133	138	143	148	173	198
60	97	102	107	112	118	123	128	133	138	143	148	153	179	204
61	100	106	111	116	122	127	132	137	143	148	153	158	185	211
62	104	109	115	120	126	131	136	142	147	153	158	164	191	218
63	107	113	118	124	130	135	141	146	152	158	163	169	197	225
64	110	116	122	128	134	140	145	151	157	163	169	174	204	232
65	114	120	126	132	138	144	150	156	162	168	174	180	210	240
66	118	124	130	136	142	148	155	161	167	173	179	186	216	247
67	121	127	134	140	146	153	159	166	172	178	185	191	223	255
68	125	131	138	144	151	158	164	171	177	184	190	197	230	262
69	128	135	142	149	155	162	169	176	182	189	196	203	236	270
70	132	139	146	153	160	167	174	181	188	195	202	207	243	278
71	136	143	150	157	165	172	179	186	193	200	208	215	250	286
72	140	147	154	162	169	177	184	191	199	206	213	221	258	294
73	144	151	159	166	174	182	189	197	204	212	219	227	265	302
74	148	155	163	171	179	186	194	202	210	218	225	233	272	311
75	152	160	168	176	184	192	200	208	216	224	232	240	279	319
76	156	164	172	180	189	197	205	213	221	230	238	246	287	328

*Each entry gives the body weight in pounds (lb.) for a person of a given height and body mass index. Pounds have been rounded off. To use the table, find the appropriate height in the left-hand column. Move across the row to a given weight. The number at the top of the column is the body mass index for the height and weight. Reprinted by permission of the *Western Journal of Medicine*, from Bray, G.A., Gray, D.S. "Obesity. Part I. Pathogenesis." (1988;149:429–41).

Meeting Goldbecks' Golden Guidelines: Goal Testing

Here is a tool that Nikki's clients find useful in measuring their progress. The chart that appears below summarizes the broad parameters of Goldbecks' Golden Guidelines. Note than within some Guidelines space is alloted for personal targets when individual needs or goals are called for. By reading the complete version of the eight Guidelines and the parallel chapters, you'll acquire the information you need to tailor them to your circumstances.

Feel free to make copies of this chart and use it to track your food intake.

GOAL TESTING

In order to meet my personal health goals based on Goldbecks' Golden Guidelines, today I ate the following:

Golden Guideline	Recommended Intake or Personal Target	Food Consumed	Amount Consumed
#1: Carbohydrate Compatibility	General: 40 to 60% of calories Personal target:	*Whole grains/cereal* Amaranth Barley Buckwheat/kasha Cornmeal Cracked wheat/bulgur Flaxseed meal Kamut Millet Oats Quinoa Rice Rye Spelt Wheat germ Whole wheat Wild Rice Whole-grain breadstuffs Vegetables, fruit, beans (see Guidelines #4 and #6)	

Golden Guideline	Recommended Intake or Personal Target	Food Consumed	Amount Consumed
#2:The Right Fat vs. Low-Fat	General: 10 to 40% of calories, with attention to ratio of omega-6 and omega-3 fats and remaining emphasis on monounsaturated fatty acids Personal target:	_Nuts/seeds and their butters_ Almonds Brazil nuts Butternuts Cashews Filberts/hazelnuts Peanuts Pecans Pine nuts/pignolia Pistachios Pumpkin seeds Sesame seeds/tahini Sunflower seeds Walnuts _Concentrated fats_ Canola oil Flaxseed oil Hemp oil Olive oil Sesame oil Other _Additional fat-providing foods_ Avocado Eggs (see Guideline #3) Fish Full-fat dairy Olives Poultry/Meat Yogurt (other than nonfat) Other	
#3: Vital Nutrient Helpers	General: Generous amounts of fresh vegetables, beans, whole grains, fruit, seeds, nuts, garlic, onions, mushrooms; up to 6 eggs per week	Eggs Garlic Mushrooms Onions/scallions/shallots For additional items see other Guidelines	

Golden Guideline	Recommended Intake or Personal Target	Food Consumed	Amount Consumed
#4: Vegetables	General: At least 6 pounds per week of produce (about 14 ounces daily), with greatest weight given to vegetables	*Vegetables* Artichokes Arugula Asparagus Beets Bok choy Broccoli Brussels sprouts Cabbage Carrots Cauliflower Celeriac Celery Chard Chicory Collards Corn Cucumbers Eggplant Endive Escarole Fennel Green beans Green peas Jicama Kale Kohlrabi Leeks Lettuce (Boston, looseleaf) Nopales (cactus) Okra Parsley Parsnips Peppers Potatoes, sweet Potatoes, white Pumpkin Radicchio Radishes Romaine	

Golden Guideline	Recommended Intake or Personal Target	Food Consumed	Amount Consumed
		Rutabagas Spinach Sprouts (alfalfa, radish, mung, clover, etc.) Summer squash (zucchini, crookneck, etc.) Sunchokes (Jerusalem artichokes) Tomatoes Turnips Watercress Winter squash (acorn, Hubbard, etc.) Yucca (cassava) Other vegetables	
#4: (and Fruit)	General: 2 to 4 servings of fruit per day, with individual modifications Personal target:	*Fruit* Apples Apricots Bananas Berries Cherries Cranberries Dates Figs Grapefruit Grapes Guavas Kiwis Lemons Limes Mangoes Melon Nectarines Oranges Papayas Peaches Pears Persimmons Pineapple	

Golden Guideline	Recommended Intake or Personal Target	Food Consumed	Amount Consumed
		Plantains Plums Pomegranates Prunes Raisins Rhubarb Tangerines Watermelon Other fruits	
#5: Super Soy Foods	General: 25 grams soy protein daily	Miso Soybeans Soy flour Soy milk Soy nuts Tempeh Tofu Other soy foods	
#6: Beans	General: A generous percent of daily protein	Adzuki/aduki beans Black beans Black-eyed peas/cowpeas Cannellini beans Chickpeas Cranberry/Roman beans Fava beans Great northern Kidney beans Lentils Lima beans Mung beans Navy beans Pea beans Pigeon peas Pink beans Pinto beans Red beans Soybeans (see Guideline #5) Split peas Whole dried peas Other beans	

Golden Guideline	Recommended Intake or Personal Target	Food Consumed	Amount Consumed
#7: Yogurt and Yogurt Cheese	General: Include on a regular basis	Yogurt Yogurt cheese	
#8: Liquids of Life	General: Water: typical adult, at least 50 ounces (six 8-ounces glasses); as noted in Guideline, some can come from vegetables, fruit, and cooked beans and grains Personal target: Leaf tea: as desired Alcohol: limit 1 drink women, 2 drinks men	Water Leaf tea Wine (4 to 5 ounces) Beer (12 ounces) Distilled alcohol (1.5 ounces)	
Outside the Guidelines	List any other food items you eat for a complete picture and to help you decide if anything is interfering with your personal goals		

The Healthiest Diet in the World

Resources

Beans
Indian Harvest
P.O. Box 428
Bemidji, MN 56619
(800) 294-2433
A good selection of uncommon, heirloom beans.

Phipps Country
P.O. Box 349
Pescadero, CA 94060
(800) 270-0889
Beans grown without chemical spraying. Unusual varieties, with availability according to the yearly crop.

Walnut Acres
Penns Creek, PA 17862
(800) 433-3998
Selection limited to the more common bean varieties, but all are organically grown. In addition to dried beans, cooked canned organic beans are offered, including soybeans which are hard to find elsewhere.

Seaweed
Larch Hanson
P.O. Box 57
Steuben, ME 04680
(207) 546-2875

Mendocino Sea Vegetable Company
P.O. Box 1265
Mendocino, CA 95460
(707) 937-2050

[handwritten: Office of Wate]

Fish Advisories *[handwritten: Fish Consumption Advisories]*

Pollution warnings in relation to fish are available without charge. Request a free copy of the "National Listing of Fish Consumption Advisories," either in the form of a brief Fact Sheet, or on diskettes, from the U.S. Environmental Protection Agency, National Center for Environmental Publications and Information, 11029 Kenwood Rd., Cincinnati, OH 45242, (513) 489-8190. Those with internet access can download the current database of warnings at http://www.epa.gov/OW/OST/pctoc.html.

Hemp Oil
The Ohio Hempery, Inc.
7002 State Route
Guysville, OH 45735
(614) 662-HEMP [4367] or (800) BUY-HEMP [289-4367]

Yogurt Cheese Funnels and Pressure Cookers
Nutensils
P.O. Box 87HD
Woodstock, NY 12498
(888) 804-8848
(914) 679-5573
Funnels are $13 postpaid. Inquire about pressure cookers.

Goldbeck Books
Ceres Press
P.O. Box 87HD
Woodstock, NY 12498
(888) 804-8848
(914) 679-5573

Bibliography

Chapter 1: Controversial Carbohydrates

Adlercreutz, H. "Does fiber-rich food containing animal lignan precursors protect against both colon and breast cancer? An extension of the 'fiber hypothesis.' " *Gastroenterology,* 1984;86:761–66.

Adlercreutz, H., et al. "Diet and urinary estrogen profile in premenopausal omnivorous and vegetarian women and in premenopausal women with breast cancer." *Journal of Steroid Biochemistry,* 1989;34:527–30.

Anderson, James W., and Gustafson, Nancy J. "Hypocholesterolemic effects of oat and bean products." *American Journal of Clinical Nutrition,* 1988;48:749–53.

Asp, Nils-Georg. "Nutritional classification and analysis of food carbohydrates." *American Journal of Clinical Nutrition,* 1994;59(suppl):679S–81S.

Baron, A. D. "Insulin and the vasculature: old actors, new roles." *Journal of Investigative Medicine,* 1996;44:406–12.

Bennett, Fiona C., and Ingram, David M. "Diet and female sex hormone concentrations: an intervention study for the type of fat consumed." *American Journal of Clinical Nutrition,* 1990;52:808–12.

Birkett, Anne, et al. "Resistant starch lowers fecal concentrations of ammonia and phenols in humans." *American Journal of Clinical Nutrition,* 1996;63:766–72.

Björck, Inger, et al. "Food properties affecting the digestion and absorption of carbohydrates." *American Journal of Clinical Nutrition,* 1994;59(suppl):699S–705S.

Blundell, John E., et al. "Carbohydrates and human appetite." *American Journal of Clinical Nutrition,* 1994;59(suppl):728S–34S.

Brand, Janette C., et al. "Food processing and the glycemic index." *American Journal of Clinical Nutrition,* 1985;42:1192–96.

Brauten, J. T., et al. "Oat B-glucan reduces blood cholesterol concentration in hypercholesterolemic subjects." *European Journal of Clinical Nutrition,* 1994;48:465–74.

Bruce, Ake, and Asp, Nils-Georg. "Implications of recent food-carbohydrate research on nutrition recommendations and product development: summary of panel discussion."*American Journal of Clinical Nutrition,* 1994;59(suppl):770S–72S.

Burke, Louise M., et al. "Muscle glycogen storage after prolonged exercise: effect of the frequency of carbohydrate feedings." *American Journal of Clinical Nutrition,* 1996;64:115–19.

Colditz, Graham A., et al., eds. "Harvard Report on Cancer Prevention. Volume 1: Causes of Human Cancer." *Cancer Causes & Control,* 1996;7(suppl).

Collins, P., et al. "Effects of cooking on serum glucose and insulin responses to starch." *British Medical Journal,* 1981;282:1032.

Cummings, J. H., et al. "Review: A new look at dietary carbohydrate: chemistry, physiology and health." *European Journal of Clinical Nutrition,* 1997;51:417–23.

Despres, J. P., et al. "Hyperinsulinemia as an independent risk factor for ischemic heart disease." *New England Journal of Medicine,* 1996;334:952–57.

Dwyer, Johanna. "Overview: Dietary approaches for reducing cardiovascular disease risks." *Journal of Nutrition,* 1995;125:656S–65S.

Ellis, R., and Morris, E. R. "Relation between phytic acid and trace metals in wheat bran and soybean." *Cereal Chemistry,* 1981;58:367.

Escalante, David, et al. "Maximizing glycemic control: how to achieve normal glycemia while minimizing hyperinsulinemia in insulin-requiring patients with diabetes mellitus." *Clinical Diabetes,* 1993;11:3–7.

Fanelli, Carmine, et al. "Effects of recent short-term hyperglycemia on responses to hypoglycemia in humans." *Diabetes,* 1995;44:513–20.

Flatt, Jean-Pierre. "Use and storage of carbohydrate and fat." *American Journal of Clinical Nutrition,* 1995;61(suppl):952S–59S.

Foster-Powell, Kaye, and Miller, Janette Brand. "International tables of glycemic index." *American Journal of Clinical Nutrition,* 1995;62(suppl):871S–93S.

Freudenheim, Jo L., et al. "Risks associated with source of fiber and fiber components in cancer of the colon and rectum." *Cancer Research,* 1990;50:3295–300.

Frolich, W., and Asp, N. G. "Minerals and phytate in the analysis of dietary fiber from cereals. III." *Cereal Chemistry,* 1985;62:238.

Fuh, M. M-T., et al. "Metabolic effects of diuretic and beta-blocker treatment of hypertension in patients with non-insulin-dependent diabetes mellitus." *American Journal of Hypertension,* 1990;3:387–90.

Fukagawa, Naomi, et al. "High-carbohydrate, high-fiber diets increase peripheral insulin sensitivity in healthy young and old adults." *American Journal of Clinical Nutrition,* 1990;52:524–28.

Gannon, M. C., et al. "The serum insulin and plasma glucose responses to milk and fruit products in type 2 (non-insulin-dependent) diabetic patients." *Diabetologia,* 1986;29:784–91.

Giacosa, Attillio, et al. "Dietary Fibres and Cancer." *Advances in Nutrition and Cancer.* Zappia, V., Salvatore, M., and Della Ragione, F., eds. New York: Plenum, 1993:85–99.

Greenwald, Peter, Lanza, Elaine, and Eddy, Gerald A. "Dietary fiber in the reduction of colon cancer risk." *Journal of the American Dietetic Association,* 1987;87(9):1178.

Harland, Barbara F. "Dietary fibre and mineral bioavailability." *Nutrition Research Reviews,* 1989;2:133–47.

Harris, R. K., et al. "Development of stability-indicating analytical methods for flaxseed lignans and their precursors." *Food Phytochemicals for Cancer Prevention II: Tea, Spices, and Herbs.* Ho, Chi-Tang, Osawa, Toshihiko, Huang, Mou-Tuan, and Rosen,

Robert T., eds. ACS Symposium Series 547, American Chemical Society, Washington, DC, 1994:296–305.

Hasler, Clare. "Review: Oat beta-glucan, coronary heart disease risk and health claims." *Functional Foods for Health News,* March 1996;3(3):6–9.

Heijnen, Marie-Louise, et al. "Neither raw nor retrograded resistant starch lowers fasting serum cholesterol concentrations in healthy normolipidemic subjects." *American Journal of Clinical Nutrition,* 1996;64:312–18.

Hirsch, Jules. "Role and benefits of carbohydrate in the diet: key issues for future dietary guidelines." *American Journal of Clinical Nutrition,* 1995;61(suppl):996S–1000S.

Holt, S. H. A., and Miller, J. B. "Particle size, satiety, and the glycaemic response. Effect of processing on wheat re: plasma glucose, and insulin on 10 men and women." *European Journal of Clinical Nutrition,* 1994;48:496–502.

Howe, Juliette C., et al. "Dietary starch composition and level of energy intake alter nutrient oxidation in 'carbohydrate-sensitive' men." *Journal of Nutrition,* 1996;126:2120–29.

Hutchins, Andrea M., et al. "Vegetables, fruits and legumes effect on urinary isoflavonoid phytoestrogen and lignan excretion." *Journal of the American Dietetic Association,* 1995;95:769–75.

"Hypertriglyceridaemia and vascular risk." (Report of a Meeting of Physicians and Scientists, University of London Medical School) *The Lancet,* 1993;342:781–87.

Jarvi, Anette E., et al. "The influence of food structure on postprandial metabolism in patients with non-insulin-dependent diabetes mellitus." *American Journal of Clinical Nutrition,* 1995;61:837–43.

Jenab, M., and Thompson, L. U. "The influence of flaxseed and lignans on colon carcinogenesis and beta-glucoronidase activity." *Carcinogenesis,* 1996;17:1343–48.

Jenkins, David J. A., et al. "Starchy Foods and Glycemic Index." *Diabetes Care,* 1988;11(2):149–59.

———. "Exceptionally low blood glucose response to dried beans: comparison with other carbohydrate foods." *British Medical Journal,* 30 August 1980;578–80.

———. "Glycemic index of foods: a physiological basis for carbohydrate exchange." *American Journal of Clinical Nutrition,* 1981;34:362–66.

———. "Low glycemic index: lente carbohydrates and physiological effects of altered food frequency." *American Journal of Clinical Nutrition,* 1994;59(suppl):706S–9S.

Jeppesen, Jorgen, et al. "Effects of low-fat, high-carbohydrate diets on risk factors for ischemic heart disease in postmenopausal women." *American Journal of Clinical Nutrition,* 1997;65:1027–33.

———. "Postprandial triglyceride and retinyl ester responses to oral fat: effects of fructose." *American Journal of Clinical Nutrition,* 1995;61:787–92.

Keim, K. S., Holloway, C. L., and Hebsted, M. "Absorption of chromium as affected by wheat bran." *Cereal Chemistry,* 1987;64:352.

Kinsella, John E., et al. "Dietary polyunsaturated fatty acids and eicosanoids: Potential effects on the modulation of inflammatory and immune cells: An overview." *Nutrition,* 1990;6(1):24–44.

Kirkman, L. M., et al. "Urinary lignan and isoflavonoid excretion in men and women consuming vegetable and soy diets." *Nutrition and Cancer,* 1995;24(1):1–12.

Krauss, Ronald, et al. "Dietary Guidelines for Healthy American Adults." AHA Medical/Scientific Statement. *Circulation,* 1996;94:1795–800.

Kritchevsky, David. "Dietary Fiber and Cancer." *Nutrition and Disease Update—Cancer.* Carroll, Kenneth K., and Kritchevsky, D., eds. Champaign II: AOCS, 1994:1–25.

Lakka, Timo A., et al. "Hyperinsulinemia and the risk of coronary heart disease." Correspondence. *New England Journal of Medicine,* 1996;335:976–77.

Lamon-Fava, Stefania, et al. "Effects of dietary intakes on plasma lipids, lipoproteins and apolipoproteins in free-living elderly men and women." *American Journal of Clinical Nutrition,* 1994;59:32–41.

Lavin, J. H., French, S. J., and Read, N. W. "The effect of sucrose- and aspartame-sweetened drinks on energy intake, hunger and food choice of female, moderately restrained eaters." *International Journal of Obesity and Related Metabolic Disorders,* 1997;21(1):37–42.

Mayer, E. J., et al. "Genetic and environmental influences on insulin levels and the insulin resistance syndrome: an analysis of women twins." *American Journal of Epidemiology,* 1996;143:323–32.

Mayes, Peter A., "Intermediary metabolism of fructose." *American Journal of Clinical Nutrition,* 1993;58(suppl):754S–66S.

McLaren, Donald S. "Is insulin resistance becoming a global epidemic?" *Nutrition,* 1997;13:64–66.

Mennen, Louise I., et al. "The association of dietary fat and fiber with coagulation factor VII in the elderly: The Rotterdam Study." *American Journal of Clinical Nutrition,* 1997;65:732–36.

Miller, Janette Brand. "Importance of glycemic index in diabetes." *American Journal of Clinical Nutrition,* 1994;59(suppl):747S–52S.

Miller, Janette C. Brand, et al. "Rice: A high or low glycemic index food?" *American Journal of Clinical Nutrition,* 1992;56:1034–36.

Morris, Eugene R. "Inositol phosphate content of selected dry beans, peas, and lentils, raw and cooked." *Journal of Food Composition and Analysis,* 1996;9(1):2–12.

Mykkanen, Leena, et al. "Low insulin sensitivity is associated with clustering of cardiovascular disease risk factors." *American Journal of Epidemiology,* 1997;146:315–21.

NIH Consensus Development Panel on Triglyceride, High-Density Lipoprotein, and Coronary Heart Disease. "Triglyceride, high-density lipoprotein, and coronary heart disease." *Journal of the American Medical Association,* 1993;269(4):505–10.

Noakes, Manny, et al. "Effect of high-amylose starch and oat bran on metabolic variables and bowel function in subjects with hypertriglyceridemia." *American Journal of Clinical Nutrition,* 1996;64:944–51.

"Nutrition and Your Health." *Dietary Guidelines for Americans.* Fourth Edition, U.S. Department of Agriculture, 1995.

"Nutritive Value of Flaxseed." Nutrient Data Laboratory, USDA/ARS/BHNRC, Riverdale, MD, 1997.

O'Dea, Kerin, et al. "Physical factors influencing postprandial glucose and insulin responses to starch." *American Journal of Clinical Nutrition,* 1980;33:760–65.

Phillips, Jodi, et al. "Effect of resistant starch on fecal bulk and fermentation-dependent events in humans." *American Journal of Clinical Nutrition,* 1995;62:121–30.

Phipps, William R. "Effect of flaxseed ingestion on the menstrual cycle." *Journal of Clinical Endocrinology and Metabolism,* 1993;77(5):1215–19.

Plaami, Sirkka. "Contents of dietary fiber and inositol phosphates in some foods consumed in Finland." Academic Dissertation, Department of Biochemistry and Food Chemistry, University of Turku, 1996.

Plaami, Sirkka, and Kumpulainen, Jorma. "Soluble and insoluble dietary fiber contents of various breads, pastas and rye flours on the Finnish market, 1990–1991." *Journal of Food Composition and Analysis,* 1994;7:134–43.

Raben, Anne, et al. "Decreased postprandial thermogenesis and fat oxidation but increased fullness after a high-fiber meal compared with a low-fiber meal." *American Journal of Clinical Nutrition,* 1994;59:1386–94.

Rassmussen, Ole. "Day-to-day variation of the glycemic response in subjects with insulin-dependent diabetes with standardized premeal glucose and prandial insulin concentrations." *American Journal of Clinical Nutrition,* 1993;57:908–11.

Reaven, Gerald M. "Role of insulin resistance in human disease." *Diabetes,* 1988; 37:1595–607.

Reaven, Gerald, et al. "Hypertension and associated metabolic abnormalities: The role of insulin resistance and the sympathoadrenal system." *New England Journal of Medicine,* 1996;334(6):374–81.

Rendleman, J. A., and Grobe, C. A. "Cereal complexes: Binding of zinc by bran and components of bran." *Cereal Chemistry,* 1982;59:310.

Retzlaff, Barbara M., et al. "Changes in plasma triacylglycerol concentrations among free-living hyperlipidemic men adopting different carbohydrate intakes over 2 y: The Dietary Alternatives Study." *American Journal of Clinical Nutrition,* 1995;62:988–95.

Riccardi, G., and Ciardullo, A. "Dietary fiber in the prevention of cardiovascular disease." *Advances in Nutrition and Cancer.* Zappia, V., Salvatore, M., and Della Ragione, F., eds. New York: Plenum, 1993:99–104.

Rimm, Eric, et al. "Vegetable, fruit, and cereal fiber intake and risk of coronary heart disease among men." *Journal of the American Medical Association,* 1996;275(6):447–51.

Salmeron, Jorge, et al. "Dietary fiber, glycemic load, and risk of non-insulin-dependent diabetes mellitus in women." *Journal of the American Medical Association,* 1997; 277(6):472–77.

Serraino, M., and Thompson, L. U. "The effect of flaxseed supplementation on early risk markers for mammary carcinogens." *Cancer Letter,* 1991;60:135–42.

———. "The effect of flaxseed supplementation on the initiation and promotional stages of mammary tumorigenesis." *Nutrition and Cancer,* 1992;17:153–59.

Shah, B. G., et. al. "Effect of dietary cereal brans on the metabolism of trace elements in a long term rat study." *Cereal Chemistry,* 1991;68:190–94.

Shannon, Jackilen, et al. "Relationship of food groups and water intake to colon cancer risk." *Cancer Epidemiology, Biomarkers & Prevention,* 1996;5:495–502.

Smith, Ulf. "Carbohydrates, fat, and insulin action." *American Journal of Clinical Nutrition,* 1994;59(suppl):686S–89S.

Stephen, Alison M., et al. "Intake of carbohydrate and its components: international comparisons, trends over time, and effects of changing to low-fat diets." *American Journal of Clinical Nutrition,* 1995;62:851S–67S.

Stolk, Ronald P., et al. "Diabetes mellitus, impaired glucose tolerance, and hyperinsulinemia in an elderly population. The Rotterdam Study." *American Journal of Epidemiology,* 1997;145:24–32.

"Taking a Closer Look at Nutrition, Genetics and Cancer." American Institute for Cancer Research. Washington, DC.

Thompson, L. U. "Antioxidants and hormone-mediated health benefits of whole grains." *Scientific Nutrition,* 1994;34:473–97.

———. "Antitumorigenic effect of a mammalian lignan precursor from flaxseed." *Nutrition and Cancer,* 1996;26:159–65.

———. "Mammalian lignan production from various foods." *Nutrition and Cancer,* 1991;16(1):43–52.

Thornberry, Suzanne. "Varying carbohydrates in the type II diet." *Real Living with Diabetes,* 1994;1:6–9.

Thorne, Mary Jane, et al. "Factors affecting starch digestibility and the glycemic response with special reference to legumes." *American Journal of Clinical Nutrition,* 1983;38:481–88.

Thun, Michael J., et al. "Risk Factors for Fatal Colon Cancer in a Large Prospective Study." *Journal of the National Cancer Institute,* 1992;84(9):1491–500.

Tillotson, Jeanne L., et al. "Relation of dietary fiber to blood lipids in the special intervention and usual care groups in the Multiple Risk Factor Intervention Trial." *American Journal of Clinical Nutrition,* 1997;65(suppl):327S–37S.

Topping, David L. "Soluble fiber polysaccharides: Effects on plasma cholesterol and colonic fermentation." *Nutrition Reviews,* 1991;49(7):195–203.

Tovar, Juscelino, Granfeldt, Y., and Björck, I. "Effect of processing on metabolic response to legumes." *American Journal of Clinical Nutrition,* 1994;59(suppl):783S.

Truswell, A. Stewart. "Food carbohydrates and plasma lipids: an update." *American Journal of Clinical Nutrition,* 1994;59(suppl):710S–18S.

Uusitupa, Matti. "Fructose in the diabetic diet." *American Journal of Clinical Nutrition,* 1994;59(suppl):753S–57S.

Van Itallie, Theodore B. "Short-term and long-term components in the regulation of food intake: evidence for a modulatory role of carbohydrate status." *American Journal of Clinical Nutrition,* 1997;30:742–57.

West, Clive E., et al. "Boys from populations with high-carbohydrate intake have higher fasting triglyceride levels than boys from populations with high-fat intake." *American Journal of Epidemiology,* 1990;131:271–82.

Witte, John S., et al. "Relation of vegetable, fruit, and grain consumption to colorectal adenomatous polyps." *American Journal of Epidemiology,* 1996;144:1015–25.

Wolever, Thomas M. S. "Glycaemic index of 102 complex carbohydrate foods in patients with diabetes." *Nutrition Research,* 1994;14(5):651–69.

———. "The glycemic index: Flogging a dead horse?" *Diabetes Care,* 1997;20(3):452–56.

———, and Miller, Janette Brand. "Sugars and blood glucose control." *American Journal of Clinical Nutrition,* 1995;62(suppl):212S–27S.

———, et al. "The glycemic index: methodology and clinical implications." *American Journal of Clinical Nutrition,* 1991;54:846–54.

———. "Glycemic index of fruits and fruit products in patients with diabetes." *International Journal of Food Sciences and Nutrition,* 1993;43:205–12.

———. "Glycemic index of some fruit and fruit products in patients with diabetes." *International Journal of Food Sciences and Nutrition,* 1993;43:205–12.

The Healthiest Diet in the World

Wynder, E., et al. "Editorial: High fiber intake indicator of a healthy lifestyle." *Journal of the American Medical Association,* 1996;275(6):447–51.

Chapter 2: Walking the Dietary Fat Tightrope

Addis, Paul B., and Park, Seok-Won. "Role of Lipid Oxidation Products in Atherosclerosis." *Food Toxicology: A Perspective on the Relative Risks.* Taylor, Steven, and Scanlan, Richard, eds. New York: Marcel Dekker, 1989:297–330.

Allman, M. A., Pena, M. M., and Pang D. "Supplementation with flaxseed oil versus sunflowerseed oil in healthy young men consuming a low fat diet: effects on platelet composition and function." *European Journal of Clinical Nutrition,* 1995;49(3):169–78.

Aro, Antti, et al. "Stearic acid, trans fatty acids, and dairy fat: effects on serum and lipoprotein lipids, apolipoproteins, lipoprotein(a), and lipid transfer proteins in healthy subjects." *American Journal of Clinical Nutrition,* 1997;65:1419–26.

Beckstrom-Sternberg, Stephen M., and Duke, James A. "Plants containing arginine." Agricultural Research Service. Phytochemeco Database, USDA.

Belury, Martha Ann. "Conjugated dienoic linoleate: A polyunsaturated fatty acid with unique chemoprotective properties." *Nutrition Reviews,* 1995;53(4):83–89.

Berdanier, Carolyn D., "Omega-3 fatty acids: A panacea?" *Nutrition Today,* 1994; 29: 28–33.

Berry, Elliot M. "Dietary fatty acids in diabetes." First International Conference on Fats and Oil Consumption in Health and Disease. Rockefeller University, NY, April 24–25, 1995.

Blackburn, George L., et al. "Dietary fat and the risk of breast cancer." *New England Journal of Medicine,* 1996;334(24):1606–7.

Bracco, Umberto. "Effect of triglyceride structure on fat absorption." *American Journal of Clinical Nutrition,* 1994;60(suppl):1002S–10S.

Callahan, Maureen. "Flaxseed: A Naturally Nutritious Food." The Flax Council of Canada, Winnipeg, Manitoba, Canada.

Canadian Recommended Nutrient Intakes (RNI). *Nutrition Recommendations, 1990.* Health and Welfare Canada Scientific Review Committee, 1990.

Carroll, Kenneth K. "Chapter 5: Lipids and Cancer." *Nutrition and Disease Update—Cancer.* Carroll, Kenneth K., and Kritchevsky, D., eds. Champaign, IL: AOCS, 1994: 235–96.

Caughey, Gillian, et al. "The effect on human tumor necrosis factor and interleukin production of diets enriched in n-3 fatty acids from vegetable oil or fish oil." *American Journal of Clinical Nutrition,* 1996;63:116–22.

Chin, S. F., et al. "Dietary sources of conjugated dienoic isomers of linoleic acid, a newly recognized class of anticarcinogens." *Journal of Food Composition and Analysis,* 1992;5:185–97.

Christen, Stephan. "Gamma-tocopherol traps mutagenic electrophiles such as NO_2 and complements alpha-tocopherol: Physical implications." *Proceedings of the National Academy of Science, USA,* 1997;94:manuscript.

Clarke, Robert, et al. "Dietary lipids and blood cholesterol: Quantitative meta-analysis of metabolic ward studies." *British Medical Journal,* 97;314:112–17.

Colditz, Graham A., et al., eds. "Harvard Report on Cancer Prevention. Volume 1: Causes of Human Cancer." *Cancer Causes & Control,* 1996;7(suppl).

Colquhoun, David M., et al. "Comparison of the effects on lipoproteins and apolipoproteins of a diet high in monounsaturated fatty acids, enriched with avocado, and a high-carbohydrate diet." *American Journal of Clinical Nutrition,* 1992;56:671–77.

Cuchel, M., et al. "Impact of hydrogenated fat consumption on endogenous cholesterol synthesis and susceptibility of low-density lipoprotein to oxidation in moderately hypercholesterolemic individuals." *Metabolism,* 1996;45:241–47.

Cunane, S. C., et al. "Nutritional attributes of traditional flaxseed in healthy young adults." *American Journal of Clinical Nutrition,* 1995;61:62–68.

Dawson-Hughes, Bess. "Calcium and vitamin D nutritional needs of elderly women." *Journal of Nutrition,* 1996;126:1165S–67S.

De Bruin, W. A., et al. "Different postprandial metabolism of olive oil and soybean oil: A possible mechanism of the high-density lipoprotein-conserving effect of olive oil." *American Journal of Clinical Nutrition,* 1993;58:477–84.

Decker, Eric A., Ph.D. "The role of phenolics, conjugated linoleic acid, carnosine, and pyrroloquinoline quinone as nonessential dietary antioxidants." *Nutrition Reviews,* 1995;53(3):49–58.

De Lorgeril, Michel, et al. "Mediterranean alpha-linolenic acid–rich diet in secondary prevention of coronary heart disease." *The Lancet,* 1994;343:1454–60.

Dempster, David W. "Bone Remodeling." *Osteoporosis: Etiology, Diagnosis, and Management: Second Edition.* Riggs, Lawrence B., and Melton, Joseph L., III, eds. Philadelphia: Lippincott-Raven, 1995:67–75.

———. "Pathogenesis of osteoporosis." *The Lancet,* 1993;341:797–801.

De Waard, Fritz. "On the Nutritional Etiology of Breast Cancer." *Advances in Nutrition and Cancer.* Zappia, V., Salvatore, M., and Della Ragione, F., eds. New York: Plenum, 1993:119–222.

Dorgan, Joanne, et al. "Effects of dietary fat and fiber on plasma and urine concentrations of androgens and estrogens in men: a controlled feeding study." *American Journal of Clinical Nutrition,* 1996;64:850–55.

———. "Relation of energy, fat, and fiber intake to plasma concentrations of estrogens and androgens in premenopausal women." *American Journal of Clinical Nutrition,* 1996;64:25–31.

Dupont, Jacqueline, et al. "Fatty acid–related functions." *American Journal of Clinical Nutrition,* 1996;63:991S–93S.

Dwyer, Johanna. "Overview: Dietary approaches for reducing cardiovascular disease risks." *Journal of Nutrition,* 1995;125(suppl):656S–65S.

"Effects of Reducing Carotenoid Levels on Humans," transcript of discussion. The Olestra Project: Potential Effects of Reducing Carotenoid Levels on Human Health. Harvard School of Public Health, January 17, 1996.

Faivre, Jean, et al. "Diet and Large Bowel Cancer." *Advances in Nutrition and Cancer.* Zappia, V., Salvatore, M., and Della Ragione, F., eds. Plenum Press, NY 1993: 107–18.

Ferro-Luzzi, Anna, and Chiselli, A. "Protective Aspects of the Mediterranean Diet." *Advances in Nutrition and Cancer.* Zappia, V., Salvatore, M., and Della Ragione, F., eds. New York: Plenum, 1993:137–44.

Fidanza, Flaminio. "Nutrition and Cancer: General Considerations." *Advances in Nutrition and Cancer.* Zappia, V., Salvatore, M., and Della Ragione, F., eds. New York: Plenum, 1993:65–67.

Fischer, Susan M., et al. "Arachidonate has protumor-promoting action that is inhibited by linoleate in mouse skin carcinogenesis." *Journal of Nutrition,* 1996;126: 1099S–1104S.

Flatt, Jean-Pierre. "Use and storage of carbohydrate and fat." *American Journal of Clinical Nutrition,* 1995;61(suppl):952S–59S.

Fraser, Gary. "Diet and coronary heart disease: Beyond dietary fats and low-density-lipoprotein cholesterol." *American Journal of Clinical Nutrition,* 1994;59(suppl): 1117S–23S.

———, et al. "A possible protective effect of nut consumption on risk of coronary heart disease." *Archives of Internal Medicine,* 1992;152:1416–24.

Freedman, Laurence S., et al. "Analysis of dietary fat, calories, body weight, and the development of mammary tumors in rats and mice: A review." *Cancer Research,* 1990;50:5710–19.

Fukuda, Y., et al. "Chemistry of Lignan Antioxidants in Sesame Seed and Oil." *Food Phytochemicals for Cancer Prevention II: Tea, Spices, and Herbs.* Ho, Chi-Tang, Osawa, Toshihiko, Huang, Mou-Tuan, and Rosen, Robert T., eds. ACS Symposium Series 547, American Chemical Society, Washington, DC, 1994:269–74.

Garg, Abhimany, et al. "Effects of varying carbohydrate content of diet in patients with non-insulin-dependent diabetes mellitus." *Journal of the American Medical Association,* 1994;271(18):1421–28.

Gey, K. Fred, et al. "Increased risk of cardiovascular disease at suboptimal plasma concentrations of essential antioxidants: An epidemiological update with special attention to carotene and vitamin C." *American Journal of Clinical Nutrition,* 1993;57(suppl): 787S–97S.

Giese, James. "Olestra: Properties, regulatory concerns, and applications." *Food Technology,* March 1996:130–31.

Gillman, M. W., et al. "Margarine intake and subsequent coronary heart disease." *Circulation,* 1995;91:925.

Giovannucci, Edward, et al. "A prospective study of dietary fat and risk of prostate cancer." *Journal of the National Cancer Institute,* 1993;85(19):1571–79.

Griffiths, John A. "Immediate metabolic availability of dietary fat in combination with carbohydrate." *American Journal of Clinical Nutrition,* 1994;59:53–59.

"Guidelines on Diet, Nutrition and Cancer Prevention: Reducing the Risk of Cancer with Healthy Food Choices and Physical Activity." American Cancer Society, Dietary Guidelines Advisory Committee, 1996.

Gustafson, Inga-Britt, et al. "Sunflower seed oil: A diet rich in monounsaturated rapeseed oil reduces the lipoprotein cholesterol concentration and increases the relative content of n-3 fatty acids in serum in hyperlipidemic subjects." *American Journal of Clinical Nutrition,* 1994;59:667–75.

Handelman, Garry. "Physiological Effects of Carotenoids in Humans." The Olestra Project: Potential Effects of Reducing Carotenoid Levels on Human Health. Harvard School of Public Health, January 17, 1996.

Hatala, Mary Ann, et al. "Comparison of linoleic acid and ecosapentaenoic acid incorporation into human breast cancer cells." *Lipids,* 1994;29(12):831–37.

Haumann, Barbara Fitch. "Conjugated linoleic acid offers research promise." *INFORM,* 1996;7(2):155–59.

Havel, Richard. "McCollum Award Lecture, 1993: Triglyceride-rich lipoproteins and atherosclerosis—new perspectives." *American Journal of Clinical Nutrition,* 1994;59: 795–99.

"Healthy People 2000: National Health Promotion and Disease Prevention Objectives." U.S. Department of Health and Human Services Public Health Service Publication No. (PHS) 91-50213. U.S. Government Printing Office, Washington, DC, 1990.

Hepburn, Frank N. "Provisional tables on the content of omega-3 fatty acids and other fat components of selected foods." *Journal of the American Dietetic Association,* 1986;86(6):788–93.

Hibbeln, Joseph R., and Salem, Norman. "Dietary polyunsaturated fatty acids and depression: When cholesterol does not satisfy." *American Journal of Clinical Nutrition,* 1995;62:1–9.

Hill, Michael J. "Diet and Precancerous Lesions." *Advances in Nutrition and Cancer.* Zappia, V., Salvatore, M., and Della Ragione, F., eds. New York: Plenum, 1993: 69–74.

Hirose, N., et al. "Inhibition of cholesterol absorption and synthesis in rats by sesamin." *Journal of Lipid Research,* 1991;32:629.

Hodgson, Jonathan, et al. "Can linoleic acid contribute to coronary artery disease?" *American Journal of Clinical Nutrition,* 1993;58:228–34.

Holub, Bruce J. "Flax, omega-3 fatty acids, and heart health." *Flax Growers Western Canada Newsletter,* June 1990:11–12.

Hudgins, L. C., et al. "Human fatty acid synthesis is stimulated for a eucaloric low fat, high carbohydrate diet." *Journal Clinical Investigation,* 1996;97:2081–91.

Hunter, David, et al. "Cohort studies of fat intake and the risk of breast cancer: A pooled analysis." *New England Journal of Medicine,* 1996;334(6):356–61.

Hunter, J. Edward. "Omega-3 fatty acids from vegetable oils." *American Journal of Clinical Nutrition,* 1990;51:809–14.

Ip, Clement, Scimeca, Joseph A., and Thompson, Henry J. "Conjugated linoleic acid: A powerful anticarcinogen from animal fat sources." *Cancer,* 1994;74:1050–55.

Jialal, Ishwarlal, and Devaraj, Sridevi. "The role of oxidized low density lipoprotein in atherogenesis." *Journal of Nutrition,* 1996; 126(suppl):1053S–57S.

Jones, Peter J. H., et al. "Effect of dietary fat selection on plasma cholesterol synthesis in older, moderately hypercholesterolemic humans." *Arteriosclerosis and Thrombosis,* 1994;14(4):542–48.

Jonnalagadda, Satya, et al. "Effects of individual fatty acids on chronic diseases." *Nutrition Today,* 1996;31(3):90–106.

Kalmijn, S., et al. "Polyunsaturated fatty acids, antioxidants, and cognitive function in very old men." *American Journal of Epidemiology,* 1997;145:33–41.

Katan, Martijn. "Cons of high-carbohydrate versus high oil diets." First International Conference on Fats and Oil Consumption in Health and Disease. Rockefeller University, NY, April 24–25, 1995.

———. "Fats for diabetics." *The Lancet,* 1994;343:1518–19.

Katsuzaki, Hirotaka, et al. "Chemistry and Antioxidative Activity of Lignan Glucosides in Sesame Seed." *Food Phytochemicals for Cancer Prevention II: Tea, Spices, and Herbs.* Ho, Chi-Tang, Osawa, Toshihiko, Huang, Mou-Tuan, and Rosen, Robert T., eds. ACS Symposium Series 547, American Chemical Society, Washington, DC, 1994:274–80.

Kholsa, Pramod, et al. "Decreasing dietary lauric and myristic acids improves plasma lipids more favorably than decreasing dietary palmitic acid in rhesus monkeys fed AHA Step 1 type diets." *Journal of Nutrition,* 1997;127(suppl):525S–30S.

Krauss, Ronald, et al. "Dietary Guidelines for Healthy American Adults." AHA Medical/Scientific Statement. *Circulation,* 1996;94:1795–800.

Kretchmer, Norman, Beard, John L., and Carlson, Susan. "The role of nutrition in the development of normal cognition." *American Journal of Clinical Nutrition,* 1996; 63(suppl):997S–1001S.

Kritchevsky, David. "Conjugated linoleic acid in food: Scientists study its role as inhibitor of cancer-causing substances." *Food & Nutrition News,* 1994;66(3):22–23.

———. "Stearic acid metabolism and atherogenesis: History." *American Journal of Clinical Nutrition,* 1994;60(suppl):997S–1001S.

Lamon-Fava, Stefania, et al. "Effects of dietary intakes on plasma lipids, lipoproteins and apolipoproteins in free-living elderly men and women." *American Journal of Clinical Nutrition,* 1994;59:32–41.

Lane, Helen W., and Carpenter, John T. "Breast cancer: Incidence, nutritional concerns, and treatment approaches." *Journal of the American Dietetic Association,* 1987;87(6): 765–69.

Latif, A, and El Daly, M. A. "Search for new fixed oils. II. Edible oil from the seeds of hemp." *Agricultural Research Review,* 1973;51(5):123–29.

Layne, Kim S., et al. "Normal subjects consuming physiological levels of 18:3(n-3) and 20:5(n-3) from flaxseed or fish oils have characteristic differences in plasma lipid and lipoprotein fatty acid levels." *Journal of Nutrition,* 1996;126:2130–40.

Lehmann, J., et al. "Vitamin E in foods from high and low linoleic acid diets." *Journal of the American Dietetic Association,* 1986;86(9):1208–16.

Levine, Glenn N., et al. "Cholesterol and cardiovascular disease: Cholesterol reduction in cardiovascular disease." *New England Journal of Medicine,* 1995;332(8):312–21.

Lichtenstein, Alice H., et al. "Hypercholesterolemic effect of dietary cholesterol in diets enriched in polyunsaturated and saturated fat." *Arteriosclerosis and Thrombosis,* 1994;14(1):168–75.

London, Stephanie, J., et al. "Fatty acid composition of the subcutaneous adipose tissue and risk of proliferative benign breast disease and breast cancer." *Journal of the National Cancer Institute,* 1993;85:785–14.

Lopez-Miranda, J., et al. "Effect of apolipoprotein E phenotype on diet-induced lowering of plasma low density lipoprotein cholesterol." *Journal of Lipid Research,* 1994; 35:1965–75.

Louheranta, Anne M., et al. "Linoleic acid intake and susceptibility of very-low-density and low-density lipoproteins to oxidation in men." *American Journal of Clinical Nutrition,* 1996;63:698–703.

Lyu, Li-Ching, et al. "Relationship between dietary intake, lipoproteins, and apolipoproteins in Taipei and Framingham." *American Journal of Clinical Nutrition,* 1994; 60:765–74.

Mann, George V. "Metabolic consequences of dietary trans fatty acids." *The Lancet,* 1994;343:1268–72.

Mantzioris, E., et al. "Differences in the relationships between dietary linoleic and alpha-linoleic acids and their respective long-chain metabolites." *American Journal of Clinical Nutrition,* 1995;61:320–25.

Mantzioris, Evangeline, et al. "Dietary substitution with an alpha-linolenic acid–rich vegetable oil increases eicosapentaenoic acid concentrations." *American Journal of Clinical Nutrition,* 1994;59:1304–10.

Mattson, Fred H., Volpenhein, R. A., and Erickson, B. A. "Effect of plant sterol esters on the absorption of dietary cholesterol." *Journal of Nutrition,* 1977;107:1139–46.

McDonald, Bruce E., et al. "Comparison of the effect of canola oil and sunflower oil on plasma lipids and lipoproteins and on in vivo thromboxane A2 and prostacyclin production in healthy young men." *American Journal of Clinical Nutrition,* 1989;50: 1382–88.

McLaughin, P. J., and Weihruach, John L. "Vitamin E content of foods." *Journal of the American Dietetic Association,* 1979;75:647–65.

Mensink, Ronald P., and Katan, Martijn. "Effect of dietary trans fatty acids on high-density and low-density lipoprotein cholesterol levels in healthy subjects." *New England Journal of Medicine,* 1990;323:439–45.

Meydani, Simin N. "Dietary modulation of cytokine production and biologic functions." *Nutrition Reviews,* 1990;48(10):361–69.

Michels, Karen B., and Sack, Frank. "To the editor: Trans fatty acids in margarine." *New England Journal of Medicine,* 1995;333(2):131–32.

Mimura, A., et al. "Antioxidative and Anticancer Components Produced by Cell Culture of Sesame." *Food Phytochemicals for Cancer Prevention II: Tea, Spices, and Herbs.* Ho, Chi-Tang, Osawa, Toshihiko, Huang, Mou-Tuan, and Rosen, Robert T., eds. ACS Symposium Series 547, American Chemical Society, Washington, DC, 1994: 281–94.

Moncada, S., and Vane, J. R. "Arachidonic acid metabolites and the interactions between platelets and blood-vessel walls." *New England Journal of Medicine,* 1979;300(20): 1142–47.

Namiki, Mitsuo. "Antimutagen and Anticarcinogen Research in Japan." *Food Phytochemicals for Cancer Prevention I: Fruits and Vegetables.* Huang, Mou-Tuan, Osawa, Toshihiko, Ho, Chi-Tang, and Rosen, Robert T., eds. ACS Symposium Series 546, American Chemical Society, Washington, DC, 1994:65–81.

Nettleton, Joyce A. "Omega-3 fatty acids: Comparison of plant and seafood sources in human nutrition." *Journal of the American Dietetic Association,* 1991;91(3):331–37.

NIH Consensus Development Panel on Triglyceride, High-Density Lipoprotein, and Coronary Heart Disease. "Triglyceride, high-density lipoprotein, and coronary heart disease." *Journal of the American Medical Association,* 1993;269(4)505–10.

"Nutrition and Your Health." Dietary Guidelines for Americans, Fourth Edition. U.S. Department of Agriculture, 1995.

Oliver, Michael F. "Should the amount of fat in the diet be reduced?" First International Conference on Fats and Oil Consumption in Health and Disease. The Rockefeller University, NY, April 24–25, 1995.

Panico, Salvatore, et al. "Dietary Prevention of Chronic Diseases: The Potential for Cardiovascular Diseases." *Advances in Nutrition and Cancer.* Zappia, V., Savatore, M., and Della Ragione, F., eds. New York: Plenum, 1993:75–83.

Perez–Jimenez, Francisco, et al. "Lipoprotein concentrations in normolipidemic males consuming oleic acid–rich diets from two different sources: olive oil and oleic acid–rich sunflower oil." *American Journal of Clinical Nutrition,* 1995;62:769–75.

Pietinen, P., et al. "Intake of fatty acids and risk of coronary heart disease in a cohort of Finnish men." *American Journal of Epidemiology,* 1997;145:876–87.

Raie, M. Y., et al. "Studies of Cannabis sativa and sorghum bicolor oils." *Fett-Wissenschaft-Technologie*, 1995;97(11):428–429.

Raper, Nancy R., et al. "Omega-3 fatty acid content of the US food supply." *Journal of the American College of Nutrition*, 1992;11(3):304–8.

Rimm, Eric. "Carotenoids and Coronary Heart Disease." The Olestra Project: Potential Effects of Reducing Carotenoid Levels on Human Health. Harvard School of Public Health, January 17, 1996.

Rolls, Barbara J., et al. "Sensory properties of a nonabsorbable fat substitute did not affect regulation of energy intake." *American Journal of Clinical Nutrition*, 1997;65:1375–83.

Rose, David P. "The effects of polyunsaturated and monounsaturated fatty acids on cancer risk and outcome." The First International Conference on Fats and Oil Consumption in Health and Disease. Rockefeller University, NY, April 24–25, 1995.

———, et al. "Influence of diets containing eicosapentaenoic or docosahexaenoic acid on growth and metastasis of breast cancer cells in nude mice." *Journal of the National Cancer Institute*, 1995;87:587–93.

Sabate, Joan, et al. "Effects of walnuts on serum lipid levels and blood pressure in normal men." *New England Journal of Medicine*, 1993;328(9):603–7.

Sadowski, James A. "Structure and Mechanism of Activation of Vitamin K Antagonists." *Oral Anticoagulants*. Poller, Leon, and Hirsh, Jack, eds. New York: Oxford University Press, 1996:9–29.

Saltzman, S. S., and Roberts, S. B. "Effects of dietary fat content on energy intake and energy metabolism in identical twins." *International Journal of Obesity*, 1994;185:117.

Spiller, Gene A., et al. "Effect of a diet high in monounsaturated fat from almonds on plasma cholesterol and lipoproteins." *Journal of the American College of Nutrition*, 1992;11(2):126–30.

Stampfer, Meir. "Effects of Carotenoid Reduction on Disease Incidence: Quantitative Estimates." The Olestra Project: Potential Effects of Reducing Carotenoid Levels on Human Health. Harvard School of Public Health, January 17, 1996.

Steinhart, Carol. "Conjugated linoleic acid—the good news about animal fat." *Journal of Chemical Education*, 1996;73(12):A302–3.

Stevens, Laura J., et al. "Essential fatty acid metabolism in boys with attention-deficit hyperactivity disorder." *American Journal of Clinical Nutrition*, 1995;62:761–68.

Stone, W. L., and Papas, A. M. "Review. Tocopherols and the etiology of colon cancer." *Journal of the National Cancer Institute*, 1997;89(14):1006–14.

Sundram, Kalyana, et al. "Trans (elaidic) fatty acids adversely affect the lipoprotein profile relative to specific saturated fatty acids in humans." *Journal of Nutrition*, 1997;127(suppl):514S–20S.

Temme, Elisabeth, et al. "Comparison of the effects of diets enriched in lauric, palmitic, or oleic acids on serum lipids and lipoproteins in healthy women and men." *American Journal of Clinical Nutrition*, 1996;63:897–903.

Thompson, Frances, et al. "Sources of fiber and fat in diets of US women aged 19 to 50: implications for nutrition education and policy." *American Journal of Public Health*, 1992;892:695–702.

Thompson, Lilian U., et al. "Flaxseed and its lignan and oil components reduce mammary tumor growth at a late stage of carcinogenesis." *Carcinogenesis*, 1996;17:1373–76.

———. "Mammalian lignan production from various foods." *Nutrition and Cancer,* 1991;16(1):43–52.

"Trans Fatty Acids." IFST Position Statement. The Institute of Food Science and Technology, April 11, 1996.

Trichopoulou, Antonia, et al. "Consumption of olive oil and specific food groups in relation to breast cancer risk in Greece." *Journal of the National Cancer Institute,* 1995;87:110–16.

Ulbricht, T. L., and Southgate, D. A. T. "Coronary heart disease: seven dietary factors." *The Lancet,* 1991;338:985–92.

"Update: National Listing of Fish and Wildlife Consumption Advisories." EPA Fact Sheet. United States Environmental Protection Agency, Office of Water, June 1996.

U.S. Recommended Daily Allowances (RDA), Recommended Dietary Allowances, 10th revised edition. National Academy of Sciences, 1989.

Verschuren, W. M. Monique, et al. "Serum total cholesterol and long-term coronary heart disease mortality in different cultures: Twenty-five-year follow-up of the Seven Countries Study." *Journal of the American Medical Association,* 1995;274(2): 131–36.

"Vitamin K and Bone Health." Food & Nutrition Research Briefs. U.S. Department of Agriculture, Agricultural Research Service, October 1996.

Watts, George, et al. "Dietary fatty acids and progression of coronary artery disease in men." *American Journal of Clinical Nutrition,* 1996;64:202–9.

Weaver, Bonnie J., et al. "Dietary canola oil: Effect on the accumulation of eicosapentaenoic acid in the alkenylacyl fraction of human platelet ethanolamine phosphoglyceride." *American Journal of Clinical Nutrition,* 1990;51:594–98.

Weihrauch, John L., and Gardner, John M. "Sterol content of foods of plant origin." *Journal of the American Dietetic Association,* 1978;73:39–47.

Weststrate, J. A. "Sucrose polyester and plasma carotenoid concentrations in healthy subjects." *American Journal of Clinical Nutrition,* 1995;62:591–97.

"What We Eat in America: First Year Results from Ongoing Survey." Nutrition Research Briefs. U.S. Department of Agriculture, Agricultural Research Service, January 1996.

Whelan, Jay. "Antagonistic effects of dietary arachidonic acid on n-3 polyunsaturated fatty acids." *Journal of Nutrition,* 1996;126:1086S–91S.

Willett, Walter. "Are trans fatty acids a serious risk for disease?" The First International Conference on Fats and Oil Consumption in Health and Disease. Rockefeller University, NY, April 24–25, 1995.

———. "Dietary fat and breast cancer: prospective studies." *Cancer Researcher Weekly,* June 7, 1993:22–23.

———. "Effects of Reducing Carotenoid Levels on Humans." The Olestra Project: Potential Effects of Reducing Carotenoid Levels on Human Health. Harvard School of Public Health, January 17, 1996.

———, and Sacks, Frank. "Chewing the fat: How much and what kind." *New England Journal of Medicine,* 1991;324(2):121–23.

———, et al. "Intake of trans fatty acids and risk of coronary heart disease among women." *The Lancet,* 1993;341:581–86.

Wu, Dayong, et al. "Immunologic effects of marine- and plant-derived n-3 polyunsaturated fatty acids in nonhuman primates." *American Journal of Clinical Nutrition,* 1996;63:273–80.

The Healthiest Diet in the World

Yamashita, K., et al. "Sesame seed lignans and gamma-tocopherol act synergistically to produce vitamin E activity in rats." *Journal of Nutrition*, 1992;122:2440–46.

Ziegler, Regina G. "Carotenoids and Human Cancer." The Olestra Project: Potential Effects of Reducing Carotenoid Levels on Human Health. Harvard School of Public Health, January 17, 1996.

Chapter 3: Preventing System Breakdowns

"A Consumer's Guide to Fresh Mushrooms." American Mushroom Council. World Wide Web Site; http://www.mushroomcouncil.com/.

Adetumbi, Moses A., and Lau, Benjamin, H.S. "Allium sativum (garlic)—a natural antibiotic." *Medical Hypotheses*, 1983;12:227–37.

Amagase, Harunobu, and Milner, John A. "Impact of various sources of garlic and their constituents on 7, 12-dimethylbenz(a)anthracene binding to mammary cell DNA." *Carcinogenesis*, 1993;14(8):1627–31.

Anderson, John B. "Calcium, phosphorus and human bone development." *Journal of Nutrition*, 1996;126:1153S–58S.

Araujo, F. B., et al. "Evaluation of oxidative stress in patients with hyperlipidemia." *Atherosclerosis*, 1995;117(1):61–71.

Ardestani, Susan K., Ahadian, Mitra, and Watson, Ronald. "Chapter 11: Antioxidant Nutrients and Breast Cancer." *Nutrition and Cancer Prevention*. Watson, Ronald R., and Mufti, Siraj I., eds. Boca Raton, FL: CRC, 1996:173–204.

Beckstrom-Sternberg, Stephen M., and Duke, James A. Plants Containing Biotin. Plants Containing Choline. Plants Containing Cysteine. Plants Containing Lecithin. Plants Containing Zinc. Phytochemeco Database. Agricultural Research Service, USDA.

Bendich, Adrianne. "Carotenoids and the immune response." *Journal of Nutrition*, 1989;119:112–15.

Block, Eric. "The chemistry of garlic and onions." *Scientific American*, 1985;252(3): 114–19.

———. "Flavorants from Garlic, Onion and other Alliums and Their Cancer-Preventive Properties." *Food Phytochemicals for Cancer Prevention I: Fruits and Vegetables.* Huang, Mou-Tuan, Osawa, Toshihiko, Ho, Chi-Tang, and Rosen, Robert T., eds. ACS Symposium Series 546, American Chemical Society, Washington, DC, 1994:84–96.

———. "The organosulfur chemistry of the genus allium—implications for the organic chemistry of sulfur." *Angewante Chemie* (International Edition in English), 1992; 31:1135–78.

Block, Gladys. "Vitamin C and cancer prevention: The epidemiologic evidence." *American Journal of Clinical Nutrition*, 1991;53(suppl):270S–82S.

Boushey, Carol J., et al. "A quantitative assessment of plasma homocysteine as a risk factor for vascular disease: probable benefits of increasing folic acid intakes." *Journal of the American Medical Association*, 1995;274:1049–58.

Burk, Raymond. "Selenium." *Present Knowledge in Nutrition*, Fifth Edition. Washington, DC: Nutrition Foundation, Inc., 1984:519–27.

Calvo, Mona S., and Park, Youngmee K. "Changing phosphorus content of the U.S. diet: Potential for adverse effects on bone." *Journal of Nutrition*, 1996;126:1168S–80S.

Cao, Guohua, et al. "Antioxidant capacity of tea and common vegetables." *Journal of Agricultural and Food Chemistry*, 1996;44(11):3426–31.

———. "Automated assay of oxygen radical absorbance capacity with the COBAS FARA II." *Clinical Chemistry,* 1995;41(12):1738–44.

Chang, Mei Ling W., and Johnson, Margaret A. "Effect of garlic on carbohydrate metabolism and lipid synthesis in rats." *Journal of Nutrition,* 1980;110:931–36.

Chew, B. P. "Antioxidant vitamins affect food animal immunity and health." *Journal of Nutrition,* 1995;125(suppl):1804S–8S.

Chow, Ching K. "Vitamin E and Cancer." *Nutrition and Disease Update—Cancer.* Carroll, Kenneth K., and Kritchevsky, David, eds. Champaign, IL; AOCS, 1994:173–233.

Clark, Larry C., and Alberts, David S. "Selenium and cancer: Risk or protection?" *Journal of the National Cancer Institute,* 1995;87(7):473–75.

Cohen, Bruce M., et al. "Decreased brain choline uptake in older adults." *Journal of the American Medical Association,* 1995;272(11):902–7.

"Common garlic powder blocks potent carcinogens in cells." *Cancer Researcher Weekly,* March 14, 1994:7.

"Continuing Survey of Food Intakes by Individuals (CSFII): What We Eat in America." U.S. Department of Agriculture, Agricultural Research Service, 1994.

"The cost of too little magnesium." *Science News,* 1997;151:279.

Cowen, R. "Chromium may prevent type II diabetes onset." *Science News,* 1990; 137(4):214.

Dausch, Judith G., and Nixon, Daniel W. "Garlic: A Review of Its Relationship to Malignant Disease." Academic Press, Inc., 1990:346–61.

Dodson, Wanda L., and Sachan, Dileep S. "Choline supplementation reduces urinary carnitine excretion in humans." *American Journal of Clinical Nutrition,* 1996;63: 904–10.

Dorant, Elisabeth, et al. "Consumption of onions and a reduced risk of stomach carcinoma." *Gastroenterology,* 1996;110(1):12–20.

Dupont, Jacqueline, et al. "Fatty acid–related functions." *American Journal of Clinical Nutrition,* 1996;63:991S–93S.

Dwyer, Johanna. "Overview: Dietary approaches for reducing cardiovascular disease risks." *Journal of Nutrition,* 1995;125(suppl):656S–65S.

"Effects of Reducing Carotenoid Levels on Humans," transcript of discussion. The Olestra Project: Potential Effects of Reducing Carotenoid Levels on Human Health. Harvard School of Public Health, January 17, 1996.

Ferro-Luzzi, Anna, and Ghiselli, Andrea. "Protective Aspects of the Mediterranean Diet." *Advances in Nutrition and Cancer.* Zappia, V., Salvatore, M., and Della Ragione, F., eds. New York: Plenum, 1993:137–44.

Fisher, Jeffrey A. *The Chromium Program.* New York: Harper & Row, 1990.

"Folate Deficiency Rapidly Raises Risk." Food & Nutrition Research Briefs. U.S. Department of Agriculture, Agricultural Research Service, April 1996.

"Folate Spares Colon and Heart." Food & Nutrition Research Briefs. U.S. Department of Agriculture, Agricultural Research Service, July 1996.

Folic Acid. 1993 Report on USDA Human Nutrition Research and Education Activities. A report to Congress covering the period January–December 1993. USDA, July 1995.

"Food and Nutrient Intakes by Individuals in the United States, 1 Day, 1989–91." NFS Rep. No. 91–2. Highlights of 1989–91 CSFII/DHKS Reports. U.S. Department of Agriculture, Agricultural Research Service, Riverdale, MD.

The Food Processor® Nutrition Analysis Software, ESHA Research, Salem, OR.

Freeland-Graves, Jeanne J., Ebangit, M. Lavone, and Bodzy, Pamela W. "Zinc and copper content of foods used in vegetarian diets." *Journal of the American Dietetic Association,* 1980;77:648–54.

Gebhardt, Susan E., and Holden, Joanne M. "Provisional Table on the Selenium Content of Foods." U.S. Department of Agriculture, HNIS/PT-109, 1993.

Gey, K. Fred, et al. "Increased risk of cardiovascular disease at suboptimal plasma concentrations of essential antioxidants: An epidemiological update with special attention to carotene and vitamin C." *American Journal of Clinical Nutrition,* 1993;57(suppl): 787S–97S.

"G.I. Guard Plummets in Protein Malnutrition." Food and Nutrition Research Briefs. U.S. Department of Agriculture, Agricultural Research Service, January 1996.

Giovannucci, Edward, et al. "Folate, methionine, and alcohol intake and risk of colorectal adenoma." *Journal of the National Cancer Institute,* 1993;85(11):875–84.

Graham, I. M., et. al. "Plasma homocysteine as a risk factor for vascular disease: The European Concerted Action Project." *Journal of the American Medical Association,* 1997;277(22):175–81.

Guengerich, F. Peter. "Influence of nutrients and other dietary materials on cytochrome P-450 enzymes." *American Journal of Clinical Nutrition,* 1995;61(suppl):651S–58S.

"Guidelines on Diet, Nutrition and Cancer Prevention: Reducing the Risk of Cancer with Healthy Food Choices and Physical Activity." American Cancer Society, Dietary Guidelines Advisory Committee, 1996.

Guthrie, Najla, et al. "Inhibition of proliferation of estrogen receptor-negative MDA-MB-435 and positive MCF-7 human breast cancer cells by palm oil tocotrienols and tamoxifen, alone and in combination." *Journal of Nutrition,* 1997;127(suppl): 544S–48S.

Handelman, Garry. "Physiological Effects of Carotenoids in Humans." The Olestra Project: Potential Effects of Reducing Carotenoid Levels on Human Health. Harvard School of Public Health, January 17, 1996.

Hands, Elizabeth S. *Food Finder, Food Sources of Vitamins & Minerals,* Third Edition. Salem, OR: ESHA Research, 1995.

Harman, Denham. "Overview: Role of antioxidant nutrients in aging." *AGE,* 1994;17:21.

Harpel, Peter C., Zhang, Xiaoxia, and Borth, Wolfgang. "Homocysteine and hemostasis: Pathogenetic mechanisms predisposing to thrombosis." *Journal of Nutrition,* 1996; 126(suppl):1285S–89S.

Harrow, Benjamin, and Mazur, Abraham. *Textbook of Biochemistry,* Ninth Edition. Philadelphia: W.B. Saunders, 1966.

Hasler, Clare. "Institute for functional foods proposal." *Functional Foods for Health News,* 1996;4(2):4–5.

Hendrich, Suzanne, et al. "Defining food components as new nutrients." *Journal of Nutrition,* 1994;124:1789S–92S.

Hertog, Michael G., et al. "Flavonoid intake and long-term risk of coronary heart disease and cancer in the Seven Countries Study." *Archives of Internal Medicine,* 1995;155: 381–87.

Hong, J. Y., et al. "Inhibition of Chemical Toxicity and Carcinogenesis by Diallyl Sulfide and Diallyl Sulfone." *Food Phytochemicals for Cancer Prevention I: Fruits and Vegetables.* Huang, Mou-Tuan, Toshihiko, Osawa, Ho, Chi-Tang, and Rosen, Robert T., eds. ACS Symposium Series 546, American Chemical Society, Washington, DC, 1994:97–101.

Hunt, Sara M., and Groff, James L. *Advanced Nutrition and Human Metabolism*. St. Paul, MN: West, 1990.

Imada, Osamu. "Toxicity Aspects of Garlic." The First World Congress on the Health Significance of Garlic and Garlic Constituents. Washington, DC, August 1990.

Imai, J., et al. "Antioxidant and radical scavenging effects of aged garlic extract and its constituents." *Planta Medica* 1994;60:417–20.

Jacob, Robert A., and Burri, Betty J. "Oxidative damage and defense." *American Journal of Clinical Nutrition*, 1996;63(suppl):985S–90S.

Jacques, Paul F., and Chylack, Leo T. "Epidemiologic evidence of a role for the antioxidant vitamins and carotenoids in cataract prevention." *American Journal of Clinical Nutrition*, 1991;53:352S–55S.

Julius, Mara, et al. "Glutathione and morbidity in a community-based sample of elderly." *Journal of Clinical Epidemiology*, 1994;47(9):1021–26.

Kalayjian, Robert C., et al. "A phase I/II trial of intravenous L-2-oxothiazolidine-4-carboxylic acid (procysteine) in asymptomatic HIV-infected subjects." *Journal of Acquired Immune Deficiency Syndromes*, 1994;7:369.

Kang, Soo-Sang. "Treatment of hyperhomocysteinemia: Physiological basis." *Journal of Nutrition*, 1996;126(suppl):1273S–75S.

Kawakishi, Shunro, and Morimitsu, Y. "Sulfur Chemistry of Onions and Inhibitory Factors of the Arachidonic Acid Cascade." *Food Phytochemicals for Cancer Prevention I: Fruits and Vegetables*. Huang, Mou-Tuan, Toshihiko, Osawa, Ho, Chi-Tang, and Rosen, Robert T., eds. ACS Symposium Series 546, American Chemical Society, Washington, DC, 1994:120–27.

Kies, Constance. "Copper Bioavailability and Metabolism; Food Sources of Dietary Copper." *Advances in Experimental Medicine and Biology*, Volume 258. New York: Plenum, 1989:1–20.

Kinsella, John E., et al. "Dietary polyunsaturated fatty acids and eicosanoids: Potential effects on the modulation of inflammatory and immune cells: An overview." *Nutrition*, 1990;6(1):24–44.

Koch, Heinrich P., and Lawson, Larry, eds. *Garlic: The Science and Therapeutic Application of Allium sativum L. and Related Species*. Baltimore: Williams & Wilkins, 1996.

Kurtzweil, Paula. "How folate can help prevent birth defects." *FDA Consumer Magazine*. U.S. Food and Drug Administration, September 1996.

Lau, Benjamin H. S. "Anti-coagulant and Lipid Regulating Effects of Garlic (Allium sativum)." *New Protective Roles for Selected Nutrients*. New York: Alan R. Liss, 1989:295–325.

———, Lam, Fred, and Wang-Cheng, Rebekah. "Effect of an odor-modified garlic preparation on blood lipids." *Nutrition Research*, 1987;7:139–49.

———, Tadi, Padma P., and Tosk, Jeffrey M. "Allium sativum (garlic) and cancer prevention." *Nutrition Research*, 1990;10:937–48.

———, Yamasaki, Takeshi, and Gridley, Daila S. "Garlic compounds modulate macrophase and T-lymphocyte functions." *Molecular Biotherapy*, 1991;3:103–7.

Lembo, G., et al. "Allergic contact dermatitis due to garlic (Allium sativum)." *Contact Dermatitis*, 1991;25:330.

Lin, Robert I. "Introduction: An overview of the nutritional and pharmacological properties of garlic." First World Congress on the Health Significance of Garlic and Garlic Constituents. Washington, DC, August 1990.

———. "Myths, theories and facts about garlic's health benefits." First World Congress on the Health Significance of Garlic and Garlic Constituents. Washington, DC, August 1990.

Lonnerdal, Bo. "Bioavailability of copper." *American Journal of Clinical Nutrition,* 1996;63(suppl):821S–29S.

Makheja, Amar N. "Anti-platelet constituents of garlic and their effects on platelet aggregation and cyclo and lipoxygenase enzymes." The First World Congress on the Health Significance of Garlic and Garlic Constituents. Washington, DC, 1990.

Malinow, M. R. "Plasma homocyst(e)ine: A risk factor for arterial occlusive diseases." *Journal of Nutrition,* 1996;126(suppl):11238S–43S.

McBride, Judy. "Preventing diabetes with chromium." *Agricultural Research,* October 1990:14–17.

McLaughlin, P. J., and Weihruach, John L. "Vitamin E content of foods." *Journal of the American Dietetic Association,* 1979;75:647–65.

Mei, Xing, Lin, Xiyun, and Liu, Jinzhou. "The preventive effect of garlic against N-nitroso compounds–induced tumorigenesis." The First World Congress on the Health Significance of Garlic and Garlic Constituents. Washington, DC, August 1990.

Meydani, Simin N., and Dupont, Jacqueline. "Effect of zinc deficiency on prostaglandin synthesis in different organs of the rat." *Journal of Nutrition,* 1982;112:1098–104.

Meydani, Simin N., et al. "Dietary antioxidants and immune function." *AGE,* 1994; 17:21.

Miller, Joshua W., et al. "Vitamin B-6 deficiency vs. folate deficiency: Comparison of responses to methionine loading in rats." *American Journal of Clinical Nutrition,* 1994;59:1033–40.

Miller-Ihli, N. J. "Graphite furnace atomic absorption spectrometry for the determination of the chromium content of selected U.S. foods." *Journal of Food Composition and Analysis,* 1996;9:290–300.

Milner, John A. "Selenium: Do We Dare Neglect It?" *Nutrition and Health, Topics and Controversies.* Bronner, F., ed. Boca Raton, FL: CRC, 1995:199–227.

Mufti, Siraj. "Chapter 5: Prevention of Alcohol-Induced Disease and Cancer by Nutrition." *Nutrition and Cancer Prevention.* Watson, Ronald R., and Mufti, Siraj I., eds. Boca Raton, FL: CRC, 1996:59–80.

"Nutrient Intakes: Mean amount consumed per individual, by sex and age, 1 day, 1995." U.S. Department of Agriculture. USDA Continuing Survey of Food Intakes by Individuals, 1995.

O'Dell, Boyd. "Copper." *Present Knowledge in Nutrition,* Fifth Edition. Washington, DC: Nutrition Foundation, 1984:506–18.

Omaye, Stanley T., et al. "Blood antioxidant changes in young women following beta-carotene depletion and repletion." *Journal of the American College of Nutrition,* 1996;15(5):469–74.

Penland, James, Speaker, Karen, K., and Moulton, Patricia L. "Dietary copper and magnesium affects activity, learning, memory and anxiety in rats." *Proceedings of North Dakota Academy of Science,* 1996;50:57.

Pinto, John Thomas, et al. "Effects of garlic thioallyl derivatives on growth, glutathione concentration, and polyamine formation of human prostate carcinoma cells in culture." *American Journal of Clinical Nutrition*, 1997;66:398–405.

Pi-Sunyer, F. Xavier, and Offenbacher, Esther. "Chromium." *Present Knowledge in Nutrition*, Fifth Edition. Washington, DC: Nutrition Foundation, 1984:571–86.

"Pros and Cons on Chromium." *Food and Nutrition Research Briefs.* U.S. Department of Agriculture, Agricultural Research Service, July 1996.

Qureshi, A. A., et al. "Response of hypercholesterolemic subjects to administration of tocotrienols." *Lipids,* 1995;30(12):1171–77.

Reed, Donald J. "Glutathione and Vitamin E in Protection Against Mutagens and Carcinogens." *Food Toxicology: A Perspective on the Relative Risks.* Taylor, Steven, and Scanlon, Richard, eds. New York: Marcel Dekker, 1989:169–203.

Rogers, Adrianne E. "Methyl donors in the diet and responses to chemical carcinogens." *American Journal of Clinical Nutrition,* 1995;61(suppl):659S–66S.

Sandstead, Harold, and Evans, Gary. "Zinc." *Present Knowledge in Nutrition,* Fifth Edition. Washington, DC: Nutrition Foundation, 1984:479–505.

Selhub, Jacob, et al. "Association between plasma homocysteine concentrations and extracranial carotid-artery stenosis." *New England Journal of Medicine,* 1995;332(5):286–91.

———. "Relationship between plasma homocysteine, vitamin status and extracranial carotid-artery stenosis in the Framingham Study population." *Journal of Nutrition,* 1996;126(suppl):1258S–65S.

———. "Vitamin status and intake as primary determinants of homocysteinemia in an elderly population." *Journal of the American Medical Association,* 1993;270(22):2693–98.

Shubert, Anita, Holden, Joanne M., and Wolf, Wayne R. "Selenium content of a core group of foods based on a critical evaluation of published analytical data." *Journal of the American Dietetic Association,* 1987;87(3):285–99.

Sies, Helmut, and Stahl, Wilhelm. "Vitamins E and C, beta-carotene, and other carotenoids as antioxidants." *American Journal of Clinical Nutrition,* 1995;62(suppl.):1315S–21S.

Simon, Joel A. "Vitamin C and cardiovascular disease: A review." *Journal of the American College of Nutrition,* 1992;11(2):107–25.

Srivastava, Krishna. "Effect of some garlic components on arachidonic acid metabolism and platelet aggregation." The First World Congress on the Health Significance of Garlic and Garlic Constituents. Washington, DC, 1990.

———. "Onion exerts antiaggregatory effects by altering arachidonic acid metabolism in platelets." *Prostaglandins Leukot. Med.,* 1986;24:43–50.

Stampfer, Meir J., and Willett, Walter C. "Homocysteine and marginal vitamin deficiency: The importance of adequate vitamin intake." *Journal of the American Medical Association,* 1993;270(22):2726–27.

Steiner, Manfred, et al. "A double-blind crossover study in moderately hypercholesterolemic men that compared the effect of aged garlic extract and placebo administration on blood lipids." *American Journal of Clinical Nutrition,* 1996;64:866–70.

Steinmetz, Kristi A., and Potter, John D. "Vegetables, fruit, and cancer prevention: A review." *Journal of the American Dietetic Association,* 1996;96(10):1027–39.

Tadi, Padma P., Teel, Robert W., and Lau, Benjamin H. S. "Organosulfur compounds of garlic modulate mutagenesis, metabolism, and DNA binding of aflatoxin B1." *Nutrition and Cancer,* 1991;15:87–95.

Talalay, Paul, et al. "Chemoprotection against cancer by Phase 2 enzyme induction." *Elsevier Science Toxicology Letters,* 1995;82/83:173–79.

"Trace Element Has Far-Flung Influence." *Food and Nutrition Research Briefs.* U.S. Department of Agriculture, Agricultural Research Service, April 1995.

Tsuda, H., et al. "Chemopreventive effects of beta-carotene, alpha-tocopherol and five naturally occurring antioxidants on initiation of hepatocarcinogensis by 2-amino-3-methylimidazo[4,5-f]quinoline in the rat." *Japanese Journal of Cancer Research,* 1994; 85(12):1214–19.

Tucker, Katherine L., et al. "Folic acid fortification of the food supply: Potential benefits and risks for the elderly population." *Journal of the American Medical Association,* 1996;276(23):1879–85.

Ubbink, Johan B., et al. "Vitamin B-12, vitamin B-6, and folate nutritional status in men with hyperhomocysteinemia." *American Journal of Clinical Nutrition,* 1993;57:47–54.

Wang, Hong, Gao, Guohua, and Prior, Ronald L. "Total antioxidant capacity of fruits." *Journal of Agricultural and Food Chemistry,* 1996;44(3):701–5.

Warshafsky, Stephen. "Effect of garlic on total serum cholesterol." *Annals of Internal Medicine,* 1993;119(7):599–605.

Weisburger, John H. "Nutritional approach to cancer prevention with emphasis on vitamins, antioxidants, and carotenoids." *American Journal of Clinical Nutrition,* 1991; 53:226S–37S.

"What We Eat in America: First Year Results from Ongoing Survey." Nutrition Research Briefs. U.S. Department of Agriculture, Agricultural Research Service, January 1996.

Williams, David E., et al. "Anticarcinogens and Tumor Promoters in Foods." *Food Toxicology: A Perspective on the Relative Risks.* Taylor, Steven, and Scanlon, Richard, eds. New York: Marcel Dekker, 1989:101–50.

Winker, Margaret A., and Fontanarosa, Phil. "Letters re: Folic acid fortification of food." *Journal of the American Medical Association,* 1996;275(9):681–83.

Witte, John S., et al. "Relation of vegetable, fruit, and grain consumption to colorectal adenomatous polyps." *American Journal of Epidemiology,* 1996;144:1015–25.

Wood, Richard J., and Zheng, Jia Ju. "High dietary calcium intakes reduce zinc absorption and balance in humans." *American Journal of Clinical Nutrition,* 1997;65: 1083–89.

Wu, Dayong, et al. "Immunologic effects of marine- and plant-derived n-3 polyunsaturated fatty acids in nonhuman primates." *American Journal of Clinical Nutrition,* 1996;63:273–80.

Yeh, Yu-Yan, and Yeh, Shaw-mei. "Hypolipidemic effects of garlic extracts in vivo and in vitro." The First World Congress on the Health Significance of Garlic and Garlic Constituents. Washington, DC, 1990.

You, Wei-Cheng, et al. "Allium vegetables and reduced risk of stomach cancer." *Journal of the National Cancer Institute,* 1989;81(2):162–64.

———. "Diet and high risk of stomach cancer in Shandong, China." *Cancer Research,* 1988;48:3518–23.

"Your Cheated Heart." Food and Nutrition Research Briefs. U.S. Department of Agriculture, Agricultural Research Service, April 1995.

Zeisel, Steven H. "Choline: An important nutrient in brain development, liver function

Bibliography

and carcinogenesis." *Journal of the American College of Nutrition,* 1992;11(5): 473–81.

Chapter 4: A Foundation of Vegetables (and Fruit)

Akagi, K., et al. "Modulating effects of ellagic acid, vanillin and quercetin in a rat medium term multi-organ carcinogenesis model." *Cancer Letter,* 1995;94(1):113–21.

Aldoori, Walid H., et al. "A prospective study of diet and the risk of symptomatic diverticular disease in men." *American Journal of Clinical Nutrition,* 1994;60:757–64.

Anderson, J. J., Rondano, P., and Holmes, A. "Roles of diet and physical activity in the prevention of osteoporosis." *Scandinavian Journal of Rheumatology Supplements,* 1996;103:65–74.

Anderson, Todd J. "The effect of cholesterol lowering and antioxidant therapy on endothelium-dependent coronary vasomotion." *New England Journal of Medicine,* 1995;332(8):488–93.

Appel, Lawrence J., et al. "A clinical trial of the effects of dietary patterns on blood pressure." *New England Journal of Medicine,* 1997;336(16):1117–24.

Ascherio, Alberto, et al. "A prospective study of nutritional factors and hypertension among US men." *Circulation,* 1992;86(5):1475–84.

———. "A prospective study of nutritional factors and hypertension among US women." *Hypertension,* 1996;27(5):1065–72.

Attaway, John A. "Citrus Juice Flavonoids with Anticarcinogenic and Antitumor Properties." *Food Phytochemicals for Cancer Prevention I: Fruits and Vegetables.* Huang, Mou-Tuan, Toshihiki, Osawa, Ho, Chi-Tang, and Rosen, Robert T., eds. ACS Symposium Series 546, American Chemical Society, Washington, DC, 1994:240–48.

Barch, D. H., Rundhaugen, L. M., and Pillay, N. S. "Ellagic acid induces transcription of the rat glutathione S-transferase-Ya gene." *Carcinogenesis,* 1995;16(3):665–68.

Betz, J. M., and Fox, W. D. "High-Performance Liquid Chromatographic Determination of Glucosinolates in Brassica Vegetables." *Food Phytochemicals for Cancer Prevention I: Fruits and Vegetables.* Huang, Mou-Tuan, Toshihiko, Osawa, Ho, Chi-Tang, and Rosen, Robert T., eds. ACS Symposium Series 546, American Chemical Society, Washington, DC, 1994:181–96.

Block, Gladys. "Dietary guidelines and the results of food consumption surveys." *American Journal of Clinical Nutrition,* 1991;53(suppl):365S–67S.

———. "Vitamin C and cancer prevention: The epidemiologic evidence." *American Journal of Clinical Nutrition,* 1991;53(suppl):270S–82S.

Brandi, Maria Luisa. "Flavonoids: Biochemical effects and therapeutic applications." *Bone and Mineral* (Suppl) 1992;19:S3–S19.

Buiatti, Eva, et al. "A case-control study of gastric cancer and diet in Italy." *International Journal of Cancer,* 1989;44:611–16.

Bunker, V. W., "The role of nutrition in osteoporosis." *British Journal of Biomedical Science,* 1994;51(3):228–40.

Burk, Raymond. "Selenium." *Present Knowledge in Nutrition,* Fifth Edition. Washington, DC: Nutrition Foundation, 1984:519–27.

Carotenoid Research Interactive Group (CARIG). "Beta-carotene and the carotenoids: Beyond the intervention trials." *Nutrition Reviews,* 1996;54(6):185–88.

"Carotenoids in individual fruits and vegetables." USDA Carotenoid Database.

Castonguay, Andre, Boukharta, Mohamed, and Jalbert, Guylaine. "Comparative Study of Ellagic Acid and Its Analogues as Chemopreventive Agents against Lung Tumorigenesis." *Food Phytochemicals for Cancer Prevention I: Fruits and Vegetables.* Huang, Mou-Tuan, Toshihiki, Osawa, Ho, Chi-Tang, and Rosen, Robert T., eds. ACS Symposium Series 546, American Chemical Society, Washington, DC, 1994:294–302.

Colditz, Graham A., et al., eds. "Harvard Report on Cancer Prevention. Volume I: Causes of Human Cancer." *Cancer Causes & Control,* 1996;7(suppl).

Constantinou, A., et al. "The dietary anticancer agent ellagic acid is a potent inhibitor of DNA topoisomerases in vitro." *Nutrition and Cancer,* 1991;23(2):121–30.

"Continuing Survey of Food Intakes by Individuals (CSFII): What We Eat in America." U.S. Department of Agriculture, Agricultural Research Service, 1994.

Cozzi, R., et al. "Taurine and ellagic acid: Two differently-acting natural antioxidants." *Environmental Molecular Mutagen,* 1995;26(3):248–54.

"Data Tables: Results from USDA's 1995 Continuing Survey of Food Intakes by Individuals and 1995 Diet and Health Knowledge Survey." U.S. Department of Agriculture, Agricultural Research Service, December 1996.

Decker, Eric A., Ph.D. "The role of phenolics, conjugated linoleic acid, carnosine, and pyrroloquinoline quinone as nonessential dietary antioxidants." *Nutrition Reviews,* 1995;53(3):49–58.

Dennison, Barbara A., Rockwell, Helen L., and Baker, Sharon L. "Excess fruit juice consumption by preschool children is associated with short stature and obesity." *Pediatrics,* 1997;99(1):15–22.

"Effects of Reducing Carotenoid Levels on Humans," transcript of discussion. The Olestra Project: Potential Effects of Reducing Carotenoid Levels on Human Health. Harvard School of Public Health, January 17, 1996.

Fahey, Jed W., and Talalay, Paul. "The Role of Crucifers in Cancer Chemoprotection." *Phytochemicals and Health.* Gustine, D. L., and Flores, H. E., eds. American Society of Plant Physiologists, 1995:87–93.

Folts, John D. "To the editor: Fruits, vegetables and stroke risk." *Journal of the American Medical Association,* 1995;274:1197–99.

"Food and Nutrient Intakes by Individuals in the United States, 1 Day, 1989–91." NFS Rep. No. 91–2. Highlights of 1989–91 CSFII/DHKS Reports. U.S. Department of Agriculture, Agricultural Research Service, Riverdale, MD.

The Food Processor®, Nutrition Analysis Software, ESHA Research, Salem, OR.

Franceschi, S., et al. "Tomatoes and risk of digestive-tract cancers." *International Journal of Cancer,* 1994;59(2):181–84.

Freudenheim, Jo L., et al. "Premenopausal breast cancer risk and intake of vegetables, fruits and related nutrients." *Journal of the National Cancer Institute,* 1996;88(6): 340–48.

Fukagawa, Naomi, et al. "High-carbohydrate, high-fiber diets increase peripheral insulin sensitivity in healthy young and old adults." *American Journal of Clinical Nutrition,* 1990;52:524–48.

Fulder, Stephen, and Tenne, Meir. "Ginger as an anti-nausea remedy in pregnancy: The issue of safety." *HerbalGram,* 1996;38:47–50.

Gärtner, Christine, Stahl, Wilhelm, and Sies, Helmet. "Lycopene is more bioavailable from tomato paste than from fresh tomatoes." *American Journal of Clinical Nutrition,* 1997;66:116–22.

Gey, K. Fred, et al. "Increased risk of cardiovascular disease at suboptimal plasma concentrations of essential antioxidants: An epidemiological update with special attention to carotene and vitamin C." *American Journal of Clinical Nutrition,* 1993; 57(suppl):787S–97S.

Gillman, Matthew, et al. "Protective effect of fruits and vegetables on development of stroke in men." *Journal of the American Medical Association,* 1995;273:1113–18.

Giovannucci, Edward. "Carotenoids and Prostate Cancer." The Olestra Project: Potential Effects of Reducing Carotenoid Levels on Human Health. Harvard School of Public Health, January 17, 1996.

———, et al. "Carotenoids and retinol in relation to risk of prostate cancer." *Journal of the National Cancer Institute,* 1995;87:1767–76.

———, et al. "Folate, methionine, and alcohol intake and risk of colorectal adenoma," *Journal of the National Cancer Institute,* 1993;85(11):875–84.

Goldfinger, Stephen E. "Hypertension: An elemental finding." *Harvard Health Letter,* 1992;7(7):5.

Goldin, Barry R. "Nonsteroidal estrogens and estrogen antagonists: Mechanism of action and health implications." *Journal of the National Cancer Institute,* 1994;86(23):1741–42.

Goodman, Marc T., et. al. "Association of soy and fiber consumption with the risk of endometrial cancer." *American Journal of Epidemiology,* 1997;146:294–306.

Greenberg, Robert E. "Editorial: Antioxidant vitamins, cancer, and cardiovascular disease." *New England Journal of Medicine,* 1996;334:1189–90.

Guengerich, F. Peter. "Influence of nutrients and other dietary materials on cytochrome P-450 enzymes." *American Journal of Clinical Nutrition,* 1995;61(suppl):651S–58S.

"Guidelines on Diet, Nutrition and Cancer Prevention: Reducing the Risk of Cancer with Healthy Food Choices and Physical Activity." American Cancer Society, Dietary Guidelines Advisory Committee, 1996.

Handelman, Garry. "Physiological Effects of Carotenoids in Humans." The Olestra Project: Potential Effects of Reducing Carotenoid Levels on Human Health. Harvard School of Public Health, January 17, 1996.

Hankinson, Susan. "Carotenoids and Age-Related Macular Degeneration." The Olestra Project: Potential Effects of Reducing Carotenoid Levels on Human Health. Harvard School of Public Health, January 17, 1996.

———. "Nutrient intake and cataract extraction in women: a prospective study." *Journal of the American Medical Association,* 1993;269:350–51.

Harrow, Benjamin, and Mazur, Abraham. *Textbook of Biochemistry,* Ninth Edition. Philadelphia: W. B. Saunders, 1966.

Hasler, Clare. "Tomatoes may lower prostate cancer risk." *Functional Foods for Health News,* 1996;4(2):11.

Hendrich, Suzanne, et al. "Defining food components as new nutrients." *Journal of Nutrition,* 1994;124:1789S–92S.

Hertog, Michael G., Hollman, Peter C. H., and Katan, Martijn B. "Content of potentially anticarcinogenic flavonoids of 28 vegetables and 9 fruits commonly consumed in the Netherlands." *Journal of Agricultural and Food Chemistry,* 1992;40:2379–83.

Hertog, Michael G., et al. "Dietary antioxidant flavonoids and risk of coronary heart disease: The Zutphen Elderly Study." *The Lancet,* 1993;342:1007–11.

———, et al. "Flavonoid intake and long-term risk of coronary heart disease and cancer in the Seven Countries Study." *Archives of Internal Medicine,* 1995;155:381–87.

Holmberg, Lars, et al. "Diet and breast cancer risk: Results from a population-based, case-control study in Sweden." *Archives of Internal Medicine,* 1994;154:1805–12.

Hunt, Curtiss D., Shuler, Terrence R., and Mullen, LoAnne M. "Concentration of boron and other elements in human foods and personal-care products." *Journal of the American Dietetic Association,* 1991;91(5):558–68.

Hunt, Sara M., and Groff, James L. *Advanced Nutrition and Human Metabolism.* St. Paul, MN: West Publishing Company, 1990.

Hutchins, Andrea M., et al. "Vegetables, fruits and legumes effect on urinary isoflavonoid phytoestrogen and lignan excretion." *Journal of the American Dietetic Association,* 1995;95:769–75.

"It's just natural: Flavor enhancers that may enhance health." *American Institute for Cancer Research Newsletter,* Winter 1997;54:10.

Jacob, Robert A., and Burri, Betty J. "Oxidative damage and defense." *American Journal of Clinical Nutrition,* 1996;63(suppl):985S–90S.

Jacques, Paul. "Carotenoids and Cataracts." The Olestra Project: Potential Effects of Reducing Carotenoid Levels on Human Health. Harvard School of Public Health, January 17, 1996.

Kensler, T. W., et al. "Chemoprotection by 1,2-Dithiole-3-thiones." *Food Phytochemicals for Cancer Prevention I: Fruits and Vegetables.* Huang, Mou-Tuan, Toshihiko, Osawa, Ho, Chi-Tang, and Rosen, Robert T., eds. ACS Symposium Series 546, American Chemical Society, Washington, DC, 1994:154–63.

Khachik, Fredrick, Beecher, Gary R., and Smith, J. Cecil Jr. "Lutein, lycopene, and their oxidative metabolites in chemoprevention of cancer." *Journal of Cellular Biochemistry,* 1995; 22(suppl):236–46.

Khaw, Kay-Tee, and Woodhouse, Peter. "Interrelation of vitamin C, infection, haemostatic factors, and cardiovascular disease." *British Medical Journal,* 1995;310:1559–64.

Kikuzaki, Hiroe, and Nakatani, Nobuji. "Antioxidant effects of some ginger constituents." *Journal of Food Science,* 1993;58(6):1407–10.

Kim, Young-In, et al. "Folate deficiency in rats induces DNA strand breaks and hypomethylation within the p53 tumor suppressor gene." *American Journal of Clinical Nutrition,* 1997;65:46–52.

Knekt, Paul. "Flavonoid intake and coronary mortality in Finland: A cohort study." *British Medical Journal,* 1996;312:478–81.

Kohlmejer, Martin, et al. "Transport of vitamin K to bone in humans." *Journal of Nutrition,* 1996;126(suppl):1992S–96S.

Kotchen, Theodore A., and Kotchen, Jane Morley. "Dietary sodium and blood pressure: Interactions with other nutrients." *American Journal of Clinical Nutrition,* 1997;65(suppl):708S–11S.

Krebs-Smith, Susan M., et al. "Fruit and vegetable intakes of children and adolescents in the United States." *Archives of Pediatric and Adolescent Medicine,* 1996;150: 81–86.

———. "US adults' fruit and vegetable intakes, 1989 to 1991: A revised baseline for the Healthy People 2000 Objective." *American Journal of Public Health,* 1995;85(12): 1623–29.

Krinsky, Norman I. "Carotenoids: Structure and Functions." The Olestra Project: Potential Effects of Reducing Carotenoid Levels on Human Health. Harvard School of Public Health, January 17, 1996.

Le Marchand, Loic, et al. "An ecological study of diet and lung cancer in the South Pacific." *International Journal of Cancer,* 1995;63:18–23.

Levy, J., et al. "Lycopene is a more potent inhibitor of human cancer cell proliferation than either alpha-carotene or beta-carotene." *Nutrition and Cancer,* 1996;24(3): 257–66.

"Life may not be in a bowl of cherries, says environmental group." *Nutrition Week,* 1997;27(24):6.

Mangels, Ann Reed, et al. "Carotenoid content of fruits and vegetables: An evaluation of analytic data." *Journal of the American Dietetic Association,* 1993;93(3):284–96.

Manson, JoAnn. "Carotenoids and Stroke." The Olestra Project: Potential Effects of Reducing Carotenoid Levels on Human Health. Harvard School of Public Health, January 17, 1996.

Martin, Keith R., et al. "Beta-carotene and lutein protect HepG2 human liver cells against oxidant-induced damage." *Journal of Nutrition,* 1996;126:2098–106.

Martini, M. C., et al. "Plasma carotenoids as biomarkers of vegetable intake: The University of Minnesota Cancer Prevention Research Unit Feeding Studies." *Cancer Epidemiology, Biomarkers and Prevention,* 1995;4(5):491–96.

Marwick, Charles. "Learning how phytochemicals fight disease." *Journal of the American Medical Association,* 1995;274(17):1328–30.

Mayes, Peter A., "Intermediary metabolism of fructose." *American Journal of Clinical Nutrition,* 1993;58(suppl):754S–66S.

McCarron, David A. "Role of adequate dietary calcium intake in the prevention and management of salt-sensitive hypertension." *American Journal of Clinical Nutrition,* 1997;65(suppl):712S–16S

Michnovicz, Jon J., and Bradlow, H. Leon. "Dietary Cytochrome P-450 Modifiers in the Control of Estrogen Metabolism." *Food Phytochemicals for Cancer Prevention I: Fruits and Vegetables.* Huang, Mou-tuan, Toshihiki, Osawa, Ho, Chi-Tang, and Rosen, Robert T., eds. ACS Symposium Series 546, American Chemical Society, Washington, DC, 1994:282–91.

———. "Induction of estradiol metabolism by dietary indole-3-carbinol in humans." *Journal of the National Cancer Institute,* 1990;82(11):947–49.

Micozzi, Marc. S., et al. "Carotenoid analyses of selected raw and cooked foods associated with a lower risk for cancer." *Journal of the National Cancer Institute,* 1990; 82(4):282–85.

Morris, Dexter L., Kritchevsky, Stephen B., and David, C. E. "Serum carotenoids and coronary heart disease: The Lipid Research Clinics coronary primary prevention trial and follow-up study." *Journal of the American Medical Association,* 1994;272: 1439–42.

Morris, Eugene R., and Hill, A. David. "Inositol phosphate content of selected dry beans, peas, and lentils, raw and cooked." *Journal of Food Composition and Analysis,* 1996;9(1):2–12.

Nielsen, Forrest H. "The Element Boron." *Nutrition and Health, Food and Nutrition Research News Briefs.* October 1–December 31, 1987.

Nijhoff, W. A., and Peters, W. H. "Quantification of induction of rat oesophageal, gastric and pancreatic glutathione and glutathione s-transferases by dietary anticarcinogens." *Carcinogenesis,* 1994;15(9):1769–72.

Nutrition and Your Health: Dietary Guidelines for Americans, Fourth Edition. U.S. Department of Agriculture, 1995.

O'Dell, Boyd. "Copper." *Present Knowledge in Nutrition,* Fifth Edition. Washington, DC: Nutrition Foundation, 1984:506–18.

Okai, Y., Higashi-Okai, K., and Nakamura, S. "Identification of heterogenous antimutagenic activities in the extract of edible brown seaweeds, Laminaria japonica (makonbu) and Undaria pinnatifida (Wakame) by the umu gene expression system in Salmonella typhimurium." *Mutation Research,* 1993;393:63–70.

Olson, James Allen, and Krinsky, Norman I. "Introduction: The colorful, fascinating world of the carotenoids: important physiologic modulators," *FASEB Journal,* 1995;9:1547–50.

"Orange peel extract's ability to stop tumor growth solved." *Cancer Research Weekly,* September 13, 1993:2–4.

Pi-Sunyer, Xavier F., and Offenbacher, Esther. "Chromium." *Present Knowledge in Nutrition,* Fifth Edition. Washington, DC: Nutrition Foundation, 1984:571–86.

Raloff, Janet. "Nutrition: Juicy anticancer prospects." *Science News,* 1996;149:997.

"A recipe for lower blood pressure." *Johns Hopkins Medical Letter,* 1992;4(3):1–2.

Reddy, Bandaru S., and Rao, Chinthalapally V. "Chemoprevention of Colon Cancer by Thiol and Other Organosulfur Compounds." *Food Phytochemicals for Cancer Prevention I: Fruits and Vegetables.* Huang, Mou-Tuan, Toshihiko, Osawa, Ho, Chi-Tang, and Rosen, Robert T., eds. ACS Symposium Series 546, American Chemical Society, Washington, DC, 1994:164–72.

Ribaya-Mercado, Judy D., et al. "Skin lycopene is destroyed preferentially over beta-carotene during ultraviolet irradiation in humans." *Journal of Nutrition,* 1995; 125:1854–59.

Rimm, Eric. "Carotenoids and Coronary Heart Disease." The Olestra Project: Potential Effects of Reducing Carotenoid Levels on Human Health. Harvard School of Public Health, January 17, 1996.

———, et al. "Vegetable, fruit, and cereal fiber intake and risk of coronary heart disease among men." *Journal of the American Medical Association,* 1996;275(6):447–51.

Rogers, Mary A. M., and Thomas, David B. "Chapter 12: Vitamin C and Cancer Prevention: An Assessment of Analytic Studies in Humans." *Nutrition and Cancer Prevention.* Watson, R. R., and Mufti, Siraj I., eds. Boca Raton, FL: CRC, 1996:205–37.

Ross, A. Catherine. "Chapter 2: Vitamin A and Cancer." *Nutrition and Disease Update— Cancer.* Carroll, Kenneth K., and Kritchevsky, David, eds. Champaign, IL: AOCS, 1994:27–109.

Rucker, Robert. "Improved functional endpoints for use in vitamin K assessment: Important implications for bone disease." *American Journal of Clinical Nutrition,* 1997; 65:883–84.

Sadowski, James A. "Structure and mechanism of activation of vitamin K antagonists." *Oral Anticoagulants.* Poller, Leon, and Hirsh, Jack, eds. Oxford University Press, NY, 1996:9–29.

———, et al. "Phylloquinone in plasma from elderly and young adults: factors influencing its concentration." *American Journal of Clinical Nutrition,* 1989;50:100–108.

Sandstead, H., and Evans, G. "Zinc." *Present Knowledge in Nutrition,* Fifth Edition. Washington, DC: Nutrition Foundation, 1984:479–505.

Sauberlich, Howerde E. "Chapter 3: Vitamin C and Cancer." *Nutrition and Disease*

Bibliography

Update—Cancer. Carroll, Kenneth K., and Kritchevsky, David, eds. Champaign, IL: AOCS, 1994:111–72.

Seddon, Johanna, et al. "Dietary carotenoids, vitamins A, C, and E, and advanced age-related macular degeneration." *Journal of the American Medical Association,* 1994; 272(18):1413–20.

Shamsuddin, Abulkalam M., et al. "Phytate and colon-cancer risk." *American Journal of Clinical Nutrition,* 1992;55:478–85.

Shannon, Jackilen, et al. "Relationship of food groups and water intake to colon cancer risk." *Cancer Epidemiology, Biomarkers & Prevention,* V.5:495–502, July 1996.

Shearer, Martin, et al. "Chemistry, nutritional sources, tissue distribution and metabolism of vitamin K with special reference to bone health." *Journal of Nutrition,* 1996; 126(suppl):1181S–86S.

Simon, Joel A. "Vitamin C and cardiovascular disease: A review." *Journal of the American College of Nutrition,* 1992;11(2):107–25.

Singh, Ram B., et al. "Effect of antioxidant-rich foods on plasma ascorbic acid, cardiac enzyme, and lipid peroxide levels in patients hospitalized with acute myocardial infarction." *Journal of the American Dietetic Association,* 1995;95(7):775–80.

Smith, Ulf. "Carbohydrates, fat, and insulin action." *American Journal of Clinical Nutrition,* 1994;59(suppl):686S–89S.

Sokoll, Lori J., et al. "Changes in serum osteocalcin, plasma phylloquinone, and urinary gamma-carboxyglutamic acid in response to altered intakes of dietary phylloquinone in human subjects." *American Journal of Clinical Nutrition,* 1997;65:779–84.

Srivastava, K. C. "Ginger (zingiber officinale) and rheumatic disorders." *Medical Hypotheses,* 1989;29(1):25–28.

———. "Ginger (zingiber officinale) in rheumatism and musculoskeletal disorders." *Medical Hypotheses,* 1992;39(4):342–48.

———. "Isolation and effects of some ginger components of platelet aggregation and eicosanoid biosynthesis." *Prostaglandins Leukot Med,* 1986;25:187–98.

Stahl, Wilhelm, and Sies, Helmut. "Uptake of lycopene and its geometrical isomers is greater from heat-processed than from unprocessed tomato juice in humans." *Journal of Nutrition,* 1992;122:2161–66.

Stampfer, Meir J., and Maliando, M. Rene. "Can lowering homocysteine levels reduce cardiovascular risk?" *New England Journal of Medicine,* 1995;332(5):328–29.

Steinmetz, Kristi A., and Potter, John D. "Vegetables, fruit, and cancer prevention: A review." *Journal of the American Dietetic Association,* 1996;96(10):1027–39.

Stoner, G. D., et al. "Inhibition of Esophageal Tumorigenesis by Phenethyl Isothiocyanate." *Food Phytochemicals for Cancer Prevention I: Fruits and Vegetables.* Huang, Mou-Tuan, Toshihiko, Osawa, Ho, Chi-Tang, and Rosen, Robert T., eds. ACS Symposium Series 546, American Chemical Society, Washington, DC, 1994:173–80.

Street, D. A., et al. "Serum antioxidants and myocardial infarction: Are low levels of carotenoids and alpha-tocopherol risk factors for myocardial infarction?" *Circulation,* 1994;90(3):1154–61.

Talalay, Paul, et al. "Chemoprotection against cancer by Phase 2 enzyme induction." *Elsevier Science Toxicology Letters,* 1995;82/83:173–79.

Tavani, Allesandra, and La Vecchia, Carlo. "Fruit and vegetable consumption and cancer risk in a Mediterranean population." *American Journal of Clinical Nutrition,* 1995; 61(suppl):1374S–77S.

Thompson, Lilian U., et al. "Mammalian lignan production from various foods." *Nutrition and Cancer,* 1991;161(1):43–52.

Thun, Michael J., et al. "Risk factors for fatal colon cancer in a large prospective study." *Journal of the National Cancer Institute,* 1992;84(19):1491–1500.

Tobian, Louis. "Dietary sodium chloride and potassium have effects on the pathophysiology of hypertension in humans and animals." *American Journal of Clinical Nutrition,* 1997;65(suppl):606S–11S.

Treasure, Charles B. "Beneficial effects of cholesterol-lowering therapy on the coronary endothelium in patients with coronary artery disease." *New England Journal of Medicine,* 1995;332(8):481–87.

Trichopoulou, Antonia, et al. "Consumption of olive oil and specific food groups in relation to breast cancer risk in Greece." *Journal of the National Cancer Institute,* 1995;87(2):110–16.

Trock, Bruce, Lanza, Elaine, and Greenwald, Peter. "Dietary fiber, vegetables, and colon cancer: Critical review and meta-analyses of the epidemiologic evidence." *Journal of the National Cancer Institute,* 1990;82(8):650–61.

Tseng, Marilyn, et al. "Micronutrients and the risk of colorectal adenomas." *American Journal of Epidemiology,* 1996;144:1005–14.

Tucker, Katherine L. "Dietary intake pattern relates to plasma folate and homocysteine concentrations in the Framingham Heart Study." *Journal of Nutrition,* 1996;126: 3025–31.

Uusitupa, Matti. "Fructose in the diabetic diet." *American Journal of Clinical Nutrition,* 1994;59(suppl):753S–57S.

Vermeer, Cees, et al. "Effects of vitamin K on bone mass and bone metabolism." *Journal of Nutrition,* 1996;126(suppl):1187S–91S.

Verschuren, W. M. Monique, et al. "Serum total cholesterol and long-term coronary heart disease mortality in different cultures: Twenty-five-year follow-up of the Seven Countries Study." *Journal of the American Medical Association,* 1995;274(2): 131–36.

"Vitamin K and Bone Health." Food & Nutrition Research Briefs. U.S. Department of Agriculture, Agricultural Research Service, October 1996.

"Vitamin K Laboratory: Recent Research Accomplishments." Tufts Human Nutrition Research Center, Tufts University home page, 1997.

Wang, Hong, et al. "Oxygen radical absorbing capacity of anthocyanins." *Journal of Agricultural and Food Chemistry,* 1997;45(2):304–9.

Watada, Alley E. Treatment for cut fruit and vegetables. Personal communication, February 1997.

Weisburger, John H. "Nutritional approach to cancer prevention with emphasis on vitamins, antioxidants, and carotenoids." *American Journal of Clinical Nutrition,* 1991; 53:226S–37S.

Williams, Carol. "Healthy eating: clarifying advice about fruit and vegetables." *British Medical Journal,* 1995;310:1453–56.

Williams, David E., et al. "Anticarcinogens and Tumor Promoters in Foods." *Food Toxicology: A Perspective on the Relative Risks.* Taylor, Steven, and Scanlon, Richard, eds. New York: Marcel Dekker, 1989:101–50.

Witte, John S., et al. "Relation of vegetable, fruit, and grain consumption to colorectal adenomatous polyps." *American Journal of Epidemiology,* 1996;144:1015–25.

You, Wei-Chang, et al. "Diet and high risk of stomach cancer in Shandong, China." *Cancer Research*, 1988;48:3518–23.

Zhang, Yuesheng, et al. "Anticarcinogenic activities of sulforaphane and structurally related synthetic norbornyl isothiocyanates." *Proceedings of the National Academy of Science USA*, 1994;91:3147–50.

Ziegler, Regina G. "Carotenoids and Human Cancer." The Olestra Project: Potential Effects of Reducing Carotenoid Levels on Human Health. Harvard School of Public Health, January 17, 1996.

———. "Vegetables, fruits and carotenoids and the risk of cancer." *American Journal of Clinical Nutrition*, 1991;53(suppl):251S–59S.

Chapter 5: In Praise of Soybeans

Adlercreutz, Herman, et al. "Diet and plasma androgens in postmenopausal vegetarian and omnivorous women and postmenopausal women with breast cancer." *American Journal of Clinical Nutrition*, 1989;49:433–42.

———. "Urinary excretion of lignans and isoflavonoid phytoestrogens in Japanese men and women consuming a traditional Japanese diet." *American Journal of Clinical Nutrition*, 1991;54:1093–100.

Akiyama, Tetsu, et al. "Genistein, a specific inhibitor of tyrosine-specific protein kinases." *Journal of Biological Chemistry*, 1987;262(12):5592–96.

Anderson, James W. "Health Benefits of Soy Protein." Soy and Human Health Home Page, http://www.aq.uiuc.edu/~stratsoy/soyhealth/.

Anderson, J. J., Ambrose, W. W., and Garner, S. C. "Orally dosed genistein from soy and prevention of cancellous bone loss in two ovariectomized rat models." *Journal of Nutrition*, 1995;125(suppl):799S.

Anthony, M. S., et al. "Soybean isoflavones improve cardiovascular risk factors without affecting the reproductive system of peripubertal rhesus monkeys." *Journal of Nutrition*, 1996;126:43–50.

Arjmandi, B. H., et al. "Soy protein prevents bone loss due to ovariectomy in rats." *Journal of Nutrition*, 1996;126:176–82.

———. "A soy protein–containing diet prevents bone loss due to ovarian hormone deficiency." Second International Symposium on the Role of Soy in Preventing and Treating Chronic Disease. September 15–18, 1996, Brussels, Belgium. U.S. Soyfoods Directory, http://soyfoods.com/.

Baird, Donna Day, et al. "Dietary intervention study to assess estrogenicity of dietary soy among postmenopausal women." *Journal of Clinical Endocrinology and Metabolism*, 1995;80(5):1685–90.

Bakhit, Raga M., et al. "Intake of 25g. of soybean protein with or without soybean fiber alters plasma lipids in men with elevated cholesterol concentrations." *Journal of Nutrition*, 1994;124:213–22.

Barnes, S. "Effect of genistein on in vitro and in vivo models of cancer." *Journal of Nutrition*, 1995;125(suppl):777S–83S.

———, et al. "Rationale for the use of genistein-containing soy matrices in chemoprevention trials for breast and prostate cancer." *Journal of Cell Biochemistry Supplement*, 1995;22:181–87.

Beckstrom-Sternberg, Stephen M., and Duke, James A. Plants Containing Biotin. Plants Containing Lecithin. Phytochemeco Database. Agricultural Research Service, USDA.

Brandi, Maria Luisa. "Flavonoids: Biochemical effects and therapeutic applications." *Bone and Mineral,* 1992;19(suppl):S3–S19.

Carroll, Kenneth K. "Review of clinical studies on cholesterol-lowering response to soy protein." *Journal of the American Dietetic Association,* 1991;91(7):820–87.

Cassidy, A., Bingham, S., and Setchell, K. "Biological effects of isoflavones in young women." *British Journal of Nutrition,* 1995;74(4):487–601.

Clarkson, Thomas B., Anthony, Mary S., and Hughes, Claude L., Jr. "Estrogenic soybean isoflavones and chronic disease. Risks and benefits." *Trends in Endocrinological Metabolism,* 1995;6(1):11–16.

Coward, L., et al. "Chemical modification of isoflavones in soy foods during cooking and processing." Second International Symposium on the Role of Soy in Preventing and Treating Chronic Disease. September 15–18, 1996, Brussels, Belgium. U.S. Soyfoods Directory, http:soyfoods.com/.

Coward, Lori, et al. "Genistein, daidzein, and their B-glycoside conjugates: Antitumor isoflavones in soybean foods from American and Asian diets." *Journal of Agricultural and Food Chemistry,* 1993;41(11):1961–67.

Cruz, Maria Lourdes, et al. "Effects of infant nutrition on cholesterol synthesis rates." *Pediatric Research,* 1994;35(2):135–40.

Dalais, F. S., et al. "Dietary soy supplementation increases vaginal cytology maturation index and bone mineral content in postmenopausal women." Second International Symposium on the Role of Soy in Preventing and Treating Chronic Disease. September 15–18, 1996, Brussels, Belgium. U.S. Soyfoods Directory, http:soyfoods.com/.

Dwyer, Johanna T., et al. "Tofu and soy drinks contain phytoestrogens." *Journal of the American Dietetic Association,* 1994;94:739–44.

Erdman, John W., Jr., and Fordyce, Elizabeth. "Soy products and the human diet." *American Journal of Clinical Nutrition,* 1989;49:725–37.

Erdman, J. W., Jr., et al. "Soy and bone health. Short-term effects of soybean isoflavones on bone in postmenopausal women." Second International Symposium on the Role of Soy in Preventing and Treating Chronic Disease. September 15–18, 1996, Brussels, Belgium. U.S. Soyfoods Directory, http:soyfoods.com/.

Esaki, H., Onozaki, H., and Osawa, Toshihiko. "Antioxidative Activity of Fermented Soybean Products." *Food Phytochemicals for Cancer Prevention I: Fruits and Vegetables.* Huang, Muo-Tuan, Toshihiko, Osawa, Ho, Chi-Tang, and Rosen, Robert T., eds. ACS Symposium Series 546, American Chemical Society, Washington, DC, 1994:353–60.

Evans, B. A., Griffiths, K., and Morton, M. S. "Inhibition of 5 alpha-reductase in genital skin fibroblasts and prostate tissue by dietary lignans and isoflavonoids." *Journal of Endocrinology,* 1995;147(2):295–302.

Forsythe, William A., III. "Soy protein, thyroid regulation and cholesterol metabolism." *Journal of Nutrition,* 1995;125(suppl):619S–23S.

Fotsis, Theodore, et al. "Genistein, a dietary ingested isoflavonoid, inhibits cell proliferation and in vitro angiogenesis." *Journal of Nutrition,* 1995;125(suppl):790S–97S.

Franke, Adrian A., et al. "Rapid HPLC analysis of dietary phytoestrogens from legumes and from human urine." *Proceedings of the Society for Experimental Biological Medicine,* 1995;208:18–26.

Fukutake, M., et al. "Quantification of genistein and genistin on soybeans and soybean products." *Food and Chemical Toxicology,* 1996;34:457–61.

Gaddi, Antonio, et al. "Dietary treatment for familial hypercholesterolemia—differential

Bibliography

effects of dietary soy protein according to the apolipoprotein E phenotypes." *American Journal of Clinical Nutrition,* 1991;53:1191–96.

Goldberg, Anne Carol. "Perspectives on soy protein as a nonpharmacological approach for lowering cholesterol." *Journal of Nutrition,* 1995;125(suppl):675S–78S.

Goodman, Marc T., et al. "Association of soy and fiber consumption with the risk of endometrial cancer." *American Journal of Epidemiology,* 1997;146:294–306.

Harding, C., et al. "Dietary soy supplementation is oestrogenic in menopausal women." Second International Symposium on the Role of Soy in Preventing and Treating Chronic Disease. September 15–18, 1996, Brussels, Belgium. U.S. Soyfoods Directory, http:soyfoods.com/.

Hasler, Clare. "Institute for functional foods proposal." *Functional Foods for Health News,* 1996;4(2):5.

Heaney, Robert P., Weaver, Connie M. and Fitzsimmons, Mary Lee. "Soybean phytate content: Effect on calcium absorption." *American Journal of Clinical Nutrition,* 1991;53:745–47.

Hempstock, J., Kavanagh, J. P., and George, N. J. R. "Growth inhibition of human prostatic cell lines by phyto-oestrogens." Second International Symposium on the Role of Soy in Preventing and Treating Chronic Disease. September 15–18, 1996, Brussels, Belgium. U.S. Soyfoods Directory, http:soyfoods.com/.

Herman, C., et al. "Soybean phytoestrogen intake and cancer risk." *Journal of Nutrition,* 1995;125(suppl):757S–70S.

Hutchins, Andrea M., Slavin, Joanne L., and Lampe, Johanna W. "Urinary isoflavonoid phytoestrogen and lignan excretion after consumption of fermented and unfermented soy products." *Journal of the American Dietetic Association,* 1995;95(5):545–51.

"Infant Mortality Rates & Life Expectancy at Birth, by Sex." Table 010. U.S. Bureau of the Census, International Data Base, 1997.

Irvine, Cliff, et al. "The potential adverse effects of soybean phytoestrogens in infant feeding." *New Zealand Medical Journal,* 1995;108(1000):208–9.

Kanazawa, Takemichi, et al. "Protective effects of soy protein on the peroxidizability of lipoproteins in cerebrovascular diseases." *Journal of Nutrition,* 1995;125(suppl): 639S–46S.

Kaufman, Peter B., et al. "A comparative survey of leguminous plants as sources of the isoflavones genistein and daidzein: Implications for human nutrition and health." *Journal of Alternative and Complementary Medicine,* 1997;3(1):7–12.

Kennedy, A. R. "The evidence for soybean products as cancer preventive agents." *Journal of Nutrition,* 1995;125(suppl):733S–43S.

Keung, W. M. "Dietary estrogenic isoflavones are potent inhibitors of beta-hydroxysteroid dehydrogenase of P. testosteronii." *Biochemical and Biophysical Research Communications,* 1995;215(3):1137–44.

"Key reasons to buy protein-rich soy." *Natural Foods Merchandiser,* December 1992. Soyfoods 2000 insert.

Koury, Suzanne Davis, and Hodges, Robert E. "Soybean proteins for human diets?" *Journal of the American Dietetic Association,* 1968;52:480–84.

Kudou, et al. "Structural Elucidation and Physiological Properties of Genuine Soybean Saponins." *Food Phytochemicals for Cancer Prevention I: Fruits and Vegetables.* Huang, Mou-Tuan, Toshihiko, Osawa, Ho, Chi-Tang, and Rosen, Robert T., eds. ACS Symposium Series 546, American Chemical Society, Washington, DC, 1994:340–48.

The Healthiest Diet in the World

Lee, H. P., et al. "Dietary effects on breast-cancer risk in Singapore." *The Lancet,* 1991;337:1197–200.

Liener, Irvin E. "Possible adverse effects of soybean anticarcinogens." *Journal of Nutrition,* 1995;125(suppl):744S–50S.

Lock, Margaret. "Contested meanings of the menopause." *The Lancet,* 1991;337: 1270–72.

Lu, L. J., et al. "Altered time course of urinary daidzein and genistein excretion during chronic soya diet in healthy male subjects." *Nutrition and Cancer,* 1995;24(3):311–23.

Madar, Zacharia. "Effect of brown rice and soybean dietary fiber on the control of glucose and lipid metabolism in diabetic rats." *American Journal of Clinical Nutrition,* 1983;38:388–93.

Martin, Pierre M., et al. "Phytoestrogen interaction with estrogen receptors in human breast cancer cells." *Endocrinology,* 1978;103(5):1860–67.

McLaughlin, P. J., and Weihruach, John L. "Vitamin E content of foods." *Journal of the American Dietetic Association,* 1979;75:647–65.

Messina, Mark, and Messina, Virginia. "Increasing use of soyfoods and their potential role in cancer prevention." *Journal of the American Dietetic Association,* 1991; 91(7):836–40.

Natarajan, V., et al. "Oxidized low density lipoprotein-mediated activation of phospholipase D in smooth muscle cells: A possible role in cell proliferation and atherogenesis." *Journal of Lipid Research,* 1995;36(9):2005–16.

Okubo, Kazuyoshi, et al. "Soybean Saponin and Isoflavonoids." *Food Phytochemicals for Cancer Prevention I: Fruits and Vegetables.* Huang, Mou-Tuan, Toshihiko, Osawa, Ho, Chi-Tang, and Rosen, Robert T., eds. ACS Symposium Series 546, American Chemical Society, Washington, DC, 1994:330–39.

Pariza, Michael W. "Fermentation-Derived Anticarcinogenic Flavor Compound." *Food Phytochemicals for Cancer Prevention I: Fruits and Vegetables.* Huang, Mou-Tuan, Toshihiko, Osawa, Ho, Chi-Tang, and Rosen, Robert T., eds. ACS Symposium Series 546, American Chemical Society, Washington, DC, 1994:349–52.

Potter, S. M. "Overview of proposed mechanisms for the hypocholesterolemic effect of soy." *Journal of Nutrition,* 1995;125(suppl):606S–11S.

Raines, E. W., and Ross, R. "Biology of atherosclerotic plaque formation: Possible role of growth factors in lesion development and the potential impact of soy." *Journal of Nutrition,* 1995;125(suppl):624S–30S.

Rao, A. V., and Sung, M. K. "Saponins as anticarcinogens." *Journal of Nutrition,* 1995;125(suppl):717S–24S.

Reinli, Kathrin, and Block, Gladys. "Phytoestrogen content of foods—a compendium of literature values." *Nutrition and Cancer,* 1996;26(2):123–48.

Santiago, L. A., Hiramatsu, M., and Mori, A. "Japanese soybean paste miso scavenges free radicals and inhibits lipid peroxidation." *Journal of Nutritional Science,* 1992;38(3):297–304.

Setchell, K. D., et al. "Exposure of infants to phyto-estrogens from soy-based infant formula." *The Lancet,* 1997;350:23–27.

Shamsuddin, Abulkalam M. "Letters to the editor: Phytate and colon-cancer risk." *American Journal of Clinical Nutrition,* 1992;55:478.

———, Elsayed, A. M., and Ulla, A. "Suppression of large intestinal cancer in F-344 rats by inositol hexaphosphate." *Carcinogenesis,* 1989;10:625–26.

Sirtori, C. R., et al. "Soy and cholesterol reduction: Clinical experience." *Journal of Nutrition,* 1995;125(suppl):598S–605S.

———. "Soybean-protein diet in the treatment of type-II hyperlipoproteinaemia." *The Lancet,* February 5, 1977:275–77.

Slavin, Joanne. "Nutritional benefits of soy protein and soy fiber." *Journal of the American Dietetic Association,* 1991;91(7):816–19.

Song, Tontong, et al. "Soy isoflavone analysis: Quality control and new internal standard." Unpublished, provided by authors (Patricia Murphy).

Spence, Paddy. "Demographics drive sales of soy products." *National Foods Merchandiser,* March 1996:114.

Steele, Vernon E., et al. "Cancer chemoprevention agent development strategies for genistein." *Journal of Nutrition,* 1995;125(suppl):713S–16S.

Takahama, Akihiro, et al. "Anti-hypertensive peptides derived from fermented soybean paste—miso." *INFORM,* 1993;4(4):525.

Thompson, Lilian U., et al. "Mammalian lignan production from various foods." *Nutrition and Cancer,* 1991;16(1):43–52.

Tsai, Alan C., et al. "Effects of soy polysaccharide on postprandial plasma glucose, insulin, glucagon, pancreatic polypeptide, somatostatin, and triglyceride in obese diabetic patients." *American Journal of Clinical Nutrition,* 1987;45:596–601.

Versphol, E. J., Tollkuhn, B., and Kloss, H. "Role of tyrosine kinase in insulin release in an insulin secreting cell line." *Cell Signal,* 1995;7(5):505–12.

Wang, Huei-ju, and Murphy, Patricia A. "Isoflavone composition of American and Japanese soybeans in Iowa: Effects of variety, crop year, and location." *Journal of Agricultural and Food Chemistry,* 1994;42(8):1674–77.

———. "Isoflavone content in commercial soybean foods." *Journal of Agricultural and Food Chemistry,* 1994;42(8):1666–73.

———. "Mass balance study of isoflavones during soybean processing." *Journal of Agricultural and Food Chemistry,* 1996;44(8):2377–83.

Wang, T. T. Y., Sathyamoorthy, N., and Phang, J. M. "Molecular effects of genistein on estrogen receptor mediated pathways." *Carcinogenesis,* 1996;17(2):271–75.

Wei, H., et al. "Antioxidant and antipromotional effects of the soybean isoflavone genistein." *Proceedings of the Society for Experimental Biological Medicine,* 1995;208(1):124–30.

Whitten, Patricia L., et al. "Potential adverse effects of phytoestrogens." *Journal of Nutrition,* 1995;125(suppl):771S–76S.

Wilcox, Gisela, et al. "Oestrogenic effects of plant foods in postmenopausal women." *British Medical Journal,* 1990;301:905–6.

Wilcox, J. N., and Blumenthal, B. F. "Thrombotic mechanisms in atherosclerosis: Potential impact of soy proteins." *Journal of Nutrition,* 1995;125(suppl):631S–38S.

Witte, John S., et al. "Relation of vegetable, fruit, and grain consumption to colorectal adenomatous polyps." *American Journal of Epidemiology,* 1996;144:1015–25.

Woods, M. N., Senie, R., and Kronenberg, F. "Effect of a Dietary Soy Bar on Menopausal Symptoms." Second International Symposium on the Role of Soy in Preventing and Treating Chronic Disease. September 15–18, 1996, Brussels, Belgium. U.S. Soyfoods Directory, http:soyfoods.com/.

Wu, Anna H., et al. "Tofu and risk of breast cancer in Asian-Americans." *Cancer Epidemiology, Biomarkers & Prevention,* 1996;5:901–6.

The Healthiest Diet in the World

Xu, X., et al. "Bioavailability of soybean isoflavones depends upon gut microflora in women. *Journal of Nutrition,* 1995;125:2307–15.

Yassin, R. R., and Little, K. M. "Early signalling mechanism in colonic epithelial cell response to gastrin." *Biochemistry Journal,* 1991;311(Pt. 3):945–50.

Young, Vernon R. "Soy protein in relation to human protein and amino acid nutrition." *Journal of the American Dietetic Association,* 1991;91(2):828–35.

Chapter 6: The Beauty of Beans

Anderson, J. J., Rondano, P., and Holmes, A. "Roles of diet and physical activity in the prevention of osteoporosis." *Scandinavian Journal of Rheumatology Supplements,* 1996;103:65–74.

Anderson, James W., and Gustafson, Nancy J. "Hypocholesterolemic effects of oat and bean products." *American Journal of Clinical Nutrition,* 1988;48:749–53.

Björck, Inger, et al. "Food properties affecting the digestion and absorption of carbohydrates." *American Journal of Clinical Nutrition,* 1994;59(suppl):699S–705S.

Breslau, Neil A., et al. "Relationship of animal protein–rich diet to kidney stone formation and calcium metabolism." *Journal of Clinical Endocrinology and Metabolism,* 1988;66(1):140–46.

Bunker, V. W. "The role of nutrition in osteoporosis." *British Journal of Biomedical Science,* 1994;51(3):228–40.

Campbell, Wayne W. "Increased protein requirements in elderly people: New data and retrospective reassessments." *American Journal of Clinical Nutrition,* 1994;60:501–9.

Curhan, Gary C., et al. "Comparison of dietary calcium with supplemental calcium and other nutrients as factors affecting the risk for kidney stones in women." *Annals of Internal Medicine,* 1997;126(7):497–504.

"Folate Deficiency Rapidly Raises Risk." *Food & Nutrition Research Briefs.* U.S. Department of Agriculture, Agricultural Research Service, April 1996.

Food & Nutrition Research News Briefs. U. S. Department of Agriculture, Agricultural Research Service, October 1–December 31, 1987.

Franke, Adrian A., et al. "Rapid HPLC analysis of dietary phytoestrogens from legumes and from human urine." *Proceedings of the Society for Experimental Biological Medicine,* 1995;208:18–26.

"Guidelines on Diet, Nutrition and Cancer Prevention: Reducing the Risk of Cancer with Healthy Food Choices and Physical Activity." The American Cancer Society, Dietary Guidelines Advisory Committee, 1996.

Hunt, Sara M., and Groff, James L. "Energy-Producing Nutrients." *Advanced Nutrition and Human Metabolism,* St. Paul, MN: West, 1990:160–67.

Hutchins, Andrea A., et al. "Vegetables, fruits and legumes: Effect on urinary isoflavonoid phytoestrogen and lignan excretion." *Journal of the American Dietetic Association,* 1995;95(7):769–74.

Jenkins, David J. A., et al. "Exceptionally low blood glucose response to dried beans: Comparison with other carbohydrate foods." *British Medical Journal,* 30 August 1980:578–80.

Kaufman, Peter B., et al. "A comparative survey of leguminous plants as sources of the isoflavones genistein and daidzein: Implications for human nutrition and health." *Journal of Alternative and Complementary Medicine,* 1997;3(1):7–12.

Kudou, et al. "Structural Elucidation and Physiological Properties of Genuine Soybean

Saponins." *Food Phytochemicals for Cancer Prevention I: Fruits and Vegetables.* Huang, Mou-Tuan, Toshihiko, Osawa, Ho, Chi-Tang, and Rosen, Robert T., eds. ACS Symposium Series 546, American Chemical Society, Washington, DC, 1994:340–48.

Kurtzweil, Paula. "How folate can help prevent birth defects." *FDA Consumer Magazine,* U.S. Food and Drug Administration, September 1996.

Thomas, Diane E., Brotherhood, J. R., and Miller, J. C. Brand. "Carbohydrate feeding before exercise and the glycemic index." *American Journal of Clinical Nutrition,* 1994;59(suppl):791S.

Thompson, Lilian U., et al. "Mammalian lignan production from various foods." *Nutrition and Cancer,* 1991;16(1):43–52.

Thorne, Mary Jane, et al. "Factors affecting starch digestibility and the glycemic response with special reference to legumes." *American Journal of Clinical Nutrition,* 1983;38: 481–88.

Tovar, Juscelino, Granfeldt, Y., and Björck, I. "Effect of processing on metabolic response to legumes." *American Journal of Clinical Nutrition,* 1994;59(suppl):783S.

Witte, John S., et al. "Relation of vegetable, fruit, and grain consumption to colorectal adenomatous polyps." *American Journal of Epidemiology,* 1996;144:1015–25.

Wood, Richard. "Potassium bicarbonate supplementation and calcium metabolism in postmenopausal women: Are we barking up the wrong tree?" *Nutrition Reviews,* 1995;52(8):278–80.

Young, Vernon R. "Soy protein in relation to human protein and amino acid nutrition." *Journal of the American Dietetic Association,* 1991;91(2):828–35.

Zemel, Michael B. "Calcium utilization: Effect of varying level and source of dietary protein." *American Journal of Clinical Nutrition,* 1988;48:880–83.

Chapter 7: Yogurt: Beyond Milk

Anderson, John B. "Calcium, phosphorus and human bone development." *Journal of Nutrition,* 1996;126:1153S–58S.

———. "Chapter 4: Diet and Osteoporosis." *Nutritional Concerns of Women.* Wolinsky, Ira, and Klimis-Tavantzis, D. eds. Boca Raton, FL: CRC, 1996:35–39.

Anderson, J. J., Rondano, P., and Holmes, A. "Roles of diet and physical activity in the prevention of osteoporosis." *Scandinavian Journal of Rheumatology Supplements,* 1996;103:65–74.

Appel, Lawrence J., et al. "A clinical trial of the effects of dietary patterns on blood pressure." *New England Journal of Medicine,* 1997;336(16):1117–24.

Ascherio, Alberto, et al. "A prospective study of nutritional factors and hypertension among US men." *Circulation,* 1992;86(5):1475–84.

———. "A prospective study of nutritional factors and hypertension among US women." *Hypertension,* 1996;27(5):1065–72.

Baer, R. J., et al. "Composition and flavor of milk produced by cows injected with recombinant bovine somatotropin." *Journal of Dairy Science,* 1989;72:1424–34.

Belury, Martha Ann. "Conjugated dienoic linoleate: A polyunsaturated fatty acid with unique chemoprotective properties." *Nutrition Reviews,* 1995;53(4):83–89.

Blanchfield, Ralph, J., IFST Web Editor. "Bovine Somatotropin (BST): The Institute of Food Science & Technology (IFST) Position Statement." Public Affairs and Technical & Legislative Committees, http://www.easynet.co.uk/ifst/, March 27, 1996.

Bovee-Oudenhoven, I., et al. "Calcium in milk and fermentation by yoghurt bacteria increase the resistance of rats to Salmonella infection." *Gut,* 1996;38(1):59–65.

Bunker, V. W. "The role of nutrition in osteoporosis." *British Journal of Biomedical Science,* 1994;51(3):228–40.

Calvo, Mona S., and Park, Youngmee K. "Changing phosphorus content of the U.S. diet: Potential for adverse effects on bone." *Journal of Nutrition,* 1996;126:1168S–80S.

"Cancer Facts & Figures 1996." American Cancer Society, 1996.

Chin, S. F., et al. "Dietary sources of conjugated dienoic isomers of linoleic acid, a newly recognized class of anticarcinogens." *Journal of Food Composition and Analysis,* 1992;5:185–97.

Curhan, Gary C., et al. "Comparison of dietary calcium with supplemental calcium and other nutrients as factors affecting the risk for kidney stones in women." *Annals of Internal Medicine,* 1997;126(7):497–504.

Dawson-Hughes, Bess. "Calcium and vitamin D nutritional needs of elderly women." *Journal of Nutrition,* 1996;126(suppl):1165S–67S.

Dempster, David W. "Bone Remodeling." *Osteoporosis: Etiology, Diagnosis, and Management: Second Edition.* Riggs, Lawrence B., and Melton, Joseph L., III, eds. Philadelphia: Lippincott-Raven, 1995:67–75.

Eichholzer, Monika, and Stahelin, Hannes. "Is there a hypocholesterolemic factor in milk and milk products?" *International Journal of Vitamin and Nutrition Research,* 1993;63:159–67.

Epstein, Samuel S. "Unlabeled milk from cows treated with biosynthetic growth hormones: A case of regulatory abdication." *International Journal of Health Services,* 1996;26(1):173–85.

Feldman, M., et al. "Evidence that the growth hormone receptor mediates differentiation and development of the mammary gland." *Endocrinology,* 1993;133(4):1602–8.

Freudenheim, J. L., et al. "Calcium intake and blood pressure in blacks and whites." *Ethnicity and Disease,* 1991;1(2):114–22.

Giovannucci, E. "Diet and colon cancer." *Cancer Researcher Weekly,* December 13, 1993:21–23.

Goldin, Barry R., and Gorback, Sherwood L. "The effect of milk and lactobacillus feeding on human intestinal bacterial enzyme activity." *American Journal of Clinical Nutrition,* 1984;39:756–61.

Ha, Yeong L., et al. "Newly recognized anticarcinogenic fatty acids: Identification and quantification in natural and processed cheeses." *Journal of Agricultural Food Chemistry,* 1989;37:75–81.

Hata, Yoshiya, et al. "A placebo-controlled study of the effect of sour milk on blood pressure in hypertensive subjects." *American Journal of Clinical Nutrition,* 1996;64:767–71.

Haumann, Barbara Fitch. "Conjugated linoleic acid offers research promise." *INFORM,* 1996;7(2):155–59.

Heaney, Robert P. "The role of nutrition in prevention and management of osteoporosis." *Clinical Obstetrics and Gynecology,* 1987;50(4):833–46.

Hilton, E., et al. "Ingestion of yogurt containing Lactobacillus acidophilus as prophylaxis for candidal vaginitis." *Annals of Internal Medicine,* 1992;116(5)353–57.

Hitchins, Anthony D., and McDonough, Frank E. "Prophylactic and therapeutic aspects of fermented milk." *American Journal of Clinical Nutrition,* 1989;49:675–84.

527

Holick, Michael F. "Vitamin D and bone health." *Journal of Nutrition,* 1996;126: 1159S–64S.

Hunt, Sara M., and Groff, James L. "Hypertension: Another Reason for an Adequate Intake of Calcium?" *Advanced Nutrition and Human Metabolism.* St. Paul, MN: West, 1990:282–84.

Ip, C., Scimeca, J. A., and Thompson, H. "Effect of timing and duration of dietary conjugated linoleic acid on mammary cancer prevention." *Nutrition and Cancer,* 1995;24(3):241–47.

Ip, Clement, et al. "Conjugated linoleic acid." *Cancer Supplement,* 1994;74(3):1050–54.

Juskevich, J. C., and Geyer, C. G. "Bovine growth hormone: Food safety evaluation." *Science,* 1990;249:875–84.

Kotchen, Theodore A., and Kotchen, Jane Morley. "Dietary sodium and blood pressure: Interactions with other nutrients." *American Journal of Clinical Nutrition,* 1997; 65(suppl):708S–11S.

Kritchevsky, David. "Chapter 4: Cholesterol and Cardiovascular Disease: How Can Nutrition Help?" *Modern Nutrition.* Wolinsky, Ira, and Hickson, James F., eds. Boca Raton, FL: CRC, 1995;89–112.

———. "Conjugated linoleic acid in food: Scientists study its role as inhibitor of cancer-causing substances." *Food & Nutrition News,* 1994;66(3):22–23.

Krokan, H. E., et al. "The inhibitory effect of conjugated dienoic derivatives (CLA) of linoleic acid on the growth of human tumor cell lines is part due to increased lipid peroxidation." *Anticancer Research,* 1995;15(4):1241–46.

Lee, K. N., Kritchevsky, D., and Pariza, M. W. "Conjugated linoleic acid and atherosclerosis in rabbits." *Atherosclerosis,* 1994;108(1):19–25.

Liew, C., et al. "Protection of conjugated linoleic acids against 2-amino-3-methyl-imidazo[4,5-f]quinoline-induced colon carcinogenesis in the F344 rat: A study of inhibitory mechanisms." *Carcinogenesis,* 1995;16(12):3037–43.

Massey, Linda K., et al. "Effect of dietary oxalate and calcium on urinary oxalate and risk of formation of calcium oxalate kidney stones." *Journal of the American Dietetic Association,* 1993;93(8):901–6.

McCarron, David A. "Role of adequate dietary calcium intake in the prevention and management of salt-sensitive hypertension." *American Journal of Clinical Nutrition,* 1997;65(suppl):712S–16S.

———, and Morris, Cynthia D. "The calcium deficiency hypothesis of hypertension." *Annals of Internal Medicine,* 1987;107:919–22.

Mepham, T. B. "Public health implications of bovine somatotrophin use in dairying: Discussion paper." *Journal of the Royal Society of Medicine,* 1992;85:736–39.

Nadathur, S. R., Gould, S. J., and Bakalinsky, A. T. "Antimutagenicity of an acetone extract of yogurt." *Mutation Research,* 1995;334(2):213–24.

National Institutes of Health. "Technology Assessment Conference statement on bovine somatotropin." *Journal of the American Medical Association,* 1991;265:1423–25.

"No wonder they love cheese." *Journal of the National Cancer Institute,* 1995; 87(7):484.

"Nutritional Content of Yogurt Cheese." ABC Research, Gainesville, FL, 5/17/86.

Perdigon, G., et al. "Immune system stimulation by probiotics." *Journal of Dairy Science,* 1995;78(7):1597–606.

Pereyra, Blanca Solis-, Aattouri, Najat, and Lemonnier, Daniel. "Role of food in the stimulation of cytokine production." *American Journal of Clinical Nutrition,* 1997; 66:521S–25S.

Peters, R. K., et al. "Diet and colon cancer in Los Angeles County, California." *Cancer Causes Control,* 1992;3(5):457–73.

Prosser, C. G. "Bovine somatotropin and milk consumption." *The Lancet,* 1988;1:1201.

Shannon, Jackilen, et al. "Relationship of food groups and water intake to colon cancer risk." *Cancer Epidemiology, Biomarkers & Prevention,* 1966;5:495–502.

Shermak, M. A., et al. "Effect of yogurt on symptoms and kinetics of hydrogen production in lactose-malabsorbing children." *American Journal of Clinical Nutrition,* 1995;62:1003–6.

Simpson, Robert. "Chapter 16: Effects of Calcium and Calcium Antagonists on Cancer Growth." *Nutrition and Cancer Prevention.* Watson, Ronald R., and Mufti, Siraj I., eds. Boca Raton, FL: CRC, 1996:299–315.

Steinhart, Carol. "Conjugated linoleic acid—the good news about animal fat." *Journal of Chemical Education,* 1996;73(12):A302–3.

Tseng, Marilyn, et al. "Micronutrients and the risk of colorectal adenomas." *American Journal of Epidemiology,* 1996;144:1005–14.

"USDA Data Tables: Results from USDA's 1995 Continuing Survey of Food Intakes by Individuals and 1995 Diet and Health Knowledge Survey." U.S. Department of Agriculture, Agriculture Research Service, 1996.

Van den Berg, J. J., et al. "Reinvestigation of the antioxidant properties of conjugated linoleic acids." *Lipids,* 1995;30(7):599–605.

Varela-Moreiras G., et al. "Effects of yogurt and fermented-then-pasteurized milk on lactose absorption in an institutionalized elderly group." *Journal of the American College of Nutrition,* 1992;11(2):168–71.

Weisburger, John H. "Nutritional approach to cancer prevention with emphasis on vitamins, antioxidants, and carotenoids." *American Journal of Clinical Nutrition,* 1991; 53:226S–37S.

Witsell, D. L., et al. "Effect of Lactobacillus acidophilus on antibiotic-associated gastrointestinal morbidity: A prospective randomized trial." *Journal of Otolaryngology,* 1995;24(4):230–13.

You, Wei-Chang, et al. "Diet and high risk of stomach cancer in Shandong, China." *Cancer Research,* 1988;48:3518–23.

Chapter 8: Drink Up

"Alcohol and bone disorders." *ORBD-NRC News,* Osteoporosis and Related Bone Diseases, National Resource Center, September 5, 1995.

"Alcohol, Vitamin C, and Blood Cholesterol." Food & Nutrition Research Briefs, U.S. Department of Agriculture, Agricultural Research Service, April 1995.

Anderson, J. J., Rondano, P., and Holmes, A. "Roles of diet and physical activity in the prevention of osteoporosis." *Scandinavian Journal of Rheumatology Supplements,* 1996;103:65–74.

Austoker, Joan. "Reducing alcohol intake. (Cancer prevention in primary care, part 3)." *British Medical Journal,* 1994;308:1549–53.

Barger-Lux, M. J., and Heaney, R. P. "Caffeine and the calcium economy revisited." *Osteoporosis Int.,* 1995;5(2):97–102.

Barrett-Connor, E., Chang, J. C., and Edelstein, S. L. "Coffee-associated osteoporosis offset by daily milk consumption: The Rancho Bernardo Study." *Journal of the American Medical Association,* 1994;271(4):280–83.

Boden, Guenther. "Effects of ethanol on carbohydrate metabolism in the elderly." *Diabetes,* 1993;42:28–34.

"Bottled Water," 21 CFR 103.35. Updated by 61 FR 14478, 04/02/96. U.S. Food and Drug Administration, Washington, DC.

Bunker, V. W., "The role of nutrition in osteoporosis." *British Journal of Biomedical Science,* 1994;51(3):228–40.

"Caffeine and Health." International Food Information Council Foundation, Washington, DC, March 1997.

Carotenoid Research Interactive Group (CARIG). "Beta-carotene and the carotenoids: Beyond the intervention trials." *Nutrition Reviews,* 1996;54(6):185–88.

Chidester, June C., et al. "Fluid intake in the institutionalized elderly." *Journal of the American Dietetic Association,* 1997;97(1):23–28.

Clifford, Andrew J., et al. "Delayed tumor onset in transgenic mice fed an amino acid–based diet supplemented with red wine solids." *American Journal of Clinical Nutrition,* 1996;64:748–56.

Colditz, Graham A., et al. "Alcohol, height, and adiposity in relation to estrogen and prolactin levels in postmenopausal women." *Journal of the National Cancer Institute,* 1995;87:1297–303.

———, eds. "Harvard Report on Cancer Prevention. Volume 1: Causes of Human Cancer." *Cancer Causes & Control,* 1996:7(suppl).

Cooper C., et al. "Is caffeine consumption a risk factor for osteoporosis?" *Journal of Bone Mineral Research,* 1992;7(4):465–71.

Cummings, Steven R., et al. "Risk factors for hip fracture in white women." *New England Journal of Medicine,* 1995;332(12):767–73.

Decker, Eric A., Ph.D. "The role of phenolics, conjugated linoleic acid, carnosine, and pyrroloquinoline quinone as nonessential dietary antioxidants." *Nutrition Reviews,* 1995;53(3):49–58.

Dwyer, Johanna. "Overview: Dietary approaches for reducing cardiovascular disease risks." *Journal of Nutrition,* 1995;125(suppl):656S–65S.

Evers, Connie. "Kids' drinking habits a problem." *Feeding Kids,* March/April 1997:X.

"Everything You Need to Know About . . . Caffeine." *International Food Information Council Foundation,* Washington, DC, March 1997.

Felson, D. T., et al. "Alcohol intake and bone mineral density in elderly men and women: The Framingham Study." *American Journal of Epidemiology,* 1995;42:485–92.

"Fluoride." Fact Sheet. International Bottled Water Association, Alexandria, VA.

Forman, M. R., et al. "Effect of alcohol consumption on plasma carotenoid concentrations in premenopausal women: A controlled dietary study." *American Journal of Clinical Nutrition,* 1995;62:131–35.

Frankel, E. N., et al. "Inhibition of oxidation of human low-density lipoprotein by phenolic substances in red wine." *The Lancet,* 1993;341:454–57.

Fuchs, Charles G., et al. "Alcohol consumption and mortality among women." *New England Journal of Medicine,* 1995;332:1245–52.

Fuhrman, Bianca, et al. "Consumption of red wine with meals reduces the susceptibility of human plasma and low-density lipoprotein to lipid peroxidation." *American Journal of Clinical Nutrition,* 1995;61:549–55.

The Healthiest Diet in the World

Gao, Yu Tang, et al. "Reduced risk of esophageal cancer associated with green tea consumption." *Journal of the National Cancer Institute*, 1994;86(11):855–58.

Gillespy, T., III, and Gillespy, M. P. "Osteoporosis." *Radiologic Clinics of North America*, 1991;29:(1)77–84.

Ginsburg, Elizabeth S., M.D., et al. "Effects of alcohol ingestion on estrogens in postmenopausal women." *Journal of the American Medical Association*, 1996;276:1747–51.

Giovannucci, Edward, et al. "Alcohol, low-methionine-low-folate diets, and risk of colon cancer in men." *Journal of the National Cancer Institute*, 1995;87:265–74.

———. "Folate, methionine, and alcohol intake and risk of colorectal adenoma." *Journal of the National Cancer Institute*, 1993;85(11):875–84.

Graham, Harold N., Ph.D. "Green tea composition, consumption, and polyphenol chemistry." *Preventive Medicine*, 1992;21:334–350.

Guengerich, F. Peter. "Influence of nutrients and other dietary materials on cytochrome P-450 enzymes." *American Journal of Clinical Nutrition*, 1995;61(suppl):651S–58S.

"Guidelines on Diet, Nutrition and Cancer Prevention: Reducing the Risk of Cancer with Healthy Food Choices and Physical Activity." American Cancer Society, Dietary Guidelines Advisory Committee, 1996.

Gutman, Robert L., and Ryu, Beung-Ho. "Rediscovering tea." *HerbalGram*, July 1996;37(suppl):34–48.

Hallfrisch, J., et al. "Effect of moderate alcohol or wine consumption on vitamin B_{12} and folate status in men and women consuming two levels of fat." *Journal of the American College of Nutrition*, 1995;14:551.

Hansen, M. A. "Assessment of age and risk factors on bone density and bone turnover in healthy premenopausal women." *Osteoporosis Int.*, 1994;4(3):123–28.

———, et al. "Potential risk factors for development of postmenopausal osteoporosis—examined over a 12-year period." *Osteoporosis Int.*, 1991;1(2):95–102.

Harland, Barbara F. "Dietary fibre and mineral bioavailability." *Nutrition Research Reviews*, 1989;2:133–47.

Harris, Susan S., and Dawson-Hughes, Bess. "Caffeine and bone loss in healthy postmenopausal women." *American Journal of Clinical Nutrition*, 1994;60:573–78.

Heaney, Robert P. "The role of nutrition in prevention and management of osteoporosis." *Clinical Obstetrics and Gynecology*, 1987;50(4):833–46.

Hernandez-Avila, M., et al. "Caffeine, moderate alcohol intake, and risk of fractures of the hip and forearm in middle-aged women." *American Journal of Clinical Nutrition*, 1991;54:157–63.

Hertog, Michael G. L., et al. "Content of potentially anticarcinogenic flavonoids of tea infusions, wines, and fruit juices." *Journal of Agricultural and Food Chemistry*, 1993;41:1242–46.

———. "Dietary antioxidant flavonoids and risk of coronary heart disease: the Zutphen Elderly Study." *The Lancet*, 1993;342:1007–11.

———. "Flavonoid intake and long-term risk of coronary heart disease and cancer in the Seven Countries Study." *Archives of Internal Medicine*, 1995;155:381–87.

Holbrook, Troy L., and Barrett-Connor, Elizabeth. "A prospective study of alcohol consumption and bone mineral density." *British Medical Journal*, 1993;306:1506–9.

Holmberg, Lars, et al. "Diet and breast cancer risk: Results from a population-based, case-control study in Sweden." *Archives of Internal Medicine*, 1994;154:1805–12.

Bibliography

Hunter, David J., et al. "A prospective study of the intake of vitamins C, E, and A and the risk of breast cancer." *New England Journal of Medicine,* 1993;329:234–41.

Imai, K., and Nakachi, K. "Cross sectional study of effects of drinking on cardiovascular and liver diseases." *British Medical Journal,* 1995;310:693–97.

Ishikawa, Toshisugu, et al. "Effect of tea flavonoid supplementation on the susceptibility of low-density lipoprotein to oxidative modification." *American Journal of Clinical Nutrition,* 1997;66:261–66.

Jang, Meishiang, et al. "Cancer chemopreventive activity of resveratrol, a natural product derived from grapes," *Science,* 1997;275:218–20.

Kendall, Cyril W. C., "Health Effects Associated with Tea Consumption." Tea Council of Canada, Toronto, May 1994.

Kerr, David, et al. "Effect of caffeine on the recognition of and responses to hypoglycemia in humans." *Annals of Internal Medicine,* 1993;119:799–805.

Kiel, D. P., et al. "Caffeine and the risk of hip fracture: The Framingham Study." *American Journal of Epidemiology,* 1990;132(4):675–84.

Knight, E. M., et al. "Effect of moderate alcohol or wine consumption on homocysteine and vitamin status of men and women fed diets containing high and low levels of fat." *FASEB Journal,* 1996;10:A197.

Krauss, Ronald, et al. "Dietary Guidelines for Healthy American Adults. AHA Medical/Scientific Statement." *Circulation,* 1996;94:1795–800.

Kuhnau, Joachim. "The Flavonoids. A Class of Semi-Essential Food Components: Their Role in Human Nutrition." *World Review of Nutrition and Dietetics,* Volume 24. Bourne, Geoffrey H., ed. Base: S. Karger, 1976:117–91.

Levine, Barbara. "Role of liquid intake in childhood obesity and related diseases." *Current Concepts and Perspectives in Nutrition,* 1996:8(2).

Lieber, Charles Saul. "Medical disorders of alcoholism." *New England Journal of Medicine,* 1995;33(16):1058–65.

Liebman, Michael, and Chai, Weiwen. "Effect of dietary calcium on urinary oxalate excretion after oxalate loads." *American Journal of Clinical Nutrition,* 1997;65: 1453–59.

Longnecker, Matthew P., and Schatzkin, Arthur. "Alcohol and breast cancer: Where are we now and where do we go from here?" *Cancer,* 1994;74:1101–11.

Longnecker, Matthew P., et al. "A meta-analysis of alcohol consumption in relation to risk of breast cancer." *Journal of the American Medical Association,* 1988;260(5): 652–56.

Massey, L. K., and Whiting, S. J. "Caffeine, urinary calcium, calcium metabolism and bone." *Journal of Nutrition,* 1993;123(9):1611–14.

Massey, Linda K., et al. "Effect of dietary oxalate and calcium on urinary oxalate and risk of formation of calcium oxalate kidney stones." *Journal of the American Dietetic Association,* 1993;93(8):901–6.

McElduff, Patrick, and Dobson, Annette J. "How much alcohol and how often? Population based case-control study of alcohol consumption and risk of a major coronary event." *British Medical Journal,* 1997;314(7088).

McKay, Donald W., et al. "Herbal tea: An alternative to regular tea for those who form calcium oxalate stones." *Journal of the American Dietetic Association,* 1995;95(3): 360–61.

Meyer, Haakon E., et al. "Dietary factors and the incidence of hip fracture in middle-aged

Norwegians: A prospective study." *American Journal of Epidemiology,* 1997;145: 117–23.

Mufti, Siraj J. "Prevention of Alcohol-Induced Disease and Cancer by Nutrition." *Nutrition and Cancer Prevention.* Watson, Ronald R., and Mufti, Siraj J., eds. Boca Raton, Fl: CRC, 1996:59–80.

Namiki, Mitsuo. "Antimutagen and Anticarcinogen Research in Japan." *Food Phytochemicals for Cancer Prevention I: Fruits and Vegetables.* Huang, Mou-Tuan, Osawa, Toshihiko, Ho, Chi-Tang, and Rosen, Robert T., eds. ACS Symposium Series 546, American Chemical Society, Washington, DC, 1994:65–81.

NIH Consensus Development Panel on Triglyceride, High-Density Lipoprotein, and Coronary Heart Disease. "Triglyceride, high-density lipoprotein, and coronary heart disease." *Journal of the American Medical Association,* 1993;269(4)505–10.

Parra-Cabrera, M. S., et al. "Risk factors in osteoporosis: Clinical and epidemiologic evidence." *Gaceta Médica Mexicana,* 1994;130(4):231–40.

Renaud, S., and de Lorgeril, M. "Wine, alcohol, platelets, and the French paradox for coronary heart disease." *The Lancet,* 1992;339:1523–26.

Rich-Edwards, Janet W., Sc.D., et al. "The primary prevention of coronary heart disease in women." *New England Journal of Medicine,* 1995;332(26):1758–66.

Rimm, Eric B., et al. "Review of moderate alcohol consumption and reduced risk of coronary heart disease: Is the effect due to beer, wine, or spirits?" *British Medical Journal,* 1996;312(7033):731–41.

Shannon, Jackilen, et al. "Relationship of food groups and water intake to colon cancer risk." *Cancer Epidemiology, Biomarkers & Prevention,* 1996;5:495–502.

Shibata, Atsuko, et al. "A prospective study of pancreatic cancer in the elderly." *International Journal of Cancer,* 1994;58:46–49.

Simon, Joel A. "Relation of smoking and alcohol consumption to serum fatty acids." *American Journal of Epidemiology,* 1996;144:325–34.

Skinner, S., et al. "Plasma homocysteine and lipid concentrations of men and women consuming moderate levels of alcohol and wine." *FASEB Journal,* 1996;10:A814.

Sohn, O. S., et al. "Effects of green and black tea on hepatic xenobiotic metabolizing systems in the male F344 rat." *Xenobiotica,* 1994;24(2):119–27.

Stoner, G. D., and Mukhtar, H. "Polyphenols as cancer chemopreventive agents." *Journal of Cell Biochemistry Supplements,* 1995;22:169–80.

Thompson, W. G. "Coffee: Brew or bane?" *American Journal of Medical Science,* 1994;308(1):49–57.

Victor, Ronald G., and Hansen, Jim. "Editorial: Alcohol and blood pressure—drink a day. . . ." *New England Journal of Medicine,* 1995;332(26):1782–83.

Wang, Hong, et al. "Oxygen radical absorbing capacity of anthocyanins." *Journal of Agricultural and Food Chemistry,* 1997;45(2):304–9.

Weidner, Gerdi, et al. "Sex differences in high density lipoprotein cholesterol among low-level alcohol consumers." *Circulation,* 1991;83:176–80.

Welsch, C. W., and VanderPloeg, L. C. "Caffeine and the Development of the Normal and Neoplastic Rodent Mammary Gland." *Nutrition and Cancer Prevention.* Watson, Ronald R., and Mufti, Siraj J., eds. Boca Raton, FL: CRC, 1996:329–51.

"Wine & Health." Department of Viticulture & Encology at UC Davis home page. With permission from *Chemistry & Industry,* May 1, 1995:338–41.

Yang, Chung S., and Wang, Zhi-Yuan. "Tea and cancer." *Journal of the National Cancer Institute*, 1993;85(13):1038–49.

Appendix

Allison, D. B., et al. "Body mass index and all-cause mortality among people age 70 and over: The longitudinal study of aging." *International Journal of Obesity and Related Metabolic Disorders*, 1997;21(6)44–31.

Berg, Frances M. "Who is dieting in the United States?" *Obesity & Health,* May/June, 1992:48–49.

French, Simone A., and Jeffery, Robert W. "Consequences of dieting to lose weight: Effects on physical and mental health." *Health Psychology,* 1994;13(3):195–212.

Levy, Alan S., and Heaton, Alan W. "Weight control practices of U.S. adults trying to lose weight." *Annals of Internal Medicine,* 1993;119(7):661–66.

Pi-Sunyer, F. X. "Medical hazards of obesity." *Annals of internal medicine,* 1993;119(7): 655–60.

———. "Short-term medical benefits and adverse effects of weight loss." *Annals of Internal Medicine,* 1993;119(7):722–26.

Serdula, Mary K., et al. "Weight control practices of U.S. adolescents and adults." *Annals of Internal Medicine,* 1993;119(7):667–71.

Shaper, Gerald A., et al. "Body weight: Implications for the prevention of coronary heart disease, stroke, and diabetes mellitus in a cohort study of middle aged men." *British Medical Journal,* 1997;314(7090):1311–17.

Troiano, R. P., et al. "Overweight prevalence and trends for children and adolescents." *Archives of Pediatric & Adolescent Medicine,* 1995;149:1085–91.

———. "The relationship between body weight and mortality: A quantitative analysis of combined information from existing studies." *International Journal of Obesity,* 1996; 20:63–75.

Recipe Index

Recipe
Index

*Recipe
Index*

Recipe
Index

Recipe
Index

Recipe
Index

545

❧✿❧

*Recipe
Index*

General Index

*General
Index*

*General
Index*

General
Index

General Index